ACSM's
Exercise Management for Persons with Chronic Diseases and Disabilities,
Second Edition

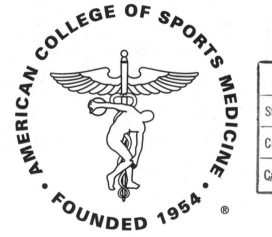

AMERICAN COLLEGE
OF SPORTS MEDICINE

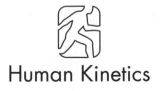

Human Kinetics

Library of Congress Cataloging-in-Publication Data

ACSM's exercise management for persons with chronic diseases and
disabilities / American College of Sports Medicine.--2nd ed.
    p. ; cm.
Includes bibliographical references and index.
  ISBN 0-7360-3872-8 (hardcover)
1. Exercise therapy. 2. Exercise tests. 3. Chronic
diseases--Exercise therapy. 4. People with
disabilities--Rehabilitation.
  [DNLM: 1. Exercise Therapy--standards. 2. Chronic
Disease--rehabilitation. 3. Disabled Persons--rehabilitation. 4.
Exercise Test--methods. WB 541 A187 2002] I. Title: Exercise
management for persons with chronic diseases and disabilities. II.
American College of Sports Medicine.
  RM725 .A3 2002
  615.8'24--dc21

2002006587

ISBN-10: 0-7360-3872-8
ISBN-13: 978-0-7360-3872-0

Acquisitions Editor: Loarn Robertson, PhD; **Developmental Editor:** D.K. Bihler; **Assistant Editors:** Jennifer L. Davis and Kathleen Bernard; **Copyeditor:** D.K. Bihler; **Proofreader:** Sue Fetters; **Indexer:** Dan Connolly; **Permission Manager:** Dalene Reeder; **Graphic Designer:** Nancy Rasmus; **Graphic Artist:** Kathleen Boudreau-Fuoss; **Photo Manager:** Leslie A. Woodrum; **Cover Designer:** Kristin A. Darling; **Photographer (interior):** Leslie A. Woodrum, except where noted; **ACSM Publications Committee Chair:** Jeffrey L. Roitman, EdD, FACSM; **ACSM Group Publisher:** D. Mark Robertson; **Printer:** Sheridan Books

Printed in the United States of America   10 9 8

Human Kinetics
Web site: www.HumanKinetics.com

United States: Human Kinetics, P.O. Box 5076, Champaign, IL 61825-5076
800-747-4457
e-mail: humank@hkusa.com

Canada: Human Kinetics, 475 Devonshire Road Unit 100, Windsor, ON N8Y 2L5
800-465-7301 (in Canada only)
e-mail: orders@hkcanada.com

Europe: Human Kinetics, 107 Bradford Road, Stanningley, Leeds LS28 6AT, United Kingdom
+44 (0) 113 255 5665
e-mail: hk@hkeurope.com

Australia: Human Kinetics, 57A Price Avenue, Lower Mitcham, South Australia 5062
08 8277 1555
e-mail: liaw@hkaustralia.com

New Zealand: Human Kinetics, Division of Sports Distributors NZ Ltd., P.O. Box 300 226, Albany
North Shore City, Auckland
0064 9 448 1207
e-mail: info@humankinetics.co.nz

Visit Human Kinetics on the Web at **www.HumanKinetics.com**.

*For more information about the American College of Sports Medicine and its programs, visit its Web site at **www.acsm.org**.*

CONTENTS

CONTRIBUTORS

Senior Editors

J. Larry Durstine, PhD, FACSM
University of South Carolina

Geoffrey E. Moore, MD, FACSM
McGill University

Section Editors

Lorraine E. Colson Bloomquist, EdD, FACSM
University of Rhode Island

Peter H. Brubaker, PhD, FACSM
Wake Forest University

Christopher B. Cooper, MD, FACSM
UCLA School of Medicine

Stephen F. Figoni, PhD, RKT, FACSM
VA Palo Alto Health Care System

Patricia L. Painter, PhD, FACSM
University of California, San Francisco

Kenneth H. Pitetti, PhD, FACSM
Wichita State University

Scott O. Roberts, PhD, FACSM
California State University, Chico

Contributors

Ann L. Albright, PhD, CDE
University of California, San Francisco

J. Edwin Atwood, MD
Palo Alto VA Medical Center
Stanford University

Stephen P. Bailey, PhD, PT, FACSM
Elon College

Connie Bayles, PhD, FACSM
University of Pittsburgh

Thomas J. Birk, PhD, MPT, FACSM
Wayne State University

Susan A. Bloomfield, PhD, FACSM
Texas A & M University

Clinton Brawner, BS
The Henry Ford Heart and Vascular Institute

Martha Canulette, MSN, RN
Presbyterian Healthplex

Christopher J. Clark, MD
Hairmyers Hospital

Thomas E. Dreisinger, PhD, FACSM, RCEP
Progressive Spine Care and Rehabilitation

Bo Fernhall, PhD, FACSM
Syracuse University

Barry A. Franklin, PhD, FACSM
William Beaumont Hospital
Wayne State University

Daniel Friedman, MD, FACSM
Presbyterian Healthplex

Andrew W. Gardner, PhD
Baltimore VA Medical Center

Adam Gitkin, MS
Arizona Heart Institute

Neil F. Gordon, MD, PhD, FACSM
The Heart and Lung Group

Kimberly B. Harbst, PhD, PT
University of Wisconsin-La Crosse

W. Guyton Hornsby, Jr., PhD, CDE, FACSM
West Virginia University

Connie C.W. Hsia, MD
University of Texas Southwestern

Kirsten L. Johansen, MD
University of California, San Francisco

Donald R. Kay, MD
University of Missouri Health Sciences Center

Steven J. Keteyian, PhD, FACSM
The Henry Ford Heart and Vascular Institute

Nancy Klimas, MD
University of Miami VA Medical Center

Joanne B. Krasnoff, MS
University of California, San Francisco

Arthur LaPerriere, PhD, FACSM
University of Miami

James J. Laskin, PhD, PT
University of Montana

Kathy Lemley, MS, PT
Milwaukee Medical Clinic

Anthony P. Marsh, PhD
Wake Forest University

Barbara Meyer, PhD
University of Wisconsin-Milwaukee

Marian A. Minor, PhD, PT
Missouri Arthritis Rehabilitation Research and Training Center

Janet A. Mulcare, PhD, FACSM
Andrews University

Jonathan N. Myers, PhD, FACSM
Palo Alto VA Medical Center
Stanford University

Patricia A. Nixon, PhD, FACSM
Wake Forest University

Karen Palmer-McLean, PhD, PT
University of Wisconsin-La Crosse

Mark H. Pedrotty, PhD
Carrie Tingley Hospital

Arlette C. Perry, PhD, FACSM
University of Miami

Elizabeth J. Protas, PhD, PT, FACSM
Texas Women's University

James H. Rimmer, PhD
University of Illinois at Chicago

William F. Riner, PhD, FACSM
John Morrison White Clinic

David J. Ross, MD
UCLA School of Medicine

Richard J. Sabath, EdD, FACSM
Children's Mercy Hospital

Anna L. Schwartz, PhD, ARNP
University of Washington

Maureen J. Simmonds, PhD, PT, MCSP
Texas Women's University

Gary S. Skrinar, PhD, FACSM
Boston University

Susan S. Smith, PhD, FACSM
Texas Women's University

Rhonda K. Stanley, PhD, PT
University of Maryland

Mark A. Tarnopolsky, MD, PhD
McMaster University Medical Center

Paul D. Thompson, MD, FACSM
Hartford Hospital

Janet P. Wallace, PhD, FACSM
Indiana University

Michael West, MD
Lovelace Health Systems

Karen Lo Nau White, PhD, PT, FACSM
Oregon State University

Christopher J. Womack, PhD, FACSM
Michigan State University

PREFACE

Preface to the First Edition

J. Larry Durstine, PhD, FACSM

Geoffrey E. Moore, MD, FACSM

Lorraine E. Colson Bloomquist, EdD, FACSM

Stephen F. Figoni, PhD, RKT, FACSM

Patricia L. Painter, PhD, FACSM

Kenneth H. Pitetti, PhD, FACSM

Carol J. Pope, PhD

Scott O. Roberts, PhD, FACSM

The fifth edition of *ACSM's Guidelines for Exercise Testing and Prescription* provides the basic principles of testing and training for normal healthy individuals and for those with cardiovascular disease. There is growing interest in the use of exercise for clients with other chronic diseases and disabilities. The purpose of this book is to provide a framework for determining functional capacity and developing appropriate exercise programming to optimize functional capacity in persons with chronic diseases and/or disabilities. The basic principles for exercise testing and training stated in *ACSM's Guidelines for Exercise Testing and Prescription* provide the foundation for this book. When not otherwise stated, these principles are assumed to apply. However, some special situations created by a disease pathology, disability, or treatment alter these basic principles. For example, exercise testing is an important aspect of the approach used in this book, but some people will not have completed an exercise test before starting an exercise program. Participation in regular physical activity can enhance functional capacity, and a primary goal of this book is to get more individuals physically active. Thus, for many people, exercise testing may not be absolutely necessary before starting a low-level physical activity program.

Exercise management for persons with a chronic disease and/or disability is now provided by a wide variety of health care and exercise professionals. Presently, management techniques depend on the provider's experience and are loosely, if at all, coordinated with other providers. A second goal of this book is to develop an integrated model of care so that everyone can work together in a program in which exercise is coordinated with other aspects of health care.

This is not an all-encompassing book on exercise testing and prescription for the populations of interest.

Rather, it is a reference manual to use as a guide for managing people with a condition outside the exercise professional's primary expertise. The editorial board and authors were chosen by virtue of their clinical and research experience in exercise programming for persons with chronic diseases and disabilities. The editors established a format for the book and then worked with the authors in writing the text. During the writing process, each chapter was peer-reviewed and then revised accordingly. Before printing, the entire book was reviewed by individuals with a broad expertise in the use of exercise. The authors have suggested reading materials for more in-depth information; these are listed at the end of each chapter and are strongly recommended. If the reader is unable to solve a clinical problem using this manual and the suggested readings, we recommend contacting the chapter author or section editor for advice.

Many people who have a chronic disease or disability enter a downward spiral toward exercise intolerance, so exercise intervention programs should be designed to resist this spiral and optimize functional capacity. Within any given population, there is a wide range of abilities determined by several factors: progression of the disease, response to treatment, and presence of other concomitant illnesses. Expected outcomes of exercise training are not always known. Realistically, optimal exercise and medical programming may yield improvements or merely prevent further deterioration. This book at times may recommend tests or programs that have not been validated, but that experience has shown to be successful. It is hoped that optimal management will bring the individual greater independence and improved quality of life.

Exercise programming must be regularly updated and adapted to the individual's clinical state. The prescription may change depending on the needs of the person, the progression/stabilization of the condition, or the therapy. As a result of disease progression, exercise programming may need to be discontinued—exercise at all costs is not our intent. Rather, we desire appropriate exercise management, including the astute clinical judgment of the exercise professional, leading to successful exercise programs.

We hope that this book will help improve the quality of life for individuals with chronic diseases or disabilities.

Preface to the Second Edition

J. Larry Durstine, PhD, FACSM

Geoffrey E. Moore, MD, FACSM

Lorraine E. Colson Bloomquist, EdD, FACSM

Peter H. Brubaker, PhD, FACSM

Christopher B. Cooper, MD, FACSM

Stephen F. Figoni, PhD, RKT, FACSM

Patricia L. Painter, PhD, FACSM

Kenneth H. Pitetti, PhD, FACSM

Scott O. Roberts, PhD, FACSM

The first edition of this book, *ACSM's Exercise Management for Persons with Chronic Diseases and Disabilities*, which we informally called CDD, was designed to be a quick reference to assist exercise professionals in managing exercise programs for persons with chronic diseases and disabilities. Existing textbooks were good reviews of scientific knowledge, but they fell short of providing guidance on *what to do*. Moreover, there were almost no sources of guidance for persons with multiple chronic diseases. We sought to provide a rational and consistent approach to helping anyone in need of an exercise program. We developed an integrated approach based on clinical experience and, working closely with the contributing authors, crafted a chapter format containing helpful tables on testing and prescription. CDD provided an overview of exercise management that addressed a wider spectrum of chronic diseases and disabilities than any other textbook on "special populations." CDD assumed that readers (1) had a strong working knowledge of exercise science and (2) sought only simple guidance in areas outside their primary expertise. CDD was about how to solve complex problems with a fairly simple set of clinical guidelines.

The second edition, *ACSM's Exercise Management for Persons with Chronic Diseases and Disabilities*, which we call CDD2, takes the same approach but with updated scientific content and improved guidance in problem solving. The biggest change is the inclusion of example cases in almost every chapter about a disease or disability. Some of these cases are simple, some complex, but all are real cases drawn from the clinical practices of the authors. These case studies strengthen this second edition because they illustrate that our recommendations are based not on academic theory but on knowledge from scientific research tempered by clinical experience. All cases are formatted to a uniform style to improve clarity and ease of use.

The limited scope of what we can achieve within our content constraints may leave some readers disappointed. We empathize with you. We would love to provide an encyclopedic book that addresses virtually all diseases and disabilities—a bona fide all-encompassing textbook— but are unable to do so for reasons of cost and (in some cases) lack of published data. We have, however, added several new diseases and disabilities as well as expanded discussion to this second edition. These include a chapter in section I on growth and development, and a new section containing five chapters on pulmonary diseases: Chronic Obstructive Pulmonary Disease, Chronic Restrictive Pulmonary Disease, Asthma, Cystic Fibrosis, and Lung and Heart-Lung Transplantation. The CDD chapter on organ transplantation has been broken into three chapters in CDD2, including the aforementioned lung and heart-lung transplant chapter as well as the chapters Cardiac Transplant and Abdominal Organ Transplant (Kidney, Liver, Pancreas). We have also added the chapters Atrial Fibrillation and Fibromyalgia. Finally, we have greatly expanded the appendix on medications, adding two appendixes on the effects of drugs on exercise capacity, and have also added a list of Web resources.

Chapter topics were chosen mainly on the basis of prevalence in the United States, although we have included some chapters because they happen to cover a relatively large knowledge base. Lack of peer-reviewed publications continues to be a problem, a fact that underscores the necessity of becoming a skilled practitioner. Historically, exercise scientists studied cardiovascular and pulmonary conditions before moving on to musculoskeletal, neurologic, and metabolic diseases. As a result, there is an uneven depth of knowledge between various diseases and disabilities. Over time, as our knowledge grows, we hope it will be possible to broaden our palette to include a wider spectrum of conditions. For now, the exercise professional must be capable of appropriately improvising to individualize exercise management.

We are truly thrilled at how well CDD has been received. Our goal is to help the reader translate the *science* of exercise physiology into the *art* of practicing exercise medicine. We hope you find CDD2 to be a substantial improvement and a worthy reference for your library.

SECTION I

Framework

J. Larry Durstine, PhD, FACSM

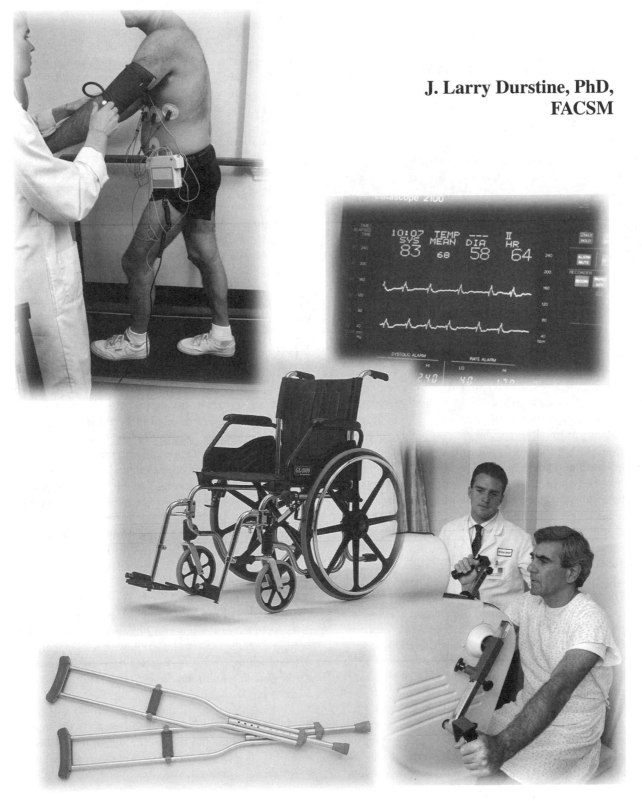

CHAPTER 1

Introduction

Geoffrey E. Moore, MD, FACSM
McGill University

J. Larry Durstine, PhD, FACSM
University of South Carolina

In general, our society has a bias toward curative rather than palliative medicine, toward making the disease go away rather than finding ways to cope with disease. An unfortunate consequence of this perspective is that for persons with chronic disease or disability, we devalue the palliative benefits of preserving functionality and well-being. Recent improvements in societal awareness of persons with disabilities, of the elderly, and of persons with terminal or end-stage disease have brought attention to medical issues surrounding individual rights of autonomy and self-determination. Since the 1960s, exercise has been promoted as a method of extending life, largely through prevention and moderation of cardiovascular disease. But in the 1980s, research and clinical applications for exercise expanded to populations with a variety of chronic diseases and disabilities, for whom exercise is perhaps more fundamentally related to *quality* of life than to *quantity* of life. Perhaps the greatest potential benefit of exercise is its ability to preserve functional capacity, freedom, and independence.

The exercise or health professional looking for guidance in managing exercise programs for people with chronic disease or disability will soon discover that most textbook chapters are grouped by diagnosis. Most chapters are written by specialists who discuss precautions and caveats for the performance of exercise in the context of a specific disease or disability. Since many diseases and disabilities have not been sufficiently studied to yield exact dose-response information, recommendations are vague, coming not from controlled trials but from empiricism and anecdote. While this approach is valid, one must recognize that its origins lie not in physiology but in the structure of academia and the perception that exercise is an adjuvant therapy.

One major shortcoming of diagnosis-oriented management is that many people have multiple concomitant problems and do not fit neatly into a single special population. Furthermore, many diseases involve multiple organ systems. Exercise professionals need a paradigm useful for anyone: a paradigm based on the effects of disease or disability on the acute response to exercise, on the adaptations to training, on the interaction of exercise with medicines, and on the expected dose-response relationship.

Problem-oriented exercise management provides a fundamental framework through which to approach any client with any combination of diseases and/or disabilities. Problem-oriented exercise management yields many advantages: it uses exercise testing to reveal physiologic dysfunction; it directs exercise therapy toward problems that might be improved by training; it integrates exercise into medical management; it assigns responsibility to the individual, thereby reinforcing the individual's sense of self-determination and autonomy; and, perhaps most importantly, it transforms problems of overwhelming complexity into components that are more manageable.

How to Use This Book

CDD2 provides an outline of how to effectively manage exercise for someone with chronic disease or disability. To use this manual, the reader should have extensive knowledge about exercise testing and training. Successful exercise management should also involve close teamwork between physicians, nurses, and allied health care providers. The editors assume that the reader is appropriately skilled in these matters and can adapt to individual circumstances. *ACSM's Resource Manual for Guidelines for Exercise Testing and Prescription* (4th edition) and *ACSM's Guidelines for Exercise Testing and Prescription* (6th edition) contain information on various exercise protocols, although some specific protocols or exercise devices may be described here. This manual does not provide detailed instruction on exercise physiology or disease, so the reader must do supplementary reading as needed to fully understand exercise management. For detailed information on diseases and disabilities, the reader should refer to standard physiology, medical, and adapted physical activity texts.

Each chapter deals with a common chronic disorder or disability that might limit functional capacity. Each chapter briefly lists the physiologic nature of the disease or disability, its effects on exercise response and adaptation, the effects of commonly used medicines, and any unique circumstances that should be considered. Recommendations for testing and programming are presented in tables for easy reference. The reader should refer to the chapter(s) relevant for each individual and use the information in those chapters as guidelines in developing an individualized exercise program.

To develop an integrated model, we have aggregated and consolidated old conventions and tried to create a comprehensive system. The first two chapters introduce these new conventions; all remaining chapters follow this model. Some terms and concepts are used interchangeably, such as *exercise prescription* and *exercise programming*. Other concepts are new, such as *family of exercise test*. These conventions were chosen not to imply correctness but to simplify.

Some concepts remain complex, for there seemed no easy approach and no substantial benefit to simplifying. For example, aerobic exercise intensity is expressed in a variety of ways: percentage of maximal oxygen consumption ($\dot{V}O_2$max), percentage peak heart rate, percentage heart rate reserve, and so on. These choices were largely left to each author's preference. One important convention in this book is the use of the words *clients* and *individuals* instead of *patients*. This convention was chosen because not all exercise managers are health care professionals in a patient–care giver relationship.

Problem-Oriented Management

A method of exercise management that uses problem-oriented techniques is presented here and is recommended by the editors. This technique uses the SOAP notes commonly employed by health care professionals. For those unfamiliar with this technique, the problem-oriented system is just an organizational tool. In brief, SOAP stands for subjective data, objective data, assessment, and plan of action. Notes, to oneself and others, are written in the SOAP outline style to clarify the thinking process and the rationale for a course of evaluation, therapy, or both. Problems and unique needs are identified and the intervention is documented, largely so that follow-up evaluations can be compared to earlier visits and success or failure can be fairly judged.

The key benefit of problem-oriented management is that several problems can be independently tracked in their own time frame but within the context of the overall situation. In healthy able-bodied persons, there is little need for this system, and there may not be much need even in persons with a single chronic disease or disability that doesn't alter the physiologic response to activity (e.g., sensory disorders such as deafness or visual impairment). But for persons in whom multiple chronic disease or disability circumstances affect exercise performance,

there can be a real need for such a system. The key to doing problem-oriented management is identifying all problems and needs and then following each problem in its own appropriate time frame. An example case, in SOAP note format, is provided in each chapter.

How to Use the Tables

Each chapter contains tables describing appropriate exercise tests and programs for the chronic disease or disability addressed in that chapter. Columns and rows are separated by lines. Columns contain categories of recommendations, and rows contain families of exercise tests, as described in chapter 2.

Each row contains recommendations regarding that family of exercise. For testing tables, the recommendation categories are Methods (to use), Measures (to take), Endpoints (and way-points) to specifically note, and general Comments. For programming tables, the categories are Modes (of training), Goals (of the program), Intensity/Frequency/Duration (in the prescription), and Time to Goal. Both testing and programming tables may have additional sections that describe appropriate Medications and Special Considerations.

How to Read the Tables

To determine which exercise test to conduct for a particular chronic disease or disability, look at the testing table in the relevant chapter. In the first column, labeled Methods, find the family of exercise test you would like to perform. Then read across to the second column, Measures, to find out which physiologic measurements are recommended during the test. Continuing to read across, within the exercise test family, look for Endpoints in the third column. Endpoints are usually indications to terminate the test, although some "endpoints" are relevant way-points, or measurements taken during the test (e.g., ventilatory threshold). The fourth column, Comments, lists relevant issues. In addition, give special attention to the sections in each table regarding appropriate Medications and Special Considerations.

Similarly, to develop an exercise program for an individual, look at the programming table. In the first column, labeled Modes, find the family of exercise test you would like to prescribe. Within each exercise family are recommended generic modes of training. Then read across to the second column, Goals, to find appropriate program objectives. Continuing to read across within the family of exercise, you will find appropriate Intensity/Frequency/Duration recommendations in the third column. The fourth column, Time to goal, provides an idea of how long it will take to reach an established goal. As with exercise testing, special note should be taken of the Medications and Special Considerations sections in each table.

What's in the Tables

Each table contains material summarized from the chapter as well as recommendations about exercise testing and programming. Protocols and programs are usually listed generically, rather than in specific terms, because detailed listing of all known protocols would be overly cumbersome. It is assumed that readers know how to conduct exercise tests and design exercise training programs.

What's Not in the Tables

Although many tables are complete and comprehensive, many are not. Some tables contain areas that are left blank, or omit mention of a particular family of exercise, usually because the author or section editor felt that insufficient data were available to justify a recommendation. Some tables list only a mode or a method because there is insufficient knowledge to recommend specific protocols, but the author's experience has been that the suggested modes/methods can be used successfully. Sometimes recommendations for exercise testing and programming of a particular disease or disability don't match; again, the reason is usually that research on exercise testing and training procedures is incomplete. Finally, in the testing and programming tables in chapters 46 through 49, some sections are combined because the disability doesn't alter the normal response to exercise or adaptations to exercise training (e.g., visual impairment).

Suggested Readings

Exercise Physiology

American College of Sports Medicine. 2001. *ACSM's resource manual for guidelines for exercise testing and prescription.* Edited by J.L. Roitman, M. Herridge, M. Kelsey, T.P. LaFontaine, L. Miller, M. Wegner, M.A. Williams, and T. York. 4th ed. Philadelphia: Lippincott Williams & Wilkins.

American College of Sports Medicine. 2000. *ACSM's guidelines for exercise testing and prescription.* Edited by B.A. Franklin, M.H. Whaley, and E.T. Howley. 6th ed. Philadelphia: Lippincott Williams & Wilkins.

American College of Sports Medicine. *ACSM's resources for clinical exercise physiology: Musculoskeletal, neuromuscular, neoplastic, immunologic, and hematologic conditions.* Edited by J.N. Myers, W.G. Herbert, and R. Humphrey. Philadelphia: Lippincott Williams & Wilkins.

Exercise in Chronic Disease and Disability

Sherrill, C. 1998. *Adapted physical activity, recreation, and sport: Cross-disciplinary and lifespan.* 5th ed. Madison, WI: Brown & Benchmark.

Skinner, J.S. 1993. *Exercise testing and exercise prescription for special cases: Theoretical basis and clinical application.* 2nd ed. Philadelphia: Lea & Febiger.

Medicine

Fauci, A.S., E. Braunwald, K.J. Isselbacher, J.D. Wilson, J.B. Martin, D.L. Kasper, S.L. Hauser, and D.L. Longo, eds. 1998. *Harrison's principles of internal medicine.* 14th ed. New York: McGraw-Hill.

Pharmacology

Kastrup, E., ed. 2001. *Drug facts and comparisons.* 5th ed. St. Louis: Facts and Comparisons.

CHAPTER 2

Framework

Geoffrey E. Moore, MD, FACSM
McGill University

J. Larry Durstine, PhD, FACSM
University of South Carolina

Anthony P. Marsh, PhD
Wake Forest University

This chapter introduces a method to manage exercise in persons with chronic disease or disability. The first section provides an overview of this model. Subsequent sections offer greater detail about factors to consider.

An exercise history should be taken from the individual to provide subjective data on aerobic ability, anaerobic ability (for athletes), endurance, strength, flexibility, neuromuscular skill, and overall functional performance. This information defines the person's problem(s), and these aspects of physical activity are easily tested in the laboratory to provide objective data. The objective data quantify the person's limitations in physiologic terms, and this information is used to assess the cause(s) of exercise intolerance. From this assessment, an exercise training plan is developed. Formulation of a plan is complex, and includes (1) medication effects; (2) exercise dose-response (desired goal; type of exercise; intensity, duration, and frequency of training; adaptability to training as well as exhaustion/overtraining limits); (3) risks of training; (4) the cost-benefit ratio; and (5) any necessary coordination among members of the health care team.

Problem-Oriented Exercise Management

Problem-oriented exercise management is the cornerstone of our approach to exercise in persons with chronic disease and disability. Problem-oriented medical management was developed in the late 1960s and has been beneficial to health care professionals. The major benefit is that this approach organizes extremely complex problems into simpler parts that are more easily tracked and solved. Given the enormous complexity of exercise in chronic disease and disability, it may not be possible to manage some persons without this technique.

Problem-oriented management consists of five steps, commonly documented in the SOAP format. SOAP is defined as the (1) collection of **S**ubjective data, (2) collection of **O**bjective data, (3) **A**ssessment and generation of a problem list, (4) formulation of a diagnostic or therapeutic **P**lan, or both, and (5) periodic reassessment (follow-up). Since the format provides a quick conceptual reminder of the situation and any progress that has been made, SOAP notes are useful not only to the manager but also to any colleagues who may be assisting.

Getting Subjective Data

Before testing someone with a chronic disease or disability, characterize his or her problem. Take a history of physical activity and medical problems to obtain the person's complaints and symptoms. With regard to exercise intolerance, symptoms might include shortness of breath, exertional chest pain, weakness, ease of fatigability, back pain, and so forth. Find out why the person is coming to you, what exercises have been done in the past, what the limitations are now, what injuries have occurred, and what medical problems (e.g., heart, lung, circulatory, gastrointestinal, metabolic, and neurological disorders) and musculoskeletal problems are present now. Determine present medicines being taken. Obtain results of any recent medical and exercise tests. Even if you are not highly skilled in physical examination, a simple physical examination is valuable in establishing the extent of obvious musculoskeletal limitations.

Learning these facts will guide you toward the exercise measures that are probably subnormal. These are the problems that limit functional capacity and they should be characterized by an exercise test. If a person cannot go to the store because he or she becomes winded or fatigued, aerobic and endurance exercise tests are indicated. If the person can't go to the store because he or she is too weak to carry the bags home, strength tests are indicated. For someone who is too clumsy to walk to the store, neuromuscular and functional performance tests are indicated. It is not helpful or cost-effective to use every exercise test on everyone; nor is it wise to use only certain tests for persons with a specific disease or disability. Subjective data help you figure out which tests to use.

Getting Objective Data

Objective data include information collected during physical examination and laboratory studies. After discerning the client's problem(s), perform tests that best characterize the exercise capacity. Appropriate medical and laboratory tests may provide measurements that confirm or refute possible causes of the symptoms. Since there are many kinds of exercise tests you could use, recommending a specific test is difficult. Furthermore, it is often not clear which test protocol is the best method. This is the main reason tests have been grouped into seven families based on what they are designed to quantify (see discussion of family of exercise test measures later in this chapter). These are the families:

1. Aerobic tests measure the ability to do exercise using high rate of oxygen consumption ($\dot{V}O_2$max).
2. Anaerobic tests measure the ability to do unsustained very high-intensity exercise.
3. Endurance tests measure the ability to sustain submaximal aerobic exercise for an extended time.
4. Strength tests measure the ability to do unsustained exercise against high resistance.
5. Flexibility tests measure the ability to move joints through their range of motion.
6. Neuromuscular tests measure the ability to do activities that require coordination and skill.
7. Functional performance tests measure the ability to do specific physical activities of daily living.

Exercise testing protocols should be individualized to suit each person and, as a result, provide the best possible information for developing the management plan. To complete this task, the exercise professional may need to develop an estimate of the individual's potential exercise capacity. That estimate, along with professional knowledge and the information presented in this book, may then be used to attain optimal test results.

Making the Assessment

Using information from the subjective and objective data-gathering steps, you should generate a list of specific problems. For example, an individual's problems may include (1) low aerobic capacity, (2) low ventilatory threshold, (3) low endurance at 75% of aerobic capacity, (4) weak hip and knee extensors, and so on. This assessment may explain the person's problem(s) or lead to further testing for problems that aren't fully explained or evident. Complete assessment may require several rounds of testing and reassessment before you have enough information to clearly identify the problem(s). Organize the assessment either by family of exercise test or by physiologic problem, and number each problem in sequence. Doing so will help you keep track of all the problems in a systematic fashion. For most people, obtaining subjective and objective data and making an assessment will not be difficult.

Formulating a Plan

The plan of action is the path that will lead to diagnosis and/or treatment of the problem(s). Making this plan is usually far more difficult than the first three steps, because exercise prescription for persons with chronic disease or disability is often complex. The initial plan for some people will require performing further assessment and obtaining additional data, but sooner or later, an overall management plan including exercise programming must be formulated. Executing this plan is difficult because part of the plan will include following a problem for a period of time. This time period can be a few days, a few weeks, or a few months. When numerous problems are present, it is possible to lose track of some of them during this time, making sequential numbering of the problems important.

First, establish an exercise prescription that has realistically achievable long-term goals. Then establish shorter-term intermediate goals that are easily achieved. This helps to develop a feeling of success. Make the goals something meaningful to the person, for example, a specific activity such as yard work. Use the exercise test measures only for your own records. Telling someone that he or she has achieved a 25% increase in aerobic capacity may mean little to him or her, but celebrating a renewed ability to do something specific like mowing the lawn is something everyone can understand.

Second, consider any unique circumstances such as prosthetics, medicines, exercise facilities, and other conditions that may require modification of a more typical program. Also, evaluate the risks, benefits, and costs of the program. Remember that anyone who exercises has some activity-dependent risks such as injuries. But persons with a chronic disease or disability have risks related to their disease or disability. The risks of exercise are commonly conceived in terms of heart attacks and sudden death, but these are really disease-dependent risks for persons with heart disease. Heart attacks and sudden death are distinctly uncommon in people who don't have heart disease, so other disease-dependent risks may prove more important. The relative risks of any activity are determined by the severity of the disease and the inherent danger of the activity. Benefits of the program will usually be an increase in physical activity, quality of life, or both, but may well be a reduction in medicines or a moderation of disease severity. Costs will generally be time and energy, particularly for people who can perform unsupervised exercise, although equipment and facility costs must also be considered. Be aware that for some, exercise training will be more of a bother than a benefit.

Third, design an exercise program incorporating each of the considerations identified. Start from the person's current fitness and choose practical levels of intensity, duration, and frequency of exercise sessions. Do not be bound to standard programs (e.g., 20-40 min, 3-4 times/wk). Such programs typically have the goal of decreasing cardiac morbidity and mortality, but these are often not the best goals for the purposes of persons with chronic disease or disability. Be careful not to exhaust the individual with work sessions that are too difficult. Choose a realistic time frame for achieving the goals, and pay attention to the necessary rate of improvement. Be careful not to overtrain the individual; there is no real purpose in overexercising a person with limited reserve who is not competing in sports. However, some persons with chronic diseases and/or disabilities can participate in athletic competition. The risk, cost, and benefit of exercise training will be discussed later in this chapter.

Fourth, develop a schedule for follow-up reassessment. Sometimes it is easy to make an assessment and a logical plan is readily apparent. More often, however, the assessment and plan are iterative processes—assessment, data collection, reassessment, more data collection, more reassessment, and so on, until the problem is solved. A therapeutic trial is a way to obtain objective data by seeing how well empiric therapy solves the problem. Once a solution has been settled upon, the appropriate time between reassessments is determined by individual circumstances. Following up too soon is a poor use of time and resources, but following up too late risks letting an old problem get out of control or a new problem go unnoticed. During follow-up, evaluate the progress and reassess the appropriateness of the prescription. Do this for each problem that is not stable and needs more attention. Problems that are not relevant may be skipped.

Organizing problems by exercise family has the advantages of maintaining the context of the exercise test and prescription, focusing strategy, and helping track minor problems. In many cases, the person in fact has several problems but really only one major problem. However, one must not lose sight of the fact that secondary problems and sedentary lifestyle compound the situation. It is easiest to keep it all straight if these problems are organized by exercise family. Organizing by physiologic problem is a good alternative. Note that the tables for recommended testing and programming found in each chapter of this book are organized by family of exercise.

Families of Exercise Tests Measures

All forms of exercise involve most of the systems found in the body, whereas different types of exercises have different physiologic effects. In this manual, exercises are grouped into seven families of laboratory measurements that characterize the capacity to perform specific activities: (1) aerobic, (2) anaerobic, (3) endurance, (4) strength, (5) flexibility, (6) neuromuscular skill, and (7) functional performance. These generic groupings provide a rationale for selecting an appropriate laboratory test and prescribing a training program. From a physiologic perspective, these groupings do overlap to an extent, but in a problem-oriented system these families of exercises are nonetheless useful for organizational purposes. Measures that characterize each family of exercise are as follows:

1. Aerobic exercise tests measure the ability to do exercise requiring high rates of oxygen consumption. Examples of aerobic test measures include $\dot{V}O_2max$, peak oxygen consumption ($\dot{V}O_2peak$), maximal steady-state oxygen consumption ($\dot{V}O_2MSS$), ventilation (e.g., spirometry), 12-lead electrocardiogram (ECG), heart rate, blood pressure, perceived exertion, metabolic equivalents (METs), time to exhaustion, and lactate threshold.

2. Anaerobic exercise tests measure the ability to exercise at an intensity that exceeds maximal ($\dot{V}O_2max$) or peak ($\dot{V}O_2peak$) oxygen consumption. Examples of anaerobic test measures include capacity for oxygen debt, 30-s peak power output, time trial performance, and peak lactate. This type of test is useful mostly for athletes.

3. Endurance exercise tests measure the ability to sustain submaximal aerobic exercise for an extended time. Examples of endurance test measures include time trial performance, 6- and 12-min walk, 1-mi (1.6K) walk, time to exhaustion or rate of perceived exertion at a constant work rate, and maximal number of repetitions.

4. Strength exercise tests measure the ability to do unsustained work against a high resistance. Examples of strength test measures include maximal number of repetitions, isokinetic work and peak torque, maximal voluntary contraction, and peak power output.

5. Flexibility exercise tests measure the ability to move joints through a prescribed range of motion (ROM). Examples of flexibility test measures include sit-and-reach distances and goniometry.

6. Neuromuscular exercise tests measure the ability to do activities that require coordination and skill. Examples of neuromuscular test measures include gait analysis, balance times, hand-eye coordination scores, and reaction time.

7. Functional performance tests measure the ability to do specific physical activities of daily living. Examples of functional performance test measures include sit-and-stand scores, lifting, timed walk, and gait.

The redundancy among the families reflects the integrated nature of physical activity and a means of characterizing specific aspects of exercise. Note that this manual usually recommends the mode of exercise (e.g., in the aerobic family—walking, jogging, cycling, rowing, combined arm/leg cycling, stair climbing, swimming, aerobic dance, and so on).

Speed of fatigability is a common complaint in people who are severely challenged by activities commonly considered routine, such as grocery shopping. Daily activities are complex physical activities that require integrated function between many of the organ systems and use all seven families of exercise. In this way, factors such as endurance and neuromuscular skill can determine daily activities and quality of life more than measures of oxygen consumption, strength, flexibility, or combinations of these measures.

Aerobic Exercise Tests

The ability to do aerobic exercise is very important for completing activities of daily living, and is commonly tested in the laboratory setting through the use of graded exercise tests. Maximal oxygen consumption is an important physiologic measurement, but many persons with a chronic disease or disability do not achieve a "true" $\dot{V}O_2$max. Rather, they reach a point at which they cannot continue. Such individuals are said to reach symptom-limited exhaustion, referred to as *peak $\dot{V}O_2$*. The distinction is important, because $\dot{V}O_2$max is limited by oxygen supply, while $\dot{V}O_2$peak is limited by some other factor, such as fatigue.

Another critical point that can be revealed during exercise testing is the point at which the person experiences a transition from an exercise intensity that can be sustained more or less indefinitely to an intensity that can be sustained for only a short time. A variety of methods are used to measure this transition, including lactate threshold, onset of blood lactate accumulation, ventilatory threshold, and Conconi heart rate threshold. Several protocols designed to detect this transition are available. For our purposes, the transition from sustainable to unsustainable exercise is the common aspect and will be referred to as $\dot{V}O_2MSS$.

Measurement of $\dot{V}O_2$ max is important in persons with chronic disease or disability. Many such people have a very low $\dot{V}O_2$peak, usually less than 25 ml $\cdot$ kg^{-1} $\cdot$ min^{-1}, and often less than 20 ml $\cdot$ kg^{-1} $\cdot$ min^{-1}. The usual range for $\dot{V}O_2MSS$ is 40 to 70% of $\dot{V}O_2$max. Many common activi-

ties of daily living, usually taken for granted by those who are healthy and able-bodied, require oxygen consumption in the range of 12 to 30 ml $\cdot$ kg^{-1} $\cdot$ min^{-1}. Many people with a chronic disease or disability have a $\dot{V}O_2$max or $\dot{V}O_2$peak below that required for activities of daily living, employment, and maintenance of individual independence, resulting in a lower quality of life.

In general, constant increment or continuously increasing (or ramp) work rate protocols are preferred over some standard protocols (e.g., Bruce protocol). Many standard protocols increase work rate in relatively large, often nonlinear increments and are effective in screening for ischemic heart disease. In exercise management, however, we are more interested in characterizing the exercise response in the submaximal range. Ramp protocols are far superior in this regard because they indicate submaximal exercise responses while still detecting coronary artery disease.

A disadvantage of using a standardized ramp protocol is that one cannot individualize exercise tests so that each subject can complete the test in 8 to 10 min. Many nonconditioned persons have low endurance exercise capacity and will be unable to exercise for this length of time. At the same time, tests lasting for 12 to 15 min or longer can give falsely low results. Therefore, one must know the client's approximate ability, estimate his or her peak exercise capacity, and design a test to yield 4 to 8 changes in work rates during an 8- to 10-min test period. Low-level ramp protocols may require special programming and manual operation, and may be difficult to reproduce on equipment that is imprecise at low exercise levels. For example, some persons can generate only 10 watts and will not be able to pedal a standard stationary cycle against any measurable resistance. Therefore, the subject must be tested by freewheel pedaling, in which only the pedaling rate is increased. With careful consideration and planning, successful exercise testing can be accomplished for nearly everyone.

Anaerobic Exercise Tests

Anaerobic tests usually consist of short-term exercise that supplements strength test data or offers data on ability to do brief periods of high-intensity exercise. In several chronic diseases, this type of test correlates closely with a variety of measures of functional capacity, including $\dot{V}O_2$max. Anaerobic tests may also be of value for athletes preparing for competition.

Endurance Exercise Tests

Endurance tests are potentially useful because many inactive persons cannot exercise longer than 5 min but can sustain exercise for 1 hour or more after training (even without an increase in $\dot{V}O_2$peak). Unfortunately, endurance tests have not been well developed and often lack test-retest reliability, well-defined endpoints, and clear physiologic meaning. Claudication tests (e.g., walk distance to onset of pain, maximal walk distance) are useful in arterial insufficiency because they satisfy these criteria.

Strength Exercise Tests

Muscular strength is a critical component of exercise capacity, particularly in persons with a chronic disease or disability. Resistance testing is essential because skeletal muscle weakness can limit functional capacity. Like aerobic exercise response, skeletal muscle function can be evaluated in myriad ways—for example, maximal repetitions for a given weight (using either free weights or a machine); isokinetic force, work, and power; and isometric force. Each of these forms of testing has its own advantages and disadvantages, and the method chosen should be carefully matched to the problems being addressed and to the person's situation. Resistance testing can reveal several important aspects of strength, including maximal force, the smoothness of contraction and relaxation (lack of spasticity), balance of strength between extensor and flexor muscle groups, symmetry between left and right sides, and resistance to fatigue. Resistance training is also an excellent addition to a rehabilitation program and is often overlooked in cardiovascular rehabilitation programs. Strength training may well belong in virtually every program for persons with a chronic disease or disability.

Flexibility Tests

Flexibility is also a critical aspect of exercise programming. Range of motion is important because muscle force, in order to be useful, must be applied through a full range of movement for the proper performance of physical work. Normal joint and spine movement can maintain symmetry of function and protect muscles, joints, and bones from strain and injury. Like other forms of exercise testing, assessment of flexibility can be performed in a variety of ways, but the easiest, most versatile, and least expensive is the use of a simple goniometer. For our purposes, goniometry is probably most worthwhile in people with neuro-musculoskeletal disability, such as those with extreme scar tissue in joints, contractures, spasticity, and so on. Many exercise programs complete flexibility training (i.e., stretching) during the warm-up and cool-down segments of an exercise training session. Some people may require more extensive stretching, perhaps in combination with specific programs, to regain and maintain flexibility.

Neuromuscular Tests

Neuromuscular tests, which assess coordination and skill, are most useful in persons with a neuromuscular disabil-

ity or those who are severely debilitated from chronic disease or are frail. As a result, these types of tests are more commonly used by physical, occupational, and kinesiology therapists than by exercise physiologists. Examples include reaction time, hand-eye coordination tests, and gait analysis. These kinds of tests should be used, for the most part, in persons with neuromuscular deficits that need specific assessment and programming.

Functional Performance Tests

A wide array of test batteries have been developed to assess functional performance. These test batteries vary in their total number of tasks, but typically the tasks are timed or ranked using a simple scale. Many functional performance measures have components that relate directly to the mobility and strength of an individual. Independent living and freedom from disability requires performance above a threshold level of function, so individuals who barely surpass these functional thresholds of mobility and strength are at risk for future disability.

Functional performance tests should mimic real tasks, be objective, and be brief as well as easy to administer. When choosing a test, one should consider its reliability, the availability of normative data, the ability to detect change over time, and clinical applicability. It is recommended that a performance-based measure be a familiar task with a distinct start and end point. This enhances the test's reliability and objectivity. The exercise specialist should become adept at administering functional performance tests, and this may require some training so that the tests are administered according to established protocols.

Several tasks are commonly used in performance-based test batteries, including time to walk a given distance (an indicator of cardiovascular endurance; e.g., 6-min walk test); time to rise from a chair and return to a seated position a given number of times (an indicator of lower extremity strength); ability/time to stand in challenging positions (an indicator of postural control; e.g., feet together in a side-by-side, semi-tandem and tandem positions, one-leg balance time); a measure of freely chosen gait speed (e.g., over a 20-ft [6.1-m] distance); and the timed "get up and go" test, which is a combination of chair rises and gait.

It is also possible to assess physical functioning using a self-report questionnaire. There are many such self-report questionnaires that measure limitations in activities, modifications in performing activities (e.g., takes longer to perform routine activities, needs assistance in performing activities), and level of difficulty in performing routine activities. As in functional performance tests, any questionnaire you choose should be valid, reliable, and tested in the population of interest. Like functional performance tests, many of these questionnaires are highly predictive of outcomes in diseased populations and can provide insight into the level of limitation and possibly the potential for future disability.

No Exercise Tests

One predicament that exercise professionals encounter is the need to design a program without having any exercise test data. It isn't necessary to have an exercise test to begin a program. By using two or more techniques to measure relative intensity (e.g., heart rate and perceived exertion), you can compare them against each other as well as prior experience. In having your client exercise, err on the low side; you'll soon discover that it's too easy and can then increase the work rates to a more appropriate level. Within a week or two, your client will be on the right track.

On the other hand, you may wish to improvise a test. It is possible to use age- and gender-predicted values as "test results," but this can lead to inappropriate prescriptions in persons who aren't close to the average values. One common example is peak heart rate in persons on beta-antagonist drugs. Many authors have attempted to refine methods to yield more accurate predictions, and if these methods work successfully for you, use them.

A more pragmatic approach, however, is to improvise an informal submaximal exercise study in the form of an exercise session, or several studies over the course of a week. The simple rules recommended in this chapter, and the protocols in each chapter's table on exercise testing, provide useful information. For example, you can perform a submaximal cycle ergometer study by using a ramped protocol and recording heart rates and rating of perceived exertion (RPE) up to a level of 17 on a 20-point scale. You would then prescribe a range of exercising heart rates based on perceived exertion.

Attitude Assessment

Behavioral medicine has made substantial advances in recent years, and there are now many instruments available that assess quality of life, self-efficacy, or readiness to change. It may be tempting to rely on one's own counseling or coaching skills, but using one of these instruments to obtain some objective data is worthwhile. Having such a measurement to gauge progress can be invaluable to a specialist managing an exercise program. Getting a client to exercise regularly at higher doses may well be the best help you can offer. Because this is largely a matter of lifestyle, having a keen appreciation of each client's barriers to change is very important for the exercise specialist. One should use instruments that are validated, reliable, well tested, and used for the special population in which you intend to use the instrument. For almost all the chapters in this book, there are quality-of-life instruments that have been uniquely designed with the specific population in mind. There are also instruments designed to be used for any population. The proper use of these instruments is beyond the scope of this text, but their use may be mentioned by some chapter authors. Many readers will find it necessary to enlist the aid of a psychologist or behavioral medicine expert.

Summary

The exercise specialist working with persons with a chronic disease or disability must be able to employ techniques from each of the seven families of exercise tests. In the past, much of the emphasis has been on aerobic exercise testing, largely because of the prevalence of cardiovascular disease and the popularity of aerobic exercise. However, many exercise professionals have long used measures of strength, flexibility, neuromuscular skill, and functional performance. Because activities of daily living are integrated functions that require some element from each family of exercise, exercise specialists working with chronically diseased or disabled populations should incorporate the various test results in developing a comprehensive exercise management plan. In addition, many of the new exercise machines are useful tools in obtaining these measurements, but exercise specialists at facilities without these specialized machines can still assess exercise intolerance by using simple tools and a little ingenuity. A thorough knowledge of testing and test devices and an ability to improvise will be required. For some exercise specialists, this success may be enhanced by collaborating with other specialists who have complementary expertise and skills.

Exercise and Medicines

Most persons with a chronic disease or disability take medicines to treat their medical problems. Unfortunately, little is known about the side effects of most medicines as they relate to exercise capacity and quality of life. Some medicines improve exercise performance in general; some improve exercise performance when used for specific chronic diseases. Some medicines reduce exercise performance and thereby can have an adverse impact on quality of life. The development of an exercise management plan includes consideration of drug-induced changes in exercise performance, as well as optimal dosing of medicines to achieve a desired exercise response. Very little is known about the effects of most medicines on adaptations to exercise training, but drug effects on exercise adaptability should be a consideration in exercise management.

It is easier to understand the effects of medicines on exercise performance if one thinks of exercise itself as a medicine. Exercise, in one sense, is an idealized "intensive care unit" in which neural, hormonal, and local factors alter heart rate and redirect blood flow to deliver oxygen and nutrients. Metabolic control of energy resources is profoundly affected while thermal, acid-base, and electrolyte regulation are altered to support exercise activity. Myriad changes constitute what we call the "exercise response," but these physiologic changes reflect biochemical alterations in the body's control of metabolism. No modern intensive care unit can match the body's extraordinary and sophisticated system for delivery of biochemical compounds during exercise, despite the fact that some natural compounds (including hormones) are often used as prescription drugs. In this way exercise is a medicine.

Part of the difficulty in prescribing exercise as a drug is that exercise doesn't allow independent control over each biochemical process. During exercise, many biochemical reactions take place and we are unable to alter the sophistication of the whole process completely to our liking. However, we can take advantage of the interactions between exercise and medicines.

First, different kinds of physical activity (e.g., aerobic, strength, flexibility) stimulate biochemical and physiologic processes in slightly different ways. Second, most medicines work by blocking or enhancing specific processes and as a result cause the desired (and undesired) effects. Drug–exercise interactions are determined by the blocked or stimulated processes common to both medicine and exercise. Thus, to understand the effect a medicine has on exercise, one must know both the biochemistry and the physiology of the exercise and the medicine. The challenge is to use these differing effects to the person's advantage.

The study of drug–exercise interactions has generally centered on high blood pressure, angina pectoris (chest pain), congestive heart failure, and ergogenic aids (drugs that improve exercise performance). Most drug–exercise studies compare exercise response on and off medication or on different medications. This is largely for two reasons: (1) these studies are easier than longitudinal drug–training studies, and (2) these kinds of studies are part of FDA approval and pharmaceutical marketing programs. As a result, the effects of drugs on aerobic exercise response are better known than are the effects of drugs on training adaptations. Most drug–exercise studies have investigated drugs that alter cardiovascular function: alpha- and beta-adrenergic antagonists (alpha and beta blockers), calcium channel antagonists (calcium-channel blockers), angiotensin converting enzyme (ACE) inhibitors, angiotensin II receptor blockers, vasoactive nitrates, and diuretics. Many neuromuscular drugs, such as antiparkinsonian drugs, have also been studied in relation to functional performance.

Paradoxical Effects

One paradox of drug–exercise interactions is that disease can alter physiologic action so that a drug can have opposite effects on exercise capacity when used in some combinations or in different disease states. Beta blockers are the most thoroughly studied drugs with regard to exercise and provide a good example of paradoxical effects. In persons with high blood pressure, beta blockers typically reduce exercise capacity. In persons with congestive heart failure, however, beta blockers can increase exercise capacity. The ACE inhibitors provide another example of paradoxical effects. In persons with high blood pressure, ACE inhibitors have no effect on exercise capacity, but in those with congestive heart failure, ACE inhibitors usually increase exercise capacity. The beta blocker example shows that drug therapy can help the person's disease but reduce exercise capacity. The mechanisms of these effects are complex and will not be discussed here, but these examples show that the effect on exercise capacity is inherent not in the drug but rather in how the drug interacts with the biochemistry of exercise.

Adverse Effects

Sometimes drugs are recommended as preferred therapy even though they reduce exercise capacity. Beta blockers and diuretics are examples. Recommended as drugs of first choice for high blood pressure, beta blockers and diuretics are proven to prevent strokes and heart attacks and to increase longevity. Furthermore, they are inexpensive in comparison to newer medicines such as calcium channel blockers, ACE inhibitors, vasodilators, and alpha blockers. However, beta blockers and diuretics often impair exercise response, aerobic capacity, and quality of life. The newer drugs generally do not have these particular side effects. Unfortunately, there are little data on efficacy in preventing strokes or heart attacks and prolonging life for most of these newer drugs. Thus, beta blockers and diuretics are recommended for high blood pressure even though newer (more expensive) drugs may make it possible to control blood pressure with fewer side effects on exercise capacity and quality of life.

Effects on Muscle

Medicines without cardiovascular action can alter exercise response through effects on skeletal muscle. Corticosteroids, beta blockers, and ACE inhibitors are examples. Corticosteroids are used for suppression of inflammatory and autoimmune diseases, as well as for immunosuppression in transplant recipients. In the absence of exercise, corticosteroids cause peripheral muscle wasting. In contrast, corticosteroids have no effect on the usual muscle adaptations to exercise training. Beta blockers also act on skeletal muscle and may attenuate skeletal muscle adaptations to training. On the other hand, long-term ACE inhibitor therapy appears to increase muscle blood flow, although this might be a result of increased physical activity. These examples suggest that the poorly understood effects of medicines on skeletal muscle may be critically important in people who are weak and lacking in endurance.

Drugs That Affect Metabolism

Use of hormones that regulate metabolism can alter functional capacity and response to training. Thyroid hormone and insulin are examples. Hyperthyroidism and hypothyroidism both reduce exercise performance, and overreplacement or underreplacement of thyroid hormone can reduce exercise capacity. However, persons on adequate thyroid replacement have normal exercise performance. In one remarkable example, sprinter Gail Devers suffered from severe hyperthyroidism but recovered after therapy to win gold medals in both the Olympic Games and world championships. Insulin is used to control blood sugar in persons with diabetes, but insulin dosing usually should be reduced (or a snack eaten before exercise) to prevent life-threatening lowering of blood sugar during exercise.

Ergogenic Aids

Ergogenic aids increase the ability to improve exercise performance. In fact, sport competitors are not allowed to use them because they provide an unfair advantage. However, it might be reasonable to make judicious use of ergogenic aids in some persons with a chronic disease or disability. For example, the use of growth hormone or anabolic steroids may someday reveal the potential for improving exercise capacity in people who are weak and frail. Other ergogenic aids, such as stimulants, might also be helpful in certain circumstances. For example, caffeinated beverages should be avoided by people with coronary artery disease but might provide benefit to other people with exercise intolerance.

Other Medications

Little is known about the effects of most other drugs on exercise performance. Notable among these are drugs with antiparkinsonian and anticholinergic activity. Almost nothing is known about the effects of polypharmacy (the use of multiple drugs). Many people take several medications several times a day and, under these circumstances, it is well known that people forget to take their medicines. Furthermore, when adherence to or timing of a medication dose varies, the exercise response may be affected. Finally, while the effects of exercise on medicines are generally unexplored, it is worth noting that

even less is known about the effects of exercise on the metabolism of medicines (i.e., whether it is increased or decreased).

The examples in this section provide no details about the interactions between medicines and exercise. (See appendixes B and C for the effects of selected medications.) Nonetheless, exercise professionals must know (or learn) about the medications their clients are taking and must be able to assess how the medicine may alter each person's physiology. A pharmacology textbook should be a standard reference for anyone attempting to manage exercise for someone who takes medicines. Exercise professionals should establish a working relationship with the individual's physician so that suggestions about changing medications or dosing schedules can be smoothly integrated into overall medical management.

Exercise Dose–Response

Prescribing exercise for persons with chronic disease or disability is a complex art. The objective is to decrease physiologic limitations and improve physical capacity through specific therapies. The biggest dilemmas are not in determining which therapies to use but in defining the goals and choosing the appropriate training intensity, duration, and frequency. The key question is: What is the dose–response relationship of exercise training for each disease and disability?

In considering exercise programming for persons with chronic disease or disability, one often has little data on which to base decisions. Recommendations for preventing death from heart disease are based on large studies, but because these studies generally have not included persons with chronic disease or disability, present data may not be applicable. Furthermore, restoring and maintaining functional capacity and independence are very different goals from preventing cardiovascular disease. Unfortunately, exercise training to optimize functional capacity has not been well studied in the context of most chronic diseases or disabilities. As a result, many exercise professionals have used clinical experience to develop their own methods for prescribing exercise. Many of the recommendations in this manual were derived in this manner.

Experience is an acceptable way to guide exercise management, but a systematic approach would be better. One logical alternative would be to model exercise in the same way that pharmacologists model medications, since exercise and medical prescriptions are similar. Medicines are prescribed by action (type of chemical), bioavailability (which determines the dose), therapeutic level (the goal of therapy), and half-life (metabolism of the medicine). Prescription of exercise is quite similar, in that the family of exercise specifies the action (e.g., aerobic training increases $\dot{V}O_2max$; strength training increases muscle strength and mass); exercise dose is a function of intensity and duration (i.e., hard workouts at high intensity or long duration yield a higher number of total MET-minutes); and exercise frequency is determined by the desired fitness level (therapeutic goal) and the length of time for recovery from an exercise session (half-life).

These principles explain some common practices in exercise science and sport. Athletes exercise daily or even twice daily, whereas wellness enthusiasts exercise 3 or 4 times/wk. People who recover quickly can exercise on the day after a big workout, whereas other people may need an intervening day of rest, particularly after a very high dose session. Like people who are sensitive to medicines and require lower doses, those with low functional capacity are easily exhausted, and it is common to prescribe short, low-intensity workouts with long rest periods (low-dose exercise). Just as a therapeutic drug level in the blood can be achieved with the use of a lower dose more frequently, conditioning can be achieved through use of lower-intensity exercise 2 or 3 times/day. Just as slowly metabolized drugs must be given less often, persons who are slow to recover and adapt need more rest between exercise sessions.

Prescribing the right dose of exercise is important because one can experience an acute "overdose" of exercise. Like marathoners "hitting the wall," persons with chronic disease or disability can suddenly become worn out, often by small amounts of exercise. Common sense suggests that one should probably avoid exhaustion (an exercise overdose), but there are few data to support or refute this notion. In comparison, overtraining is essentially a chronic overdose of exercise, and is associated with psychologic and physiologic decompensation as well as musculoskeletal injury. Acute exercise overdoses and chronic overtraining must be avoided in persons who have limited reserve because of chronic disease or disability.

One area in which pharmacologists are ahead of exercise specialists is in following the therapeutic effect of medicines. Pharmacologists can do this by measuring drug levels in the blood. This information can then be used to help guide dose frequency. Exercise specialists can try using exercise tests to assess progress, but this information is not as helpful as data on drug level in the blood are to pharmacologists. A systematic way to guide frequency of exercise training has not been developed, largely because we do not fully understand fatigue and adaptation.

The person's starting level, resistance to fatigue, and adaptability to training are probably what determine the total dose of exercise required to achieve a given fitness level. Perceived fatigue is not like perceived exertion, which is proportional to exercise intensity (e.g., the 20-point Borg scale). Fatigue seems to have a threshold. After this threshold is reached, exhaustion occurs quite rapidly. Adaptability is also poorly understood. It is possible to increase the adaptation rate by training harder (e.g., increasing the intensity or frequency of exercise sessions), but training too hard leads to decompensation or injury. Thus, all we can say at present is that high doses of exercise increase the risk of exhaustion and that high frequency of exercise superimposes more training on incomplete recovery and risks overtraining.

Risk, Cost, and Benefit

It is common to think of musculoskeletal injury, heart attack, and sudden death as the risks of exercise. In fact, persons who are healthy and able-bodied are at risk largely for musculoskeletal injuries. For example, despite highly publicized cases of sudden death, basketball players are at greater risk for spraining their ankles. Only the basketball players with heart disease are at risk for sudden death. So exercise involves two kinds of risks: disease-dependent and activity-dependent risks. Disease-dependent risks are the adverse effects of exercise that are a consequence of disease. Activity-dependent risks are the adverse effects of exercise that are a consequence of accidents occurring during an activity. Activity- and disease-dependent risks must be considered for each person with a chronic disease or disability.

In general, the most important risks are disease dependent: arthritic joints can become more inflamed, diabetics can lose control of their blood sugar, people with high blood pressure can have a stroke or heart attack, clients with heart failure can have abnormal heart rhythms, clients with poor balance can fall, prosthetics can cause skin trauma and irritation, and so on. The most common activity-dependent complications are probably musculoskeletal injury and exhaustion, while the most feared risks of heart attack and sudden death occur largely in people with heart disease. Accurate estimates of these risks are not available. Although few clinical exercise trials in persons with a chronic disease or disability have reported life-threatening complications, virtually all studies have used small, selected populations that precluded high-risk subjects. Some data suggest a high incidence of musculoskeletal injury with the use of intense exercise in weak and frail individuals, although this has not been a universal finding. Although the data on risk are generally not clear, it is prudent to monitor vigilantly for potential complications.

The costs of exercise training include time, energy, and money put into the program. Fortunately, exercise can be inexpensive compared to other modern medical therapies (particularly so for unsupervised exercise).

Even so, exercise is far from cost-free. Membership in a YMCA/YWCA, health club, or fitness center can cost hundreds of dollars per year. Some individuals may need to choose a center that caters to persons who have special medical circumstances and need medical supervision. Investment in the appropriate clothing, shoes, and assorted equipment can also be substantial. This can be particularly true for those who must invest in prosthetic equipment or sport/racing wheelchairs. Protective equipment such as pads, gloves, skin protection materials, and helmets must not be overlooked. Since very few people can participate in a lifetime of exercise and be totally free from medical complications (especially activity-dependent problems), it may be reasonable to assume that there will be at least some associated medical costs. Lastly, personal time and energy are major costs of any program, but these are difficult to quantify in monetary terms.

The various investments in an exercise program must be weighed against the probable benefits. Benefits from exercise training are usually related to functional capacity and quality of life, although some populations also benefit from decreased morbidity and mortality. Furthermore, it is sometimes possible to decrease the doses of medications and reap a direct financial return on investment. There has been some success in predicting outcome for cardiac rehabilitation clients, and this technique may be useful for other populations. Until then, an exercise trial is probably worthwhile in any person with a chronic disease or disability. In contrast, a person who has several diseases and/or disabilities may gain little or may even be adversely affected by exercise training. Thus, it is difficult to know who is too sick to benefit from exercise. In people who are too sick to improve, it usually becomes apparent that exercise is of little benefit. Unfortunately, it is not currently possible to know how much someone will benefit from a given exercise program, and in many cases it is impossible to compare the benefits to costs in monetary terms. Better methods of predicting adaptation would improve goal setting and improve risk-benefit as well as cost-benefit analyses.

Putting It All Together

Now comes the point of putting it all together. Some of the techniques suggested in this manual will be new to exercise specialists, and will require time to learn and become proficient in their use. Successful exercise management does not require the use of these principles, but thinking about exercise in the contexts presented here can help determine what exercise tests to use, how to accommodate medicines, how to develop goals, how to estimate the dose-response, and how to assess the risk-benefit and cost-benefit relationships. These considerations may be particularly complicated in persons with a low exhaustion threshold, frequent intercurrent illness, multiple-chronic diseases, and poor adherence. In someone with only one relatively minor medical problem or disability, these tasks may be simple and straight-forward. In someone with a severe chronic disease or disability or multiple chronic diseases and/or dis-abilities, these tasks are highly complex. Problem-oriented exercise management using SOAP notes is one mechanism that can be employed to solve these problems. When using this approach, be sure to follow some key steps.

When taking subjective data:

- Uncover the nature of the problem as it relates to exercise.
- Ask about old and new musculoskeletal injuries.
- Look at the person for obvious problems.

When choosing exercise tests (objective data):

- Select the families of exercise tests that provide insight into the problem.
- Use modes and protocols that can be individualized.
- Use tests that provide specific measures that either will further define the problem or will determine specific aspects of the exercise program.
- Be aware of medications that may affect the test results, and know the times they are taken.
- Be aware of concomitant conditions and any special circumstances.

When making an assessment:

- Organize the assessment either by family of exercise or by physiologic problem.
- Consider possible need for additional tests.
- Be flexible in assessing multiple problems, and attack each one independently (but watch for interactions).
- Be aware that each problem may follow its own time course.
- If unsure, consider a therapeutic trial.

When developing an exercise program:

- Choose the families and modes of exercise that best treat the problem.
- Choose goals that are realistically attainable to increase the chance of success.
- Adjust exercise doses on the basis of exercise test measures, perceived exercise intensity, and the "fatigue threshold."
- Recommend frequency of training based on the total exercise dose and the person's adaptability.

- Accommodate any need for prosthetic, orthotic, or assistive devices.
- Consider the potential interactions of exercise and medications.
- Consider the disease-dependent and activity-dependent risks.
- Be aware that most of the benefits are probably related to quality of life.

When monitoring:

- Beware the sudden onset of exhaustion, as well as insufficient recovery and overtraining.
- Monitor stability of the underlying medical problems and changes in medications.
- When in doubt about safety, or if an activity causes pain, don't do it.
- When in doubt about progression, increase in small increments.
- Do not allow clients to push themselves hard unless they are well warmed up.

When following up:

- Report progress in terms meaningful to the individual, not in exercise jargon.
- Estimate dose–response and be willing to consider failure to benefit.
- Always follow up on unresolved problems.
- Use the numbers you assign to the problems to help keep track of everything.
- Most interventions take weeks (if not months) to achieve a benefit, so be patient.

Tips on SOAP Notes

To make the process of writing SOAP notes quick and easy, follow these guidelines:

- Be concise.
- Avoid sentences; use key phrases instead.
- Discuss only currently relevant problems; leave out irrelevant information.
- Organize the problems by exercise family (i.e., aerobic, strength, flexibility, and so on).
- Assign a number to each problem, and always refer to that problem by its number.
- Always follow up unresolved problems.

Suggested Readings

Guralnik, J.M., L. Ferrucci, C.F. Pieper, S.G. Leveille, K.S. Markides, G.V. Ostir, S. Studenski, L.F. Berkman, and R.B. Wallace. 2000. Lower extremity function and subsequent disability: Consistency across studies, predictive models, and value of gait speed alone compared with the short physical performance battery. *Journal of Gerontology, Series A, Biological Sciences and Medical Sciences* 55: M221-23.

Jette, A.M., D.U. Jette, J. Ng, D.J. Plotkin, and M.A. Bach. 1999. Are performance-based measures sufficiently reliable for use in multicenter trials? Musculoskeletal Impairment (MSI) study group. *Journal of Gerontology, Series A, Biological Sciences and Medical Sciences* 54: M3-6.

Rikli, R.E., and C.J. Jones. 1999. Development and validation of a functional fitness test for community-residing older adults. *Journal of Aging and Physical Activity* 7: 129-61.

Rikli, R.E., and C.J. Jones. 1999. Functional fitness normative scores for community-residing older adults, ages 60-94. *Journal of Aging and Physical Activity* 7: 162-81.

CHAPTER 3

Considerations Regarding Physical Activity for Children and Youth

William F. Riner, PhD, FACSM
John Morrison White Clinic

Richard J. Sabath, EdD, FACSM
Children's Mercy Hospital

The inclusion of a chapter dealing with children and youth in a reference volume focused on chronic disease and disability may seem somewhat paradoxical. In our society, those conditions are associated with the older population, while children are stereotypically considered healthy. However, as much as 10% of the pediatric population may be affected by health problems throughout childhood and adolescence. These conditions include congenital and acquired conditions of the heart, lungs, kidneys, neuromuscular and skeletal systems, as well as sensory, cognitive, and central nervous system dysfunction. As the role of physical activity in medical management of chronic disease and disability in the adult population increases, it seems imperative to consider the implications for children, for whom activity is the behavioral norm. Several volumes and numerous papers have been published dealing with the role of exercise in the lives of children with medical problems.

While links between disease and disability and low levels of physical activity have been identified, it is not uncommon that excessive precautions and reactions result in unnecessary restrictions on children. Therefore, care must be taken by the physician or other health professional, as well as the parents, to avoid overprotection. When there is organic disease present, exercise can be an effective therapy in mitigating detrimental consequences of the ailment. However, there are concerns about the possibility of injury, overuse syndromes, and abnormal responses to activity in sick children as well as in the healthy pediatric population.

The purpose of this chapter is to focus on some of the issues related to the physiology of children and youth that might have bearing on the responses to exercise that might be expected. As in adults, illness and disability will influence those responses in addition to the age-specific effects. The discussion in this chapter includes the effects of disease or disability on growth and development as well as acute and adaptive responses to exercise in healthy and sick children. Exercise testing methods and the benefits and risks of exercise for children and youth with selected categories of ailments are also considered.

Effects of Health Status and Physical Activity on Growth and Development

The regulation of growth and development in all children is influenced by environmental (e.g., social, cultural, economic, geographic, nutritional) and biological (e.g., genetic, endocrine) factors. These same factors play a role in determining health status, including the presence and consequences of many chronic diseases and disabilities. Obviously, genetic abnormalities in biological mechanisms can affect metabolic function and body composition, as well as neuromuscular and circulorespiratory function. The environment in which a child lives can also be responsible for an illness or disability, whether congenital or acquired. Environment also affects the way in which those conditions are handled by children, their families, and the health care providers who treat them.

Frequently, the growth status of a child is used as the indicator of overall health status. The nutritional status of a child may also be affected by illness or its treatment, as in the case of cancer. Resulting deterioration or retarded development of bone and muscle tissue may cause a child to measure low on the growth charts, perhaps never achieving normal height and weight for his or her age. Low levels of physical activity, imposed by restriction during the acute stages of illness or treatment, may also impede growth. Although the impact may be less dramatic, otherwise healthy children may experience impaired skeletal, muscular, and functional development as well as obesity if they are not physically active. The impact of health status and physical activity on normal growth and development is well established and should be given appropriate consideration by all who treat children affected by chronic ailments.

Normal Responses to Physical Activity in Children and Youth

Although children and youth respond to exercise and physical activity in much the same way that adults would, some physiological differences between children and adults do exist. These differences should be considered when exercise testing and evaluating physiological function of children.

Aerobic Exercise

The aerobic capacity of children is measured most frequently in a laboratory setting using a treadmill or cycle ergometer. The mode of evaluation is often determined by investigator preference, size of the child, space available for testing, and the physiological parameters to be evaluated. Maximal oxygen consumption ($\dot{V}O_2$max) is generally considered the best indicator of aerobic fitness, but peak oxygen consumption ($\dot{V}O_2$peak) is perhaps more appropriate when describing this parameter in children because many of them have difficulty achieving a true plateau in $\dot{V}O_2$max during exercise testing. During childhood there is relatively little difference in absolute $\dot{V}O_2$ between the sexes. However, beginning at the time of puberty, gender differences in absolute $\dot{V}O_2$ begin to increase such that male $\dot{V}O_2$max values are approximately 20% greater by the late teen years. These differences persist even when oxygen consumption is expressed in relative terms. Significant improvements also occur in measures of cardiovascular endurance in both males and females throughout the maturational process.

The maximal heart rate of children and adolescents is generally considerably higher than that found in the adult population. Children also have higher submaximal heart rates than adults at a standard exercise intensity. Maximal heart rate remains essentially unchanged in both males and females throughout childhood (approximately 200-205 contractions/min), while resting heart rate declines. Frequently, as a sequela of correction for congenital heart defects, children will experience chronotropic deficits of approximately 20 contractions/min. This will require the practitioner to make modifications in the exercise prescription in regard to target heart rate expectations. As with adults, maximal heart rates achieved during exercise testing are dependent on both the mode and type of exercise, with treadmill running producing higher values than walking or cycle ergometer exercise.

Pulmonary parameters are important variables for health care professionals to monitor during spirometry and evaluation of maximal oxygen uptake. Children and adults differ in regard to resting respiratory rate (i.e., breaths/min). Resting breathing rate decreases progressively during childhood, resulting in lower relative minute ventilation as children age. However, absolute minute ventilation increases throughout the pediatric years. Maximal breathing frequency also declines as the child ages.

Children sweat less than adults during hot weather exercise, resulting in a decrease in evaporative cooling. Children are also slower to acclimatize to exercise in the heat than adults are. Furthermore, children experience a greater rise in core temperature during hot weather exercise due to voluntary hypohydration. This leads to possible volume depletion and an increased susceptibility to heat injuries as well as a decreased ability to exercise efficiently in the heat. From an exercise management perspective, children should be exposed to warm weather exercise gradually and given frequent opportunities (e.g., every 15-20 min) for fluid replacement. Younger children will usually need to be encouraged to drink because the need for fluids is often greater than the desire to ingest them.

The blood pressure response of children and adolescents follows the same general pattern of adults during aerobic exercise, although the magnitude of change observed in systolic blood pressure is not as great. Normal adults usually increase their systolic blood pressure 6 to 8 mmHg for each MET increase in work rate. Young children normally experience a 2 to 3 mmHg rise, while adolescents show increases in systolic blood pressure of 4 to 6 mmHg per MET increase in exercise intensity.

Regulating exercise intensity in children may be somewhat more difficult than in adults. Younger children are frequently unable or find it difficult to count heart rate accurately. Rating of perceived exertion (RPE) appears to work reasonably well in children over the age of eight, but young children are cognitively unable to use the RPE scale accurately and consistently. The use of the simple walk/talk principle seems to work satisfactorily in most children.

Anaerobic Exercise

The anaerobic capacities for children and adolescent males and females are lower than those of adults, whether expressed per unit of lean body mass or in absolute units, with children ranking lower than adolescents and adults and females lower than males. Anaerobic power increases throughout childhood and adolescence with peak values achieved in early adulthood.

Neuromuscular Function

Muscle strength increases during childhood primarily as the result of increasing muscle mass. Males demonstrate significant increases in muscle size and strength that are temporally related to the time of their peak height velocity. This maturation-driven change produces significant disparities in muscular strength between adolescent males and females and is most noticeable in terms of upper body strength. While maturation and serum testosterone levels play a major role in increasing muscular size and strength after puberty, studies have shown that strength may be improved by resistance training in both sexes prior to the onset of puberty. Maturation-enhanced local muscle endurance also occurs and leads to improved performance in endurance activities.

Psychological-Social Function

Research has shown that, in general, physical activity and fitness positively affect self-concept, self-efficacy, and self-esteem. The data are more limited and less conclusive with respect to the effect of physical activity on body image. While physical activity seems to have a positive effect on the symptoms of depression and in the reduction of stress in children, the effect of physical activity on anxiety is inconclusive. Physical activity has also been found to be positively associated with several measures of psychological well-being.

Exercise Testing Children and Youth

To achieve optimum results during exercise evaluations of children, the proper testing environment is critical. The laboratory should be physically attractive to children, containing age-appropriate pictures of interest. The lab should be a minimum of 400 to 600 ft^2 with good lighting and ventilation. Room temperature should be maintained between 20 and 22° C (~72 and 76° F) with a relative humidity of less than 60%. Enthusiastic, compassionate,

and encouraging staff who enjoy working with children are essential in performing successful pediatric exercise tests. With younger children, it will be necessary to proceed much more slowly than with adults. Age-appropriate language should be used to describe each piece of equipment and the desired objectives during the test. Pictures of children performing various aspects of the exercise test are also useful in helping younger children understand what is expected and feel more at ease. Using this approach, treadmill evaluations have been routinely performed on children as young as four years of age.

The use of appropriately sized equipment and protocols is critical. Since children achieve steady state faster than adults, treadmill protocols using 2- to 3-min stages are appropriate. The mode of exercise is also important in determining the results achieved. In children and adolescents, treadmill testing will produce $\dot{V}O_2$max values 7 to 10% greater than cycle ergometers; treadmill running has been found to elicit $\dot{V}O_2$max values 6 to 10% higher than treadmill walking. Test protocols should be designed to last between 8 and 12 min.

From a test-administration perspective, children consistently rate submaximal exercise lower on RPE charts than adolescents and adults. Younger children are often intimidated about communicating with unfamiliar adults in new situations. The test administrator must continuously monitor the child by asking frequent questions to assess his or her status as the test progresses. To avoid false positive answers and early test termination, refrain from asking leading questions or describing specific symptoms (e.g., chest or leg pain, dizziness, shortness of breath). Younger, unfit adolescent clients may require strong verbal encouragement to achieve satisfactory intensity levels during exercise evaluation.

Exercise prescriptions for children should take into consideration the attention span of the child as well as the role of the parent(s) in providing appropriate role models. Prescribed activities should be enjoyable and relatively nonspecific, with increased movement as the initial goal, especially if the child is suffering from hypoactivity syndrome.

Benefits and Risks of Exercise Testing

The potential benefits of conducting exercise tests in children with various diseases or disabilities are the following:

- Documenting any impairment in cardiac or pulmonary functional capacity
- Detecting and managing exercise-induced asthma
- Detecting myocardial ischemia
- Assessing physical work capacity

- Assessing the results of rehabilitation programs
- Documenting functional changes during the course of a progressive disease
- Providing indications for surgery, therapy, or additional tests
- Assessing cardiac rate and rhythm as well as blood pressure response
- Assessing exercise-related symptoms
- Evaluating the effects of therapy
- Increasing confidence, in the child and parents, in the ability of the child to exercise safely

Although extensive data are lacking, exercise testing in children is considered relatively safe and is generally thought to carry a much lower risk than testing in adult clients. The use of side rails and handrails can help reduce the potential risk of falling. Detailed guidelines for conducting pediatric exercise tests are available from the American Heart Association and the American College of Sports Medicine (ACSM).

General Concerns for Chronically Ill or Disabled Children Participating in Physical Activity

When working with children, it is important to realize that each individual constantly changes as he or she grows, and that each one does so at a different rate. Obviously, this means that each child, whether healthy or not, will require special consideration. When disease or disability is present, these growth and development concerns may be of even more significance due to the effect of the health status on the maturation process. Although physical activity should be expected to provide many of the same benefits to all children, there may be limitations imposed by the individual's health status. Beyond the obvious acute effects, a condition or its treatment may retard growth and affect the development of functional systems that are integral in physical performance. Because exercise is essential for normal growth and development, if the condition is so debilitating that it severely limits the individual's ability to participate in activity, additional impairment may occur. Parental apprehension about the child being involved in activity must be considered and adequate measures to address those concerns must be taken. This will require reassurance by the physician, program professionals, and activity leaders. Parents should be allowed to observe (unobtrusively) all sessions and must be fully informed of all details of the child's participation.

Assessment for children with chronic diseases or disabilities will be essentially the same as for normal children, with the addition of precautions appropriate to the condition. Besides condition-specific clinical evaluations, to facilitate appropriate exercise prescription and intervention, children with chronic diseases and disabilities should be assessed for body composition, neuromuscular function, and aerobic and anaerobic fitness. Methodologies and protocols suitable for these children are discussed in detail in numerous sources.

The benefits, risks, and precautions that apply to healthy children will generally hold for those affected by disease or disability. Of course, limitations imposed by each individual's medical status must be considered. The primary benefit of participation in physical activity for all children is improved quality of life with respect to social, psychological, and physical well-being. For the child affected by disease or disability, the therapeutic consequences of exercise can be significant. Self-esteem, self-efficacy, and self-concept, especially as the child ages, can be greatly enhanced if he or she can have a nearly normal lifestyle of activity. Furthermore, for these children, regular exercise should have the same primary preventive benefits with respect to other diseases, such as coronary artery disease, osteoporosis, hypertension, diabetes, and obesity.

Depending on the particular characteristics of a disease or disability, special consideration must be given regarding the intensity of an activity, the environmental conditions, and the risk for contact injury. Very high intensity efforts can lead to injuries in any child, but those with chronic lung disease such as cystic fibrosis, congenital heart defects, or sickle-cell disease have an increased risk of injury and must be considered accordingly. Children are less able than adults to accommodate very high or very low environmental temperatures, and those with a compromised health status may be even less able to adapt to such environmentally stressful conditions. Such activities as climbing, diving, and similar activities may not be appropriate for children with certain conditions. Each case should be evaluated on its own merits.

Selected Diseases and Disorders of Children and Youth

As indicated, all children respond and adapt to exercise somewhat differently than do older youth and adults. Those who are affected by disease or disability may display even greater variation. This section addresses response issues within selected conditions as well as how the role physical activity would play in the growth and development of normal children might also be altered by the child's health status.

Congenital and Acquired Heart Defects

In every 1,000 live births, approximately 8 infants have some type of heart defect ranging from mild to very severe. Most children with congenital heart defects (CHD) do not require activity restrictions and can participate in normal physical activity. However, some children with severe or very complex CHD may need to avoid strenuous activity or competitive sports. Refer to the Bethesda conference guidelines (Mitchell et al., 1985) for a detailed discussion of recommendations regarding athletic competition and specific congenital heart defects.

Common forms of CHD include atrial and ventricular septal defects, patent ductus arteriosus, and atrioventricular canal. These conditions can range from mild to severe. Some, as in the case of small septal defects, may repair themselves spontaneously; others may require significant surgical intervention. No special modifications in exercise testing modes are usually necessary for children with CHD. Many individuals with these defects can participate in a wide range of physical activities without modification. Those with pulmonary hypertension, arrhythmia, and/or evidence of myocardial dysfunction, however, may need to restrict their exercise to low-intensity activities, as indicated by the Bethesda conference guidelines.

Cyanotic defects result in decreased oxygen delivery to the body with a subsequent alteration in skin coloration. This coloration is dark blue or purplish when the condition is severe. Numerous defects constitute this class of CHD (e.g., tetralogy of Fallot, tricuspid atresia, pulmonary atresia, transposition of the great arteries, truncus arteriosus, and total anomalous pulmonary venous connection). However, it is beyond the scope of this chapter to describe the complex anatomy and physiology associated with each of these defects.

Children with cyanotic defects often have mild to moderate decreases in their aerobic capacity. Those with significant residual problems following surgical repair may be even more limited. Limitation in competitive sports increases as the degree of residual problems increases after surgery. Children with good surgical repair of these defects and those with no (or minimal) residual effects can often participate in various types of competitive sports (refer to the Bethesda conference guidelines for full recommendations). Post-surgery clients who experience oxygen desaturation during exercise will require individualized exercise prescriptions.

Obstructive CHD occurs when one of the heart valves or blood vessels returning or carrying blood from the heart becomes stenotic or atretic. The most common obstructive conditions are coarctation of the aorta and pulmonary and aortic stenosis. Defects or this type are classified from trivial to severe. As the severity of the defect increases, the potential for functional impairment also increases. Physical activity and competitive athletic competition restrictions are likely at the most severe levels of obstructive CHD. Children with mild to moderate obstructive CHD can normally participate in unrestricted or low-intensity levels of physical activity if the Bethesda conference guidelines are followed.

Valvular stenoses may worsen as the CHD child grows. Thus, regular assessment via echocardiography, exercise testing, and perhaps cardiac catheterization is usually necessary. Most children with obstructive CHD can perform modified Balke protocols as well as cycle ergometer protocols without significant alteration. Exercise evaluation of children with severe obstructive CHD may be contraindicated.

Obviously, any of the above conditions or their treatments can have either a temporarily or permanently deleterious effect on growth and development. This should be addressed as appropriate with the child and his or her parents. Physical activity may be among the most effective means by which those effects can be offset.

Diabetes Mellitus

Although treatment for diabetes mellitus (DM) has greatly advanced in recent years, the disease can make life difficult for children and their families. The freedom and spontaneity of childhood can be severely affected. Insulin-dependent diabetes mellitus (IDDM), the type previously associated with early onset and affecting only 5 to 10% of the population, is no longer the only concern for children. An increase in sedentary behavior, and the resulting obesity, have resulted in a marked increase in the incidence of childhood non-insulin-dependent diabetes mellitus (NIDDM), which was previously expected to occur in middle-aged persons. This means that an increasing number of young people are going to be exposed to the consequences of DM for much longer periods of time.

There is evidence regarding the benefits of exercise in the management of NIDDM, and to a lesser extent IDDM, through several mechanisms. The primary mechanisms by which exercise can be directly beneficial include an increase in sensitivity to insulin, increases in glucose transport protein (Glut-4), and glycogen synthase activity. Intestinal absorption of glucose may also be affected by exercise. A physically active lifestyle may aid in preventing or delaying the onset of NIDDM, primarily through control of obesity, in all age groups. Additional benefits of regular activity include serum lipid reduction, increased aerobic fitness, and overall improvement in quality of life. The negative impact on social and psychological well-being can be mitigated for the child by involvement in a normally active lifestyle.

Precautions that should be considered for the diabetic (IDDM) child involved in physical activity include careful attention to preventing hypoglycemia by monitoring and regulating insulin levels and glucose intake. Special attention must be given to both the intensity and duration of the activity. High-intensity activity and physical exhaustion in young people with IDDM may cause an abnormal reaction, resulting in sustained hyperglycemia. Also, careful management of wounds and other injuries must be maintained.

The stabilization of glucose levels is much more difficult in cases of IDDM than in those of NIDDM. The procedure must be much more highly structured, resulting in even more severe intrusion into the life of the child. Nevertheless, the benefits can be worth the effort. The more knowledgeable the child is about and involved in his or her daily care, the more successful the management will be. If the diabetic child can get through the adolescent years in otherwise good condition, the prognosis for his or her future is usually better.

Neuromuscular Disorders

Some limited work has been done regarding the implications of exercise testing and therapy for children affected by various progressive neuromuscular disorders, both congenital and acquired. Since the focus for this type of problem should be on the muscular system, including muscular strength, endurance, power, and the metabolic cost of movement, all testing and therapeutic procedures should address these areas. Another area of related concern is that of children with gait and coordination disorders that are frequently subclinical, thereby frequently receiving little or no attention.

Exercise testing can be effective in accessing and tracking delayed development or progressive deterioration in coordination as well as the efficacy of interventions. Although there are relatively few controlled studies, there is some evidence that therapeutic modalities involving exercise training (aerobic, anaerobic, and resistance) may be beneficial in slowing the progression of some conditions and in maintaining or improving functional abilities. The difficulties involved in designing and carrying out the type of studies necessary to provide conclusive clinical data are significant. However, it seems reasonable that having affected children involved in appropriate physical activity would do no harm. Indeed, it would most likely yield some benefits related to normalizing growth and development.

Pulmonary Disorders

It is recognized that bronchial asthma, including exercise-induced asthma, and cystic fibrosis (CF) are the most commonly occurring chronic pulmonary diseases among children. Both conditions result in limitations on exercise tolerance and cardiorespiratory responses that vary from those normally expected in children. Although chronic asthma attacks may be initiated by a number of environmental factors, such as allergens and pollution, exercise-induced asthma has been attributed to several mechanisms. These vary from the rather simple cooling, drying, and rewarming of the airways with increased ventilation to more complex concepts involving chemical inflammation mediators. CF is an inherited condition of genetically defective sodium and chloride ion transport, which results in extracellular dehydration. Multiple organs and functions are affected by the thick mucus, which blocks ducts, tubules, and small airways. The function of affected organs, especially the lungs, is impaired to the point of causing early death.

Although both conditions can be life threatening, long-term survival and a relatively normal life can be expected with well-managed asthma. CF has a poor prognosis, however. Nevertheless, the benefits of regular exercise have been demonstrated, mostly related to improvement in aerobic fitness for both and of increased ventilatory muscle endurance and strength in the CF individual. The possibility of increased mucus clearance has also been reported, although benefits in pulmonary function are limited, if present at all. Caution must be observed when individuals with CF are exposed to heat and altitude. They are usually capable of normal thermoregulation, but special attention must be paid to fluid and electrolyte replacement. There is a risk of oxygen desaturation if oxygen tension in the environment is low.

The usefulness of exercise testing in the diagnosis and/or prognosis determination for both conditions has been well documented. The determination of exercise tolerance and aerobic fitness is not only beneficial for the health care provider, but it also instills confidence in both clients and parents.

Summary

Children, like adults, are frequently affected by chronic disease and disability. Childhood afflictions can be even more tragic than adulthood onsets, simply because of the fact that the onset of a limiting condition in childhood means that the individual will have to cope with the problem for a much longer period of time. Thus, an underlying goal for the practitioner is to be sensitive to these concerns and always be alert for ways to help chronically ill children deal with their problems.

Further complicating effective management, many children may present with multiple problems. The practitioner must be creative and resourceful in using exercise testing and prescription to evaluate current status and progression, as well as to facilitate as active a lifestyle as possible for the affected child. The desired outcome will be an improved quality of life and possible mitigation of the long-term consequences of disease or disability. Being physically active is the nature of a child. This nature should be foremost in the minds of everyone working with children, whether sick or well.

Suggested Readings

Armstrong, N., and W. van Mechelen, eds. 2000. *Paediatric exercise science and medicine.* Oxford: Oxford University Press.

Bar-Or, O. 1983. *Pediatric sports medicine for the practitioner: From physiologic principles to clinical applications.* New York: Springer-Verlag.

Bouchard, C., R.M. Malina, and L. Prusse. 1997. *Genetics of fitness and physical performance.* Champaign, IL: Human Kinetics.

Canadian Society for Exercise Physiology. 1996. *Measurement in pediatric exercise science.* Edited by D. Docherty. Champaign, IL: Human Kinetics.

Goldberg, B., ed. 1995. *Sports and exercise for children with chronic health conditions.* Champaign, IL: Human Kinetics.

Malina, R.M., and C. Bouchard. 1991. *Growth, maturation, and physical activity.* Champaign, IL: Human Kinetics.

Mitchell, J.H., B.J. Maron, and S.E. Epstein. 1985. Sixteenth Bethesda Conference: Cardiovascular abnormalities in the athlete: Recommendations regarding eligibility for competition. *Journal of the American College of Cardiology* 6: 29-30.

Rowland, T.W. 1996. *Developmental exercise physiology.* Champaign, IL: Human Kinetics.

Rowland. T.W., ed. 1993. *Pediatric laboratory exercise testing: Clinical guidelines.* Champaign, IL: Human Kinetics.

Rowland, T.W. 1990. *Exercise and children's health.* Champaign, IL: Human Kinetics.

Tomassoni, T.L. 1996. Clinical Sciences Symposium: The role of exercise in the diagnosis and management of chronic disease in children and youth. *Medicine and Science in Sports and Exercise* 28 (4): 403-35.

SECTION II

Cardiovascular Diseases

Scott O. Roberts, PhD, FACSM
Peter H. Brubaker, PhD, FACSM

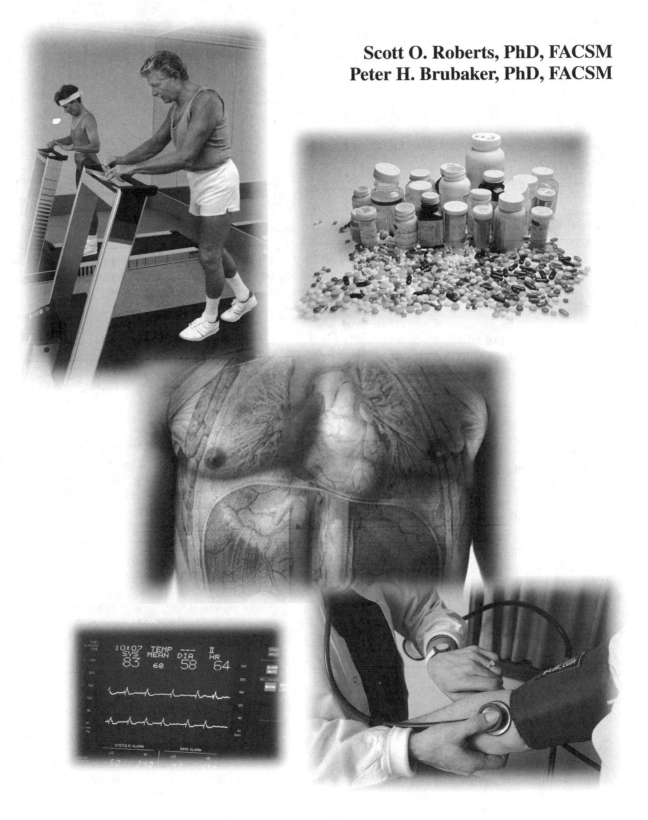

CHAPTER 4

Myocardial Infarction

Barry A. Franklin, PhD, FACSM
William Beaumont Hospital
Wayne State University

Overview of the Pathophysiology

Coronary atherosclerosis involves a localized accumulation of lipid and fibrous tissue within the coronary artery, progressively narrowing the lumen of the vessel. Fatty streaks may progress over time to fibrous plaques and eventually to atheroma. Clinically significant lesions (i.e., ≥ 75% of the vessel's cross-sectional area), producing myocardial ischemia and left ventricular dysfunction, often develop in the proximal, epicardial segments of the coronary artery at sites of abrupt curvature or branching. These lesions or lesions that are less obstructed may be complicated by hemorrhage, ulceration, calcification, or thrombosis. Plaque, which is composed of fibrous tissue and to a lesser extent lipids, can be either active and unstable or quiet and stable. If unstable, even mild- to moderate-sized plaques may fissure, rupture, and/or swell. This cascade of events at vulnerable regions can result in a sudden and complete obstruction of a coronary artery, causing an acute myocardial infarction (MI).

The plaque instability that causes these events can be dramatically decreased with reductions in total and LDL-cholesterol. Inflammation has also been linked to the atherosclerotic process as well as the triggering of acute MI. For example, C-reactive protein has been shown to reflect inflammation and strongly predicts coronary risk in middle-aged men and women. Prolonged ischemia (>60 min) causes irreversible cellular damage and muscle death, or necrosis, leading to acute MI. More than 1.5 million Americans have an MI each year, including a similar number of men and women; of these, approximately 500,000, or one-third, will die.

MI is classically characterized by a diagnostic triad of signs and symptoms:

- severe, prolonged chest pain or pressure, which may radiate to the arms, back, or neck, frequently associated with sweating, nausea, or vomiting;
- increased serum levels of cardiac enzymes released by the necrotic myocardial cells (e.g., CK-MB > 5% of total CK; CPK or CK, women > 70 U/L, men > 90 U/L; troponin I ≥ 0.5 ng/ml); and
- electrocardiographic changes in the leads overlying the area of infarction, manifested as ST-segment elevation and T-wave inversion, resulting from ischemic injury and disappearing over time.

Finally, pronounced Q waves indicate myocardial necrosis and are irreversible.

MI usually affects the left ventricle and is associated with permanent cessation of contractile function in the necrotic area of the myocardium and impaired contractility in the surrounding ischemic muscle. Two types of infarctions are generally described, depending upon the amount of myocardial tissue involved:

- transmural infarction (i.e., Q-wave MI), which involves the full thickness of the ventricular wall; and
- subendocardial infarction (i.e., non-Q-wave MI), which is limited to the inner half of the myocardium.

Infarctions are further described according to the involvement of the coronary circulation and location on the ventricular wall. For example, anterior infarctions result from lesions in the left anterior descending coronary artery and involve the anterior wall of the left ventricle, whereas inferior wall infarctions are generally the result of right coronary artery lesions. Other commonly designated infarct sites are lateral, posterior, and septal or, with extensive infarctions involving large portions of the ventricle, combinations of these locations (e.g., anteroseptal, inferolateral).

The risk of future cardiovascular morbidity and mortality after acute MI is largely determined by two variables:

- the extent of left ventricular damage or dysfunction, using ejection fraction as the reference criteria (mean normal [±SD] left ventricular ejection fraction at rest is 62.3 ± 6.1%), and
- the degree of residual myocardial ischemia (suggesting additional myocardium in jeopardy), manifested by exertional angina pectoris, ST-segment depression, technetium (Tc)-99 m Sestamibi

(Cardiolite) or thallous (thallium) chloride-201 transient perfusion abnormalities, or combinations thereof.

Effects on the Exercise Response

Acute MI may alter the client's cardiorespiratory and hemodynamic responses to submaximal and maximal exercise. Clients who have suffered a previous MI often have a subnormal aerobic capacity (50-70% of age-, gender-predicted). The reduced oxygen transport capacity is primarily due to diminished cardiac output (stroke volume and/or heart rate) rather than a reduction in peripheral extraction of oxygen. In some clients, a primary limitation appears to be the decreased contractile force of the left ventricle due to residual ischemia or necrosis, causing a progressive decrease in ejection fraction and stroke volume. This is often manifested as a blunted or decreasing systolic blood pressure response to progressive exercise (exertional hypotension). In others, cardiac output may be limited by the restriction in the rise of the heart rate due to intrinsic disease of the SA or AV node (chronotropic impairment), or the appearance of anginal symptoms, with or without ischemic ST-segment depression, which preclude exercising to a higher level. Threatening exercise-induced ventricular arrhythmias also occur more commonly in individuals with previous MI than in persons without heart disease, especially in the presence of ischemic ST-segment depression, angina pectoris, or both. In addition, since these clients are often taking medications to decrease heart rate and blood pressure (and myocardial oxygen demands), the type and dose of these medications should be noted before the client undergoes exercise testing or training.

Effects of Exercise Training

Common rationale for exercise training of clients with previous MI include:

- increased maximal oxygen consumption ($\dot{V}O_2$max) (mean ~20%), which generally varies inversely with the pretraining $\dot{V}O_2$max;
- improvement in the ventilatory response to exercise;
- relief of anginal symptoms secondary to reductions in heart rate and/or blood pressure and myocardial oxygen demand at any given somatic oxygen uptake or submaximal work rate;
- increased heart rate variability;
- modest decreases in body weight, fat stores, blood pressure (particularly in hypertensives), total blood

cholesterol, serum triglycerides, and low-density lipoprotein (LDL) cholesterol;

- increases in the "antiatherogenic" high-density lipoprotein (HDL) cholesterol subfraction;
- improved psychosocial well-being and self-efficacy; and
- protection against the triggering of MI by strenuous physical exertion (i.e., $\geq$ 6 METs).

On the other hand, conventional exercise training, as an isolated intervention, generally does little to increase left ventricular ejection fraction and myocardial perfusion. Numerous training studies have now demonstrated increased exercise tolerance in clients with impaired left ventricular function, despite the lack of improvement in resting hemodynamics or ejection fraction. However, clients who have both left ventricular dysfunction and exercise-induced myocardial ischemia show little or no increase in $\dot{V}O_2$max after early outpatient cardiac rehabilitation.

Meta-analyses of previous randomized, controlled clinical trials of rehabilitation with exercise after MI have now shown a 20 to 25% reduction in total and cardiovascular-related mortality, with no difference in the rate of nonfatal recurrent events. However, current thrombolytic and revascularization procedures, which markedly decrease early postinfarction mortality, may diminish the impact of adjunctive contemporary cardiac rehabilitation programs on survival.

The advisability of vigorous exercise training for two client subsets has been previously questioned:

- clients with exertional ST-segment depression without symptoms (silent ischemia); and
- clients recovering from MI involving a large portion of the anterior wall.

Although an isolated report suggested that vigorous exercise training in these clients may actually worsen cardiac function, recent studies suggest that increased fibrosis, infarct expansion, and a deterioration in left ventricular function are unlikely outcomes of exercise training.

Management and Medications

Medical management of the client is essentially palliative, undertaken to minimize the severity of clinical sequelae and to potentially slow, halt, or even reverse the progression of disease. Individuals at moderate to high risk may likely experience a reduction in mortality from successful percutaneous transluminal coronary angioplasty or coronary artery bypass graft surgery. Risk factor interventions aimed at smoking cessation, lipid/

lipoprotein modification, hypertension control, increasing physical activity, and efficacious drugs, including beta blockers, angiotensin-converting enzyme (ACE) inhibitors, HMG-CoA reductase inhibitors (e.g., statins), and aspirin, have produced remarkably consistent reductions (about 20-25%) in cardiovascular-related morbidity and mortality. When selectively combined, even greater reductions in subsequent cardiovascular events are likely to be achieved.

Appropriate pharmacotherapy decreases mortality after acute MI, attenuates the manifestations of acute ischemic syndromes, improves symptoms in stable angina and heart failure, suppresses worrisome atrial and ventricular arrhythmias, and inhibits platelet function and fibrin formation. Accordingly, many clients take one or more medications after acute MI, including anti-ischemic drugs (e.g., beta blockers, calcium-channel blocking agents, nitroglycerin, and longer-acting nitrate drugs), platelet inhibitors, anticoagulants, drugs for the treatment of heart failure (e.g., digitalis, diuretics, ACE inhibitors), vasodilators, antiarrhythmic drugs, and lipid-altering drugs (see chapter 22). Several of the cardiovascular medications, however, may potentially influence the responses to exercise testing and training. They are listed here:

• Diuretics do not alter chronotropic reserve or aerobic capacity (except possibly in clients with congestive heart failure). Thus, the prescribed exercise heart rate can be determined in the standard fashion. On the other hand, diuretics may precipitate ventricular ectopy if hypokalemia or hypomagnesemia occurs and a "false positive" test results.

• Beta blockers decrease submaximal and maximal heart rate and, sometimes, exercise capacity, especially with nonselective agents. These drugs may also prevent or delay signs/symptoms of myocardial ischemia and increase exercise tolerance in clients with exertional angina. Nevertheless, exercise trainability appears to be unaffected, despite therapeutic doses and a reduced training heart rate. Because beta blockers do not alter the remarkably consistent relationship between % $\dot{V}O_2$max and % HRmax, the generally prescribed metabolic load for training (60-80% $\dot{V}O_2$max) may be achieved at the conventional relative heart rate recommendation for training (70-85% HRmax).

• Vasodilators and angiotensin-converting enzyme inhibitors do not generally affect the heart rate response to exercise. Consequently, exercise training intensity can be prescribed in the usual manner. Clients on these medications may be subject to hypotensive episodes in the postexercise period, unless an adequate cool-down is performed.

• Calcium-channel blockers do not generally impair functional capacity or exercise trainability and may, in fact, increase exercise tolerance in clients with angina. However, certain calcium-channel blockers (e.g., bepridil, diltiazem, verapamil) may decrease the heart rate response at rest and during exercise, and prevent or delay manifestations of myocardial ischemia. Consequently, the prescribed training heart rate should be based on the medicated client's response to an exercise test.

• Central nervous system-active drugs, including clonidine, guanfacine, and guanabenz, can have attenuating effects on heart rate and blood pressure during exercise. Thus, the potential for hypotension, dizziness, and syncope should be carefully monitored.

• Alpha receptor blockers significantly lower systolic and diastolic blood pressure but appear to have minimal effects on heart rate and metabolic responses to exercise. Therefore, training heart rates may be prescribed in the usual manner.

• Antiarrhythmic agents can cause false negative (quinidine) or false positive (procainamide) test results; however, these do not substantially alter the heart rate response or aerobic capacity in persons with or without heart disease. In contrast, a decrease of 20 contractions/min in exercise HRmax has been reported in clients taking amiodarone.

• Digitalis appears to have little effect on the hemodynamic and metabolic responses to exercise. ST-segment depression can be induced or accentuated during exercise in persons with or without heart disease who are taking digitalis. In clients who are taking digitalis, marked ST-segment depression may indicate myocardial ischemia, particularly when it is accompanied by a prolonged QT interval. Nevertheless, exercise-induced ST-segment depression should be interpreted with caution in the presence of digitalis therapy.

Recommendations for Exercise Testing

Low-level exercise testing (generally ≤ 5 METs) of the convalescing client with uncomplicated MI is used not only to assess a client's functional status but also as a diagnostic, prognostic, and therapeutic guide. The test also serves to promote client confidence, providing reassurance that routine activities can be undertaken safely. Abnormal findings (e.g., angina, ischemic ST-segment depression) suggest that additional areas of myocardium are served by stenosed coronary vessels and remain in jeopardy.

The test protocol for peak or symptom-limited testing should be selected to accommodate the individual's ability to perform lower-extremity exercise (see the Myocardial Infarction: Exercise Testing table). Clients who are

Myocardial Infarction: Exercise Testing

Methods	Measures	Endpoints*	Comments
Aerobic Cycle (ramp protocol 17 watts/min; staged protocol 25-50 watts/3-min stage) Treadmill (1-2 METs/3-min stage)	• 12-lead ECG, HR	• Serious dysrhythmias • >2mm ST-segment depression or elevation • Ischemic threshold • T-wave inversion with significant ST change	• Use low level treadmill protocol for acute MI clients. • Important in establishing a safe training intensity. • Chronotropic impairment results in poor prognosis.** • Minimal treadmill speed should be ≤ 1.0 mph.
	• BP, rate pressure product	• SBP > 250 mmHg or DBP > 115 mmHg	• Exertional hypotension (drop of ≥ 20 mmHg or failure to rise) suggests poor prognosis.
	• RPE (6-20) • Angina scale	• +3 or earlier on +1-+4 scale (see angina scale on p. 45)	
	• Gas analysis ($\dot{V}O_2$peak or $\dot{V}O_2$max)		• Only if exact measures are indicated, ventilatory threshold is often useful.
	• Radionuclide testing		• Is more sensitive and specific than exercise ECG in assessing ischemic heart disease.
Strength Isokinetic/Isotonic	• 90% maximal voluntary contraction (MVC) greatest load lifted 2-3 times	• 3 consecutive reps	• Use 1RM (estimated from 90% MVC) to establish training work rate.

*Measurements of particular significance; do not always indicate test termination.

**A delayed decrease in the heart rate (< 12 contractions/min) during the first min of recovery is also a powerful predictor of overall mortality.

Medications	Special Considerations
• See appendixes A, B, and C. • Diuretics: May elicit ventricular ectopy and cause "false positive" test responses. • Beta blockers: Decrease submaximal and maximal HR and BP response and sometimes exercise capacity, especially with nonselective medications. • Vasodilators and ACE inhibitors: Do not generally affect exercise HR response. However, clients may be more susceptible to postexercise hypotension. • Calcium-channel blockers: May mask ischemia and decrease exercise HR response (e.g., verapamil). • Central nervous system-active drugs: Have varied effects on HR and BP during exercise. Caution for hypotension, dizziness, and syncope. • Alpha blockers: Decrease systolic and diastolic BP response but have minimal effects on HR and $\dot{V}O_2$ responses to exercise. • Digitalis: May promote spurious ST–T-wave changes (interpret with caution); sometimes used to control atrial dysrhythmias. • Nitroglycerin: May mask or attenuate ischemic responses.	• Clients with concomitant orthopedic limitations may require cycle or arm ergometry or alternatively, pharmacologic stress testing to assess cardiac function. • CAD clients are more likely to demonstrate limiting signs or symptoms, including angina, ischemic ST depression, BP abnormalities, and serious ventricular dysrhythmias. • Clients with high-grade peripheral vascular disease may not be able to achieve adequate cardiac stress (≥ 85% maximal age-predicted HR) with conventional treadmill testing. • Maximal stress testing should not be performed immediately prior to hematologic screening. • Some cardiac medications (e.g., diuretics, beta blockers, alpha agonists, vasodilators) can influence temperature regulation. • 12-hour fast or light meal is recommended prior to testing.

unable to perform treadmill or cycle ergometer exercise may, alternatively, be evaluated by arm crank ergometry or pharmacologic stress testing (e.g., dobutamine, dipyridamole, and adenosine) at rest.

The exercise test should begin at an intensity level considerably below the anticipated peak or symptom-limited capacity and increase gradually in 2- or 3-min stages, with hemodynamic measures made at each progressive stage. If possible, exercise capacity should be directly measured using gas exchange techniques rather than predicted from work rate (e.g., treadmill speed and grade or duration), which tends to overestimate aerobic fitness. Increments in work rate should be chosen so that the total test time to volitional fatigue approximates 10 ± 2 min. Contraindications to testing and indications for terminating exercise should be closely observed.

The primary objectives of exercise testing for these individuals are to evaluate quantitatively and accurately the following functions:

- chronotropic capacity, and heart rate recovery;
- aerobic capacity ($\dot{V}O_2$max);
- myocardial aerobic capacity, estimated by the peak rate-pressure product;
- exertional symptoms (e.g., increasing chest pain or lightheadedness); and
- associated changes in electrical functions of the heart (e.g., arrhythmias, ST–T-wave changes).

These data are critical to categorize risk status (e.g., low, moderate, high) and establish a safe and effective metabolic load for aerobic exercise training. Indicators of an adverse prognosis in the post-MI client include the following:

- ischemic ST-segment depression at a low level of exercise;
- functional capacity < 5 METs;
- low peak rate-pressure product (i.e., $\geq 21,700$ mmHg x contractions/min); and
- hypotensive blood pressure response to exercise.

Exercise testing for clients on "long-acting" beta blockers should be conducted at approximately the same time of day the subject will be exercising. This is because the significant reduction in exercise heart rate may dissipate over time.

Because ST-segment abnormalities that develop during exercise are not interpretable in the presence of digitalis, substantial ST-segment depression at rest, left ventricular hypertrophy, or left bundle-branch block, exercise testing with myocardial perfusion imaging is often recommended to screen for myocardial ischemia in individuals with these conditions.

Recommendations for Exercise Programming

Simple exposure to orthostatic or gravitational stress (e.g., intermittent sitting or standing during the bed rest stage of hospital convalescence [Phase I]) can obviate much of the deterioration in exercise performance that normally follows acute MI. Large muscle group exercise that is rhythmic, such as walking, cycle ergometry, rowing, or stair climbing, is appropriate for outpatient (Phase II-IV) physical conditioning. Because the training benefits do not transfer from the legs to the arms, and vice versa, both sets of limbs should be exercised. Mild to moderate resistance training can also provide a safe and effective method for improving cardiovascular function, body composition, coronary risk factors, flexibility, and muscular strength and endurance in clinically stable cardiac clients.

Mode, intensity, frequency, and duration recommendations for exercise training/physical activity can be found in the Myocardial Infarction: Exercise Programming table. They are summarized as follows:

- Intensity generally corresponds to 40 to 80% of $\dot{V}O_2$max on maximal heart rate reserve, using RPE (11 to 15 [on the Borg scale of 6-20]) as an adjunct to heart rate as an intensity guide.
- Frequency of exercise is at least three nonconsecutive days/wk.
- Duration of training involves 20 to 40 min of continuous or accumulated (interval) exercise, preceded and followed by warm-up and cool-down periods of 5 to 10 min.
- Mode of exercise should include, in addition to a formal or structured program, the recommendation to increase the adoption and maintenance of physical activity in daily living; maximum benefit requires 5 to 6 h/wk of physical activity.

Myocardial Infarction: Exercise Programming

Modes	Goals	Intensity/ Frequency/Duration	Time to Goal
Aerobic • Large muscle activities • Arm/leg ergometry	• Increase aerobic capacity • Decrease BP and HR response to submaximal exercise • Decrease submaximal myocardial $\dot{V}O_2$ demand • Decrease CAD risk factors • Increase ADLs	• RPE 11-15/20 • 40-80% $\dot{V}O_2$max or HR reserve • ≥ 3 days/wk • 20-40 min/session • 5-10 min of warm-up and cool-down activities	• 4-6 mo
Strength* • Circuit training	• Increase ability to perform leisure and occupational activities and ADLs • Increase muscle strength and endurance	• 40-50% maximal voluntary contraction (avoid Valsalva) • 2-3 days/wk • 1-3 sets of 10-15 reps • 8-10 different exercises • Resistance gradually increased over time	• 4-6 mo
Flexibility** • Upper and lower body ROM activities	• Increase risk of injury	• Static stretches: hold for 10-30 s • 2-3 days/wk	• 4-6 mo

*A single set of exercises to volitional fatigue is highly effective, at least over the initial months of training.

**Strength and flexibility training are often used, but not well researched. Typical programs are recommended here.

Medications	Special Considerations
• See appendixes A, B, and C. • Beta blockers: No major effect on exercise trainability in cardiac patients. • Calcium-channel blockers: No major effect on exercise trainability in cardiac patients.	• Low-fit clients (functional capacity ≤5 METs) can often train at 40-50% $\dot{V}O_2$peak; 70% is appropriate for most clients. • Monitor for abnormal signs and symptoms (i.e., chest pain or pressure, dizziness, and dysrhythmias). • High-intensity exercise may precipitate cardiovascular complications in post-MI patients. • Supervision is suggested for moderate- to high-risk patients (e.g., those with exercise-induced myocardial ischemia manifested as ST-segment depression and/or angina pectoris and those with poor left ventricular function [ejection fraction ≤ 30%]). • Many post-MI patients have peripheral arterial disease and/or diabetes mellitus (see tables in chapters 13 and 21 for additional guidelines). • When possible, select exercise equipment that can be adjusted in 1-MET increments. • Increasing muscular strength is an important component of an exercise program for post-MI clients, as it will improve coronary risk factors and decrease HR, BP, and myocardial $\dot{V}O_2$ demand at any given resistance (e.g., during lifting or carrying objects). • The minimum recommended frequency of training is 3 nonconsecutive days/wk.

CASE STUDY   Myocardial Infarction

A 58-year-old auto executive presented to the emergency department about six hours after shoveling heavy, wet snow. He was diaphoretic and complaining of severe substernal chest discomfort (+8/10) which radiated to his left arm and jaw. His coronary risk factors included a positive family history of coronary artery disease (his father suffered his first MI at age 60), diabetes, cigarette smoking (he quit at age 50), and a sedentary lifestyle. In addition, he was overweight. His only medication at the time of hospital admittance was an oral hypoglycemic agent.

S: "I've got bad chest pain and it's getting worse." The client was also pale and perspiring profusely.

O: Vitals: Height: 6'0" (1.83 m)   Weight: 254 lb (116 kg)   BMI: 35.8 kg/m^2
            HR: 79 contractions/min   BP: 102/68 mmHg

Middle-aged male in distress; pale; perspiring profusely

Lungs: Soft bibasilar rales

Cardiovascular: Regular rhythm, S1, S2, S3, with II/VI mitral regurgitation murmur, peripheral pulses 1+, trace edema

ECG: Junctional rhythm—marked ST-segment elevation in II, III, aVF, V_4-V_6; ST-segment depression in I, aVL, and V_2

Cardiac enzymes: Troponin I = 1.8 ng/ml

Cardiac catheterization:
  Total occlusion of the proximal LAD, 95% stenosis of the RCA
  Ejection fraction: 33%
  Percutaneous transluminal coronary angioplasty successful

Graded exercise test (post-PTCA, day 5, low level):
  Peak exercise: 4-5 METs
  Peak HR: 108 contractions/min
  No ECG changes or symptoms of cardiac ischemia

Medications: Tenormin, ASA, Glyburide, Atorvastatin

A: 1. Acute inferolateral MI

2. CAD with successful revascularization

3. Obesity

4. Diabetes

5. Deconditioning/sedentary lifestyle

P: 1. Refer to Phase II cardiac rehabilitation: comprehensive exercise and lifestyle modification.

2. Improve weight/diabetes management.

3. Initiate an 8-week program of exercise training, education, and counseling:
   Target HR: 90-102 contractions/min
   RPE: 11-13 (fairly light to somewhat hard)
   Interval or circuit training: 50-60 min/session, 3 nonconsecutive days/wk

Exercise Program
Goals:

1. Peak exercise tolerance > 6 METs
2. Increase functional capacity
3. Adjunct to diabetes/weight management
4. Reinforce lifestyle changes/medical management

Mode	Frequency	Duration	Intensity	Progression
Aerobic	3 days/wk	20 min/session	THR (90-102 contractions/min) RPE 11-13/20	Increase to 40 min @ 60-70% THR after 8 wk
Strength (all major muscle groups)	3 days/wk	1 set of ≤ 10 reps	50-70% of 1RM	Increase to 2 sets of 10-12 reps after 12 wk
Flexibility (all major muscle groups)	3 days/wk	20 s/stretch	Maintain stretch below discomfort point	Discomfort point should occur at higher ROM
Neuromuscular				
Functional				
Warm-up/Cool-down	Before and after each session	10-15 min	RPE <10/20	Maintain

Follow-Up

Approximately 14 weeks after his MI, he completed 9 min on a Bruce protocol (3.4 mph, 14% grade, 9-10 METs). Peak heart rate was 135 contractions/min. The test was terminated due to volitional fatigue, without significant ST-segment depression or anginal symptoms. Isolated PVCs were noted during and after exercise. The exercise prescription was updated and he entered a Phase III program.

Suggested Readings

American College of Sports Medicine. 2000. *ACSM's guidelines for exercise testing and prescription*. Edited by B.A. Franklin, M.H. Whaley, and E.T. Howley. 6th ed. Philadelphia: Lippincott Williams & Wilkins.

Dominguez, H., C. Torp-Pedersen, L. Koeber et al. 2001. Prognostic value of exercise testing in a cohort of patients followed for 15 years after acute myocardial infarction. *European Heart Journal* 22: 273-76.

Dorn, J., J. Naughton, D. Imamura et al. 1999. Results of a multicenter randomized clinical trial of exercise and long-term survival in myocardial infarction patients: The National Exercise and Heart Disease Project (NEHDP). *Circulation* 100: 1764-69.

Franklin, B.A., P. George, R. Henry et al. 2001. Acute myocardial infarction after manual or automated snow removal. *American Journal of Cardiology* 87: 1282-83.

Franklin, B.A., and J.K. Kahn. 1996. Delayed progression or regression of coronary atherosclerosis with intensive risk factor modification: Effects of diet, drugs, and exercise. *Sports and Medicine* 22: 306-20.

Franklin, B.A., and R.J. Shephard. 2000. Avoiding repeat cardiac events: The ABCDEs of tertiary prevention. *Physician and Sportsmedicine* 28: 31-58.

Giannuzzi, P., L. Tavazzi, P.L. Temporelli et al. 1993. Long-term physical training and left ventricular remodeling after anterior myocardial infarction: Results of the exercise in anterior myocardial infarction (EAMI) trial. *Journal of the American College of Cardiology* 22: 1821-29.

Hambrecht, R., J. Niebauer, C. Marburger et al. 1993. Various intensities of leisure time physical activity in patients with coronary artery disease: Effects on cardiorespiratory fitness and progression of coronary atherosclerotic lesions. *Journal of the American College of Cardiology* 22: 468-77.

Leon, A.S. 2000. Exercise following myocardial infarction: Current recommendations. *Sports and Medicine* 29: 301-11.

Pollock, M.L., B.A. Franklin, G.J. Balady et al. AHA Science Advisory. 2000. Resistance exercise in individuals with and without cardiovascular disease: Benefits, rationale, safety, and prescription. *Circulation* 101: 828-33.

Senaratne, M.P., G. Smith, and S.S. Gulamhusein. 2000. Feasibility and safety of early exercise testing using the Bruce protocol after acute myocardial infarction. *Journal of the American College of Cardiology* 35: 1212-20.

Shephard, R.J., and G.J. Balady. 1999. Exercise as cardiovascular therapy. *Circulation* 99: 963-72.

Stahle, A., R. Nordlander, and L. Bergfeldt. 1999. Aerobic group training improves exercise capacity and heart rate variability in elderly patients with a recent coronary event. A randomized controlled study. *European Heart Journal* 20: 1638-46.

Villella, M., A. Villella, S. Barlera et al. 1999. Prognostic significance of double product and inadequate double product response to maximal symptom-limited exercise stress testing after myocardial infarction in 6296 patients treated with thrombolytic agents. *American Heart Journal* 137: 443-52.

Wenger, N.K., E.S. Froelicher, L.K. Smith et al. 1995. *Cardiac rehabilitation*. Clinical Practice Guideline No. 17. Rockville, MD: U.S. Department of Health and Human Services, Public Health Service, Agency for Health Care Policy and Research and the National Heart, Lung, and Blood Institute. AHCPR Publication No. 96-0672.

CHAPTER 5

Coronary Artery Bypass Graft Surgery and Percutaneous Transluminal Coronary Angioplasty

Barry A. Franklin, PhD, FACSM
William Beaumont Hospital
Wayne State University

Overview of the Pathophysiology

Coronary atherosclerosis involves a localized accumulation of fibrous tissue and, to a lesser extent, lipid within the coronary artery, causing progressive narrowing of the lumen of the vessel. Clinically significant lesions, producing myocardial ischemia and ventricular dysfunction, usually obstruct over 75% of the vessel lumen. The aims of revascularization are:

- to increase blood flow and oxygen delivery to ischemic myocardium beyond an obstructive arterial lesion;
- to decrease or eliminate the potential consequences or manifestations of myocardial ischemia, including significant ST-segment depression, angina pectoris, threatening ventricular arrhythmias, or combinations thereof; and
- to potentially reduce cardiovascular-related morbidity and mortality.

Two techniques are currently utilized: coronary artery bypass graft surgery (CABGS) and percutaneous transluminal coronary angioplasty (PTCA). The surgical technique involves passing the critically obstructed coronary artery with either a saphenous vein, removed from the client's leg(s), or an internal mammary artery, one of the major arteries carrying blood to the chest wall. Recent variations of the technique include minimally invasive direct coronary artery bypass surgery, wherein the surgeon operates with fiberoptical scopes through small incisions between the ribs to work directly on a contracting heart, or off-pump coronary artery bypass, where surgeons operate on the contracting heart without the use of the heart-lung machine. With PTCA, a balloon or double-lumen dilation catheter is directed to the site of a coronary lesion until it lies within the vascular stenosis. Inflation of the balloon produces:

- plaque compression and redistribution; and
- stretching of the vessel wall with an increase in the overall vessel diameter.

Today, the majority of all persons diagnosed with ischemic heart disease who are referred for revascularization undergo PTCA (> 700,000 patients/yr).

CABGS

Current indications for CABGS, after defining coronary anatomy and left ventricular function by cardiac catheterization, are as follows:

- to relieve anginal symptoms that are refractory to pharmacologic therapy and/or when PTCA is contraindicated;

- to prolong life in clients with left main coronary artery disease, triple-vessel disease, double-vessel disease, left ventricular dysfunction, and/or proximal left anterior descending coronary artery disease; and

- to preserve left ventricular function in clients with diffuse or left main coronary artery disease and significant additional myocardium in jeopardy, particularly when previous myocardial infarction has already compromised left ventricular function.

Clients who undergo CABGS today are characteristically older, are more likely to have three-vessel disease, and have intrinsically poorer pump function. The left ventricular ejection fraction in clients who undergo CABGS averages 38%; the value for those undergoing PTCA is 55%.

Complications of CABGS, including perioperative infarction in 5 to 12% of all cases, occur more frequently in older clients, diabetics, women, obese clients, clients with left ventricular dysfunction (ejection fraction < 30%), and clients undergoing emergency bypass surgery.

Current patency rates for saphenous vein grafts are 90, 80, and 60% after 1, 5, and 11 years, respectively. The greatest incidence of graft occlusion occurs between 5 and 8 years after surgery, often heralded by recurrent angina pectoris, diminished physical work capacity, or both. In contrast, internal mammary grafts have a 93% 10-year graft patency and appear to be resistant to atherosclerosis. This fact may partially explain the impressive 10-year actuarial survival advantage in clients undergoing CABGS who received internal mammary grafts when compared with those who received saphenous vein bypass grafting. Total relief of angina pectoris typically occurs in 70% of clients undergoing CABGS at 5 years; approximately 50% are asymptomatic at 10 years.

PTCA

Although the use of PTCA was initially restricted to elective cases of low-risk individuals who had discrete, proximal, single-vessel lesions, indications for the procedure have since broadened to include clients with two-vessel or three-vessel disease, impaired left ventricular function, and acute occlusion during myocardial infarction. However, clients undergoing PTCA must be willing to undergo emergency CABGS if dilation fails or complications occur.

Compared with CABGS, which generally requires a hospital stay of 5 to 7 days, the recovery period following elective PTCA is much shorter (1-2 days) and the

cost is considerably less. However, arterial injuries, blood-clotting-related complications, and restenosis remain the major limitations of PTCA. Approximately 30% of clients undergoing PTCA will develop restenosis of the treated vessel within six months of the procedure.

In 1994, the U.S. Food and Drug Administration approved the use of the Palmaz-Schatz stent, a tiny, flexible metal cylinder inserted into the opened coronary artery to maintain patency. More recently, investigators have sought to coat stents with sirolimus, a drug that attenuates the potential for inflammation of the inner walls of blood vessels, to further reduce the likelihood of subsequent restenosis.

Effects on the Exercise Response

Successful revascularization may favorably alter the exercise response to a single exercise session in several ways. By increasing the blood flow and oxygen supply to myocardial regions beyond an obstructive coronary arterial lesion, CABGS or PTCA may reduce or eliminate electrocardiographic changes resulting from ischemia, that is, T-wave inversion and/or ST-segment depression, as well as anginal symptoms on exertion. The latter may serve to increase physical work capacity in clients who are symptomatic at low levels of exercise. Correcting the imbalance between myocardial oxygen supply and demand may also improve ventricular contractility and wall motion, favorably altering the hemodynamic response to exercise. Chronotropic impairment, a delayed heart rate recovery immediately after exercise, and/or exertional hypotension may normalize after revascularization. Ischemia-related ventricular arrhythmias may also be abolished by successful PTCA or CABGS. Indeed, silent ischemia has been suggested as the missing link between the increased risk of cardiac arrest and the lack of premonitoring symptoms during exercise-based cardiac rehabilitation.

Effects of Exercise Training

The benefits and limitations of exercise training for clients undergoing PTCA or CABGS are similar to those for survivors of acute myocardial infarction (see chapter 4). Surveillance for the development of threatening ventricular arrhythmias during exercise-based cardiac rehabilitation after CABGS may improve medical management and prognosis by facilitating the early detection and treatment of electrical instability in selected high-risk individuals. The average improvement in physical work capacity and maximal oxygen consumption ($\dot{V}O_2$max) is about 20%. Moreover, training-induced reductions in heart rate and blood pressure serve to decrease myocardial demands at rest and at any given submaximal work rate. Even short-term endurance training in clients rehabilitated after CABGS promotes favorable modification of glucose metabolism, presumably by a decrease in insulin resistance.

Although results from several meta-analyses have demonstrated a 20 to 25% reduction in fatal cardiovascular events and total mortality after myocardial infarction, the contribution of exercise training to survival of clients following CABGS and PTCA has not been evaluated. It is also unclear what role physical conditioning per se plays in maintaining graft patency, preventing restenosis, or retarding atherosclerotic coronary disease following successful revascularization. Unfortunately, studies to date generally suggest that exercise training as an isolated intervention is largely ineffective in achieving these outcomes.

Management and Medications

Treatment of the revascularization client has progressed from the use of nitrate drugs and beta-blocking agents to an aggressive multi-modality approach using coronary risk factor modification, pharmacologic therapy (e.g., calcium-channel-blocking drugs, antiarrhythmic and lipid-lowering drugs), thrombolytic enzymes, PTCA, surgical interventions, and when necessary, use of the automatic implantable cardioverter defibrillator. The exact roles of these modalities in clients undergoing PTCA or CABGS are uncertain today. Nevertheless, lifestyle interventions designed to slow, halt, or even reverse the underlying atherosclerotic disease process remain the mainstay of treatment, including:

- regular aerobic exercise;
- blood pressure control;
- smoking cessation;
- cholesterol lowering; and
- reduction of body weight and fat stores.

Smoking cessation, for example, is associated with a higher prevalence of disease-free bypass grafts over time.

Empiric experience has shown that close observation and monitoring of revascularization clients during exercise-based cardiac rehabilitation can often detect a deterioration in clinical status. Exercise-related signs or symptoms that may indicate restenosis of a treated vessel, occlusion of vein grafts, or progression of atherosclerotic disease include:

- recurring anginal pain (e.g., chest pain or pressure, an ache in the jaw or neck, pain across the shoulders or back);

- dizziness or lightheadedness; and
- threatening forms of ventricular ectopy (e.g., frequent paired or multiform ventricular premature contractions, couplets, or ventricular tachycardia).

Cardiac and lipid-lowering medications commonly used to treat revascularization clients are summarized elsewhere (see chapters 4 and 22), with specific reference to their hemodynamic and electrocardiographic effects. Unfortunately, interventions to prevent restenosis using aspirin (alone or in combination with dipyridamole), anti-coagulants (e.g., warfarin, heparin), N-3 omega fatty acids, corticosteroid hormone therapy, and calcium-channel-blocking drugs, have been largely ineffective. Repeat PTCA is the usual treatment for restenosis, and most clients experience sustained improvement after the procedure.

Recommendations for Exercise Testing

Exercise testing can follow the general protocols and procedures outlined for post-myocardial infarction (MI) clients (see CABGS and PTCA: Exercise Testing table). Treadmill or cycle ergometer testing 3 to 5 weeks after CABGS has proved valuable in assessing exercise tolerance and in prescribing levels of physical activity; in contrast, arm ergometer testing at this time may be uncomfortable because of midsternal incisional pain. Follow-up testing procedures are similar to those after acute MI (e.g., following an additional 3-6 mo of exercise training and yearly thereafter). For the purpose of risk stratification, symptomatic clients 5 years or less and all clients more than 5 years after CABGS may benefit from exercise testing with concomitant myocardial perfusion imaging. A functional capacity of 9 METs or more indicates a favorable prognosis, regardless of other responses.

Exercise testing after PTCA may be done sooner and more frequently than that typically recommended after MI or CABGS. Recently, supine cycle ergometer echocardiography has been shown to be a safe and reliable tool to detect exercise-induced wall motion abnormalities after PTCA and provide prognostic information in the risk assessment of clinical restenosis. However, among asymptomatic subjects with single-vessel disease, the detection of restenosis after PTCA via conventional exercise testing remains unreliable, especially when quantitative coronary angiography is used as a reference. On the other hand, the presence of 75% or more cross-sectional narrowing shown by intravascular ultrasound is well correlated with 1 or more mm ST-segment depression at follow-up treadmill testing after PTCA. The addition of QT dispersion (QTd = QTmax − QTmin) to

CABGS and PTCA: Exercise Testing

Methods	Measures	Endpoints*	Comments
Aerobic Cycle (ramp protocol 17 watts/min; staged protocol 25-50 watts/3-min stage) Treadmill (1-2 METs/3-min stage)	• 12-lead ECG, HR	• Serious dysrhythmias • >2mm ST-segment depression or elevation • Ischemic threshold • T-wave inversion with significant ST change	• ST-segment displacement can occur with restenosis or partial occlusion. • Important in establishing a safe training intensity. • Chronotropic impairment suggests poor prognosis. • Minimal treadmill speed should be ≤ 1.0 mph.
	• BP, rate pressure product	• SBP > 250 mmHg or DBP > 115 mmHg	• Exertional hypotension (drop of ≥ 20 mmHg or failure to rise) suggests poor prognosis.
	• RPE (6-20)		• Useful as an adjunct to HR as an exercise intensity guide.
	• Gas analysis ($\dot{V}O_2$peak or $\dot{V}O_2$max)		• Only if exact measures are indicated. • For CABGS clients, a peak work rate of ≥ 9 METs suggests good prognosis.
Strength Isokinetic/Isotonic	• 90% maximal voluntary contraction (MVC) greatest load lifted 2-3 times	• 3 consecutive reps	• Use 1RM (estimated from 90% MVC) to establish training work rate. • Should not be performed until sternum has healed.

*Measurements of particular significance; do not always indicate test termination.

Medications	Special Considerations
• See chapter 4 testing table and appendixes A, B, and C.	• See chapter 4 testing table. • Chest and leg wounds usually require 4 to 12 wk for complete healing. Upper body arm crank ergometer testing that may cause sternal tension or clicking should be avoided until healing is complete. • An extended active cool-down after peak or symptom-limited exercise testing has been suggested to reduce the risk of cardiovascular complications that are more likely to occur in the postexercise period. • Prolonged convalescence after CABGS may further serve to decrease $\dot{V}O_2$max. • After CABGS, exercise testing often increases self-confidence and self-efficacy. • Clients often resume normal or near-normal activities soon after PTCA (i.e., within 24-48 hr).

ST-segment depression during exercise testing also improves the diagnostic value and can be used as a noninvasive tool in the diagnosis of restenosis after PTCA.

Preliminary signs or symptoms of restenosis, manifested as significant ST-segment depression, the provocation of angina pectoris, or both, may be apparent with exercise testing as early as 2 to 3 days after PTCA. A more accepted time period for initial evaluation of PTCA clients is 2 to 5 weeks, followed by another exercise test at 6 months. Thereafter, exercise testing once a year is generally considered adequate.

CABGS and PTCA: Exercise Programming

Modes	Goals	Intensity/Frequency/Duration	Time to Goal
Aerobic • Large muscle activities • Arm/leg ergometry	• Increase aerobic capacity • Decrease BP and HR response to submaximal exercise • Decrease submaximal myocardial O_2 demand • Decrease CAD risk factors • Increase ADLs	• RPE 12-15/20 • 40-80% $\dot{V}O_2$max or HR reserve • Intensity must be kept below ischemic threshold • 3-5 days/wk • 20-60 min/session • 5-10 min of warm-up and cool-down activities	• 4-6 mo
Strength • Circuit training	• Increase ability to perform leisure, occupational, and ADLs • Increase muscle strength and endurance • Decrease rate-pressure product during lifting or carrying objects	• 40-50% maximal voluntary contraction (avoid Valsalva) • 2-3 days/wk • 1-3 sets* of 10-15 reps • 8-10 different exercises • 1-2 lb (0.5-0.9 kg) to start (wait 12 wk post-CABG before using heavier weights) • Resistance gradually increased over time	• 4-6 mo
Flexibility • Upper and lower body ROM activities	• Decrease risk of injury • Improve ROM in CABG patients	• 2-3 days/wk • Static stretches: hold for 10-30 s	• 4-6 mo

*A single set of exercises to volitional fatigue is highly effective, at least during the initial months of training.

Medications	Special Considerations
• See chapter 4 programming table and appendixes A, B, and C. • Beta blockers: No major effect on exercise trainability in cardiac patients. • Calcium-channel blockers: No major effect on exercise trainability in cardiac patients.	• See chapter 4 programming table. • CABGS patients typically begin inpatient rehabilitation sooner and progress at a more accelerated rate. • CABGS patients generally devote more time to upper extremity range-of-motion exercises. • Carefully monitor for signs (e.g., ischemic ST-segment depression) and symptoms (e.g., angina) of graft occlusion (CABGS) or restenosis (PTCA). Periodic intermittent or continuous ECG monitoring may be helpful in this regard. • The upper limits of early exercise prescription (i.e., inpatient) for CABGS clients include an RPE of 11-13 and an HR at standing rest of +30 contractions/min.

Recommendations for Exercise Programming

Simple exposure to orthostatic or gravitational stress during the ever-decreasing bed rest stage of hospital convalescence and soon thereafter may obviate much of the deterioration in cardiorespiratory fitness that normally follows CABGS and, to a lesser extent, PTCA. A significant increase in aerobic capacity generally occurs in the weeks after coronary revascularization, even in clients who undergo no formal exercise training. Research indicates that self-care and other out-of-hospital activities performed by cardiac clients soon after hospital discharge frequently lead to sustained increases in heart rate and oxygen uptake that exceed the minimal effective intensity (i.e., 40 to 50% heart rate or $\dot{V}O_2$max) commonly prescribed for training. These transient fluxes in cardiorespiratory activity may promote a training effect and account, at least in part, for the spontaneous improvement in aerobic capacity during the early weeks after coronary revascularization.

Walking is recommended as the primary mode of exercise soon after CABGS or PTCA. Moreover, recent studies have shown that brisk walking is of a sufficient intensity to elicit a training heart rate (defined as ≥ 70% of measured maximal heart rate) in all but the most highly fit clients with coronary disease. General recommendations for exercise training are found in the CABGS and PTCA: Exercise Programming table. Compared with MI clients, clients after CABGS typically:

- begin inpatient exercise rehabilitation sooner;

- progress at a more accelerated rate; and

- devote more attention to upper extremity range-of-motion (ROM) exercises.

Clients who undergo CABGS may experience significant soft tissue injury and bone damage of the chest wall. If these areas do not receive ROM exercise in the early postsurgical period, the musculature can become weaker and foreshorten, resulting in more discomfort for the client during convalescence and a prolonged recovery period. ROM exercises used in the inpatient program for the CABGS client typically include shoulder flexion, abduction, and internal and external rotation; elbow flexion; hip flexion, abduction, and internal and external rotation; plantar flexion and dorsiflexion; and ankle inversion and eversion. On the other hand, CABGS clients who experience sternal movement or have postsurgical sternal wound complications would not perform these exercises, unless medically cleared. Upper body ergometry or traditional resistance training exercises that may cause pulling on the sternum should be avoided until healing is complete (generally 12 weeks after CABGS and sternotomy). The sternum should be checked for stability by an experienced health care professional before a resistance training regimen is initiated or at any time that symptoms of chest discomfort or clicking develop.

Middle-aged and older clients may begin to resume normal activities, including light- to moderate-intensity exercise such as brisk walking, within 24 to 48 hours after PTCA. Appropriately selected PTCA clients who wish to initiate a resistance training program may benefit by first participating in an aerobic exercise regimen for two weeks or more, whether in a home-based or medically supervised program. Exercise-based cardiac rehabilitation (Phase II) provides close monitoring and supervision in which failures (restenosis) can be detected early.

CASE STUDY Coronary Artery Bypass Surgery

A 72-year-old retired salesman had recently experienced substernal chest discomfort while walking up a hill in cold weather, and again while climbing a flight of stairs. These symptoms were not always precipitated by physical exertion and sometimes occurred after heavy meals as well. Six years earlier, the client had experienced an anteroseptal MI. Additional coronary risk factors included a history of hypertension, hypercholesterolemia (total cholesterol consistently > 260 mg/dl), obesity, and a family history of premature coronary artery disease. He had a positive exercise stress test, and cardiac catheterization revealed triple-vessel disease with left ventricular hypokinesis and an ejection fraction of 25%. Coronary artery bypass surgery was performed, and he was referred to cardiac rehabilitation.

S: "I had bypass surgery a couple of months ago."

O: Vitals: HR: 84 contractions/min   BP: 160/96 mmHg   BMI: 32.6 kg/m^2

Elderly male, no acute distress; no jugular venous distention

Lungs: Clear

Heart: Regular rate, irregular rhythm; no gallops or murmurs; distal pulses 2+ and non-delayed; no peripheral edema

ECG: Sinus rhythm with infrequent PVCs; non-specific ST–T-wave abnormalities with Q waves in leads V_2-V_4

Graded exercise test (treadmill, modified Bruce protocol):
Rest HR: 92 contractions/min
BP: 146/90 mmHg
Peak HR: 124 contractions/min
Peak BP: 160/84 mmHg
Peak Exercise: 2.5 mph, 12% grade; test terminated due to fatigue (RPE 18/20)   *(continued)*

CASE STUDY   Coronary Artery Bypass Surgery (continued)

No significant ST-segment depression symptoms; isolated PVCs
Isotope imaging showed no evidence of ischemia-induced perfusion abnormalities
Medications: Inderal, Lipitor, Aspirin, Lanoxin

A: 1. Recent bypass surgery and prior MI

2. Deconditioning

P: Initiate a 12-week cardiac rehabilitation program.

Exercise Program
Goals:

1. Peak exercise tolerance > 6 METs
2. Increase functional capacity
3. Adjunct to diabetes/weight management
4. Reinforce lifestyle changes/medical management

Mode	Frequency	Duration	Intensity	Progression
Aerobic	3 days/wk	20 min/session	THR (96-108 contractions/min) RPE 12-15/20	Increase to 40 min @ 60-80% THR after 8 wk
Strength (lower extremity; upper extremity delayed until sternum well healed)	3 days/wk	1 set of ≤ 10 reps	40-50% of 1RM	Increase to 2 sets of 10-12 reps after 12 wk
Flexibility (shoulders, elbows, wrists, hips, knees, ankles)	3 days/wk	20 s/stretch	Maintain stretch below discomfort point	Discomfort point should occur at higher ROM
Neuromuscular				
Functional				
Warm-up/Cool-down	Before and after each sesson	10-15 min	RPE <10/20	Maintain

Follow-Up

Approximately 6 months after bypass surgery, the client completed 7 min of the conventional Bruce treadmill protocol (1 min @ 3.4 mph, 14% grade, ~ 7-8 METs) to volitional fatigue, without significant ST-segment depression or anginal symptoms. Isolated PVCs were noted during and after exercise, and the client achieved a peak heart rate of 128 contractions/min. He chose to continue cardiac rehabilitation with a home-based exercise program.

Suggested Readings

American Association of Cardiovascular and Pulmonary Rehabilitation. 1999. *Guidelines for cardiac rehabilitation and secondary prevention programs.* 3rd ed. Champaign, IL: Human Kinetics.

American College of Sports Medicine. 2000. *ACSM's Guidelines for exercise testing and prescription.* Edited by B.A. Franklin, M.H. Whaley, and E.T. Howley. 6th ed. Philadelphia: Lippincott Williams & Wilkins.

Aytemir, K., N. Ozer, S. Aksoyek et al. 1999. QT dispersion plus ST-segment depression: A new predictor of restenosis after successful percutaneous transluminal coronary angioplasty. *Clinical Cardiology* 22: 409-12.

Convertino, V.A. 1983. Effect of orthopedic stress on exercise performance after bed rest: Relation to inhospital rehabilitation. *Journal of Cardiac Rehabilitation* 3: 660-63.

Dagianti, A., S. Rosanio, M. Penco et al. 1997. Clinical and prognostic usefulness of supine bicycle exercise echocardiography in the functional evaluation of patients undergoing elective percutaneous transluminal coronary angioplasty. *Circulation* 95: 1176-84.

Dylewicz, P., S. Bienkowska, L. Szczesniak et al. 2000. Beneficial effect of short-term endurance training on glucose metabolism during rehabilitation after coronary bypass surgery. *Chest* 117: 47-51.

Franklin, B.A., P. McCullough, and G.C. Timmis. 1999. Exercise. In *Clinical trials in cardiovascular disease*, edited by C. Hennekens, J. Manson, J. Buring, and P.M. Ridker, 278-95. Philadelphia: W.B. Saunders.

Galante, A., A. Pietroiusti, C. Cavazzinei et al. 2000. Incidence and risk factors associated with cardiac arrhythmias during rehabilitation after coronary artery bypass surgery. *Archives of Physical Medicine and Rehabilitation* 81: 947-52.

Galassi, A.R., R. Foti, S. Azzarelli et al. 2000. Usefulness of exercise tomographic myocardial perfusion imaging for detection of restenosis after coronary stent implantation. *American Journal of Cardiology* 85: 1362-64.

Korpilahti, K., E. Engblom, H. Hamalainen et al. 1999. Significance of graft occlusion and coronary atherosclerosis 5 years after coronary artery bypass grafting. A quantitative angiographic study with serial exercise testing. *Journal of Internal Medicine* 245: 545-52.

Laarman, G., H.E. Luijten, L.G. van Zeyl et al. 1990. Assessment of silent restenosis and long-term follow-up after successful angioplasty in single vessel coronary artery dis-

ease: The value of quantitative exercise electrocardiography and quantitative coronary angiography. *Journal of the American College of Cardiology* 16: 578-85.

Malekianpour, M., J. Rodes, G. Cote et al. 1999. Value of exercise electrocardiography in the detection of restenosis after coronary angioplasty in patients with one-vessel disease. *American Journal of Cardiology* 84: 258-63.

The Post Coronary Artery Bypass Graft Trial Investigators. 1997. The effect of aggressive lowering of low-density lipoprotein cholesterol levels and low dose anticoagulation on obstructive changes in saphenous-vein coronary artery bypass grafts. *New England Journal of Medicine* 336: 153-62.

Wenger, N.K., E.S. Froelicher, L.K. Smith et al. 1995. *Cardiac rehabilitation*. Clinical Practice Guideline No. 17. Rockville, MD: U.S. Department of Health and Human Services, Public Health Service, Agency for Health Care Policy and Research and the National Heart, Lung, and Blood Institute. AHCPR Publication No. 96-0672.

Zellweger, M.J., H.C. Lewin, S. Lai et al. 2001. When to stress patients after coronary artery bypass surgery? Risk stratification in patients early and late post-CABG using stress myocardial perfusion SPECT: Implications of appropriate clinical strategies. *Journal of the American College of Cardiology* 37: 144-52.

CHAPTER 6

Angina and Silent Ischemia

Adam Gitkin, MS
Arizona Heart Institute

Martha Canulette, MSN, RN
Presbyterian Healthplex

Daniel Friedman, MD, FACSM
Presbyterian Healthplex

Overview of the Pathophysiology

Ischemia is a lack of blood flow and oxygen to a specific organ or region of the body. With respect to the heart, myocardial ischemia occurs when a mismatch between myocardial oxygen demand and supply exists. This may occur from an obstruction in the coronary arteries, such as atherosclerosis, or a focal spasm in the coronary arteries independent of atherosclerosis. Two types of ischemia exist: symptomatic and silent.

Symptomatic ischemia may be present in several ways. The most common is angina. Angina is typically described as a discomfort in the chest and presents with a heavy, squeezing, or constricting feeling. It is usually retrosternal and often radiates to the shoulders, arms, neck, or jaw. Some people experience shortness of breath, nausea, or diaphoresis (sweating). Atypical features may also be present. Symptoms generally last from 10 to 20 s at a time, but occasionally for as long as 30 min or more.

Not all chest pain is angina, however, and many forms of chest pain do not involve the heart. Various conditions involving other structures in the chest can occasionally cause chest discomfort. These include spasm of the esophagus; reflux of acid from the stomach; hiatal hernia; inflammation of the bones or cartilage of the chest wall or sternum; or muscular pain from muscles of the chest wall, back, shoulder, or arms.

Symptomatic angina is divided into three forms: stable, unstable, and variant (also called vasospastic or Prinzmetal's angina).

Stable angina is reproducibly associated with a specific amount of physical exertion, emotional stress, or exposure to cold and is predictably relieved promptly with rest or sublingual nitroglycerin. With stable angina, a fixed stenosis is associated with a particular segment of a coronary artery. When a coronary artery lumen diameter is narrowed by more than 70%, the reduced blood flow may be sufficient to serve the low cardiac oxygen needs at rest, but is insufficient for increases in oxygen demand. This may occur from constriction of the coronary blood vessels, due in part to dysfunction of the endothelium (inner layer of blood vessels) in releasing chemicals to dilate these vessels.

Unstable angina (USA) occurs unpredictably. It indicates intermittent complete blockage of an artery which may soon become permanent. The three principal presentations of USA are:

- angina that occurs at rest or upon awakening from sleep, lasting more than 20 min;

- new onset, or first experience, of anginal chest pain; and

- increasing severity, frequency, duration, or threshold pattern (level of activity that reproduces the pain) of previously diagnosed angina.

The pathogenesis of USA is multi-factorial and includes one or more of the following:

- platelet aggregation or thrombosis (clot) at a site of coronary artery narrowing;

- rupture and hemorrhage into an atherosclerotic plaque; and

- transient periods of vasospasm at the atherosclerotic plaque.

Often, USA is a precursor to MI. People with this form of angina must be admitted to a coronary care unit and treated immediately with anti-clotting (anticoagulant) drugs or emergency balloon angioplasty.

Variant, vasospastic, or **Prinzmetal's angina** occurs when the coronary arteries spasm, or contract suddenly. Angiograms in this type of angina show no obstruction or stenoses, and very little evidence of atheroma. Intense vasospasm (i.e., a form of cramp of the vessel wall muscles) alone reduces coronary oxygen supply and results in angina. This leads to transient narrowing. Treatments with medications that decrease spasm, such as calcium-channel antagonists, are often effective. In general, the prognosis is thought to be good.

Some people with coronary artery disease (CAD) do not have symptoms consistent with ischemia. This absence of symptoms is called silent ischemia. Laboratory techniques, such as cardiac stress testing and continuous ambulatory electrocardiography are used to determine silent ischemia. During myocardial ischemia, ST-segment and T-wave changes can be seen. Commonly, horizontal or downward sloping ST-segment depressions and T-wave flattening or inversions are seen. Silent ischemia is particularly common among diabetics, possibly related to impaired pain sensation due to peripheral neuropathy. Treatment for persons with silent ischemia is similar to that used to treat people with angina.

Effects on the Exercise Response

People with exercise-related myocardial ischemia may need to stop a single session of physical activity prematurely. This may result from abnormal hemodynamic responses. First, coronary vasoconstriction of diseased coronary arterial segments may occur. With diseased arteries, a reduction occurs in the production of nitric oxide, also known as endothelial-derived relaxing factor. This substance normally causes dilation, or widening, of the coronary blood vessels with increased physical activity. Also, with diseased arteries, increased platelet aggregation causes release of thromboxane A2, a chemical that strongly constricts blood vessels. In addition, a release of endothelin, another chemical that constricts coronary arteries, occurs in people with coronary atherosclerosis. Endothelin is released in much lower levels in people with healthy coronary arteries.

Second, since the myocardial cells are not well perfused with oxygen, they can not contract well. This reduces stroke volume (i.e., amount of blood pumping out of the heart with each beat) and subsequent left ventricular ejection fraction. This limits cardiac output (i.e., amount of blood pumped out of the heart per minute) and then limits skeletal muscle perfusion, leading to fatigue. An increase in diastolic blood pressure greater than 15 mmHg during aerobic exercise, known as diastolic hypertension, can be seen. The decreased stroke volume may lead to compensatory increases in heart rate,

known as increased chronotropic response. A longer warm-up is needed during exercise.

Effects of Exercise Training

Exercise training is generally beneficial for people with stable angina. Exercise alone, or in combination with other lifestyle behavior changes, helps to reduce overall cardiac risk and can help prevent, retard growth of, or even reverse atherosclerotic plaques. The overall goal for people with angina is to raise their ischemic threshold, or the point during physical stress at which angina symptoms occur. Optimal pharmacological therapy will help enhance exercise performance. After exercise training, people should be able to perform more leisure- and exercise-related physical activity without signs and symptoms of angina. People who develop exertional angina benefit from exercise primarily by decreasing the heart's demand for oxygen or may benefit by increasing the heart's supply of oxygen.

With exercise training, a decrease in the severity and extent of exercise-related myocardial ischemia occurs via a reduction in myocardial oxygen demand. The following physiological process explains how this is accomplished. Exercise training leads to an increase in vagal tone, which causes a decrease in heart rate. This increases the amount of time the ventricles can fill with blood, known as ventricular filling time. Increased filling time produces increased end diastolic volume, the amount of blood available to be pumped from the heart, and an increased stroke volume.

In addition, there is some drop in arterial blood pressure. The subsequent decreases in heart rate and systolic blood pressure thus decrease the **rate pressure product** (RPP), also called **double product**, which is an index of myocardial oxygen requirement. With a reduction of RPP, the exercise intensity needed to precipitate chest pain (symptomatic ischemia) or ST-segment depression (silent ischemia) becomes greater. In other words, a person will be able to perform a more intense physical activity before exceeding the RPP that elicits angina.

Some evidence suggests that exercise training increases the supply of blood and oxygen to the heart at rest and during exercise. This is achieved primarily by two mechanisms. First are changes in the coronary artery endothelium and second are changes in the smooth muscle of the coronary artery walls. With long-term exercise training (e.g., 4-7 times/wk for ≥ 12 wk), there is repeated laminar shear stress on the surface of the coronary endothelial cells of the arterioles. This stress changes the shape of the endothelial cells in the direction of the blood flow, and stimulates the production of nitric oxide. Nitric oxide diffuses out of the endothelial cells and into the surrounding coronary smooth muscle cells, which causes a chemical cascade with resultant vasodilation (i.e., relaxation and opening) of coronary arteries. The second mechanism involves the training-induced changes in coronary arterial smooth muscle function (blood vessel resistance). With repeated exercise training, there is an improvement in calcium handling of the smooth muscle cells. This leads to a decrease in coronary tone (vasoconstriction) and an increase in the vasodilatation (relaxation) of the coronary arteries.

Management and Medications

The primary goals for treatment of myocardial ischemia are to increase myocardial supply and decrease myocardial demand. Primary management used to decrease myocardial oxygen demand includes medications and exercise. Management used to increase myocardial oxygen supply includes controlling multiple CAD risk factors (e.g., smoking cessation, hypertension control, weight loss, stress management), direct revascularization of ischemic myocardium procedures (e.g., balloon angioplasty, stent placements, directional atherectomy, laser angioplasty, and rotablator), and coronary artery bypass graft surgery (CABGS). Primary drug categories used to treat angina include the following: antiplatelet drugs, beta blockers, calcium-channel antagonists, and nitrates (nitroglycerin).

• Antiplatelet drugs (e.g., aspirin) decrease the adherence of platelets to the walls of blood vessels and decrease the aggregation of platelets. This later step is accomplished by preventing the production of the cyclooxygenase enzyme in blood vessels. This inhibition will help to inhibit thromboxane A2, a potent platelet aggregator and blood vessel constrictor. The combination of the previous two mechanisms helps to inhibit the clotting process that assists in preventing ischemia. Aspirin, as low as 81 mg/day, reduces the likelihood of heart attacks. Plavix, an adenosine diphosphate binding inhibitor, is used particularly after coronary stenting.

• Beta blockers (e.g., atenolol) decrease myocardial oxygen demand by exerting a negative chronotropic (i.e., heart rate) and negative inotropic (i.e., force of contraction) effect on the heart. The negative chronotropic response occurs because adrenaline effects are blocked in the sinoatrial node.

• Calcium-channel blockers (e.g., verapamil) are also used in people with angina. These medications also decrease myocardial oxygen demand but by a different mechanism. They interfere with the calcium entry into the blood vessel smooth muscle. Because calcium is needed for coronary vasoconstriction, the resultant effect is vasodilatation.

• Nitrates (both short- and long-acting nitroglycerin) are commonly prescribed for angina. Nitrates decrease myocardial oxygen demand by two mechanisms. Nitrates dilate peripheral blood vessels (decreasing venous tone), which decreases the mean systemic filling pressure (i.e., the pressure needed to pump blood back to the heart). This decreases venous return (i.e., amount of blood returning to the heart) and leads to a decrease in cardiac preload (myocardial wall tension to achieve contraction). At the same time, nitrates increase oxygen supply by way of an increase in coronary perfusion and decrease in coronary vasospasm.

Recommendations for Exercise Testing

Evaluation of people suspected of having CAD that may cause ischemia is primarily done with graded exercise testing and may not be safe for all people with ischemia. Exercise testing is contraindicated in people with unstable angina.

A standard exercise test should monitor heart rate, blood pressure, and 12-lead ECG (see the Angina and Silent Ischemia: Exercise Testing table for test protocol). In addition to ECG changes such as ST-segment alterations, blood pressure, and provokable ventricular ectopy, important information comes from the aerobic capacity of the individual. During the test, documentation of anginal symptoms, the rating of angina, and the exact onset and duration of angina should be carefully documented. The duration of the exercise test also has important prognostic implications. Even in persons with confirmed significant CAD, the capacity to exercise into stage IV of a Bruce protocol is associated with an eight-year survival rate of 93%. In contrast, persons who can complete only stage I have an eight-year survival rate of 45%. A hypotensive response to exercise is associated with an 80% predictive value for significant CAD. A low work capacity and early onset of angina combined with marked ST-segment depression, especially continuing into recovery, are associated with very significant CAD including left main and three-vessel diseases.

Indications to terminate exercise testing include client symptoms such as anginal pain and fatigue, clinical signs such as poor perfusion, ECG signs such as dysrhythmias or ST-segment displacement (horizontal or descending) greater than 0.3 mV above or below that of the resting tracing, blood pressure abnormalities such as a fall in systolic pressure, client desire to stop, and failure of testing equipment. Reasons for terminating a test specific to CAD include indications of increasing left ventricular

Angina and Silent Ischemia: Exercise Testing

Methods	Measures	Endpoints*	Comments

Aerobic
Cycle
(ramp protocol 17 watts/
min; staged protocol 25-50
watts/3-min stage)
Treadmill
(1-2 METs/3-min stage)
	• 12-lead ECG, HR	• Serious dysrhythmias
		• > 2 mm ST-segment
		  depression or elevation
		• Ischemic threshold
		• T-wave inversion with
		  significant ST change	

	• BP, rate pressure
	  product
		• Plateau or drop in SBP
		  with increased work rate
		• SBP > 250 mmHg or
		  DBP > 115 mmHg
			• Drop in BP with exercise is
			  associated with increased
			  prognosis of ischemic heart
			  disease.

	• RPE (6-20)		• May be useful for setting exercise intensity.

	• Angina scale	• +3 or earlier on +1-
		  +4 scale (see angina
		  scale on page 45)
			• Onset of angina at low work
			  rates is predictive of ischemic
			  heart disease.

*Measurements of particular significance; do not always indicate test termination.

Medications	Special Considerations
• See appendixes A, B, and C. • Most cardiac medications can alter the hemodynamic responses to exercise and possibly reduce the sensitivity of the test.	• Clarify symptoms of angina with client before testing. • Unstable angina is a contraindication to exercise testing. • Poor left ventricular function may lead to dyspnea.

failure, myocardial ischemia, or intraventricular conduction abnormalities.

Specificity in diagnosing CAD can be further obtained by combining cardiac imaging with the test. Nuclear imaging modalities are also known as myocardial perfusion imaging, radionuclide perfusion imaging, and nuclear scans. The premise is that uptake of radioisotopes, such as thallium and sestamibi, by the myocardium should be equivalent to myocardial blood flow. Exercise echocardiography is also useful by comparing rest and exercise wall motion.

In persons unable to exercise adequately enough to perform the exercise test, pharmacological stress testing can be used in conjunction with nuclear perfusion imaging of the heart. The first of these techniques is the use of intravenous coronary vasodilators, such as Persantine (dipyridamole) and adenosine. These agents dilate normal coronary arteries more than diseased ones. Blood flow to the heart is assessed at rest and during infusion of either compound, along with simultaneous nuclear imaging with thallium or technetium. The second technique is the use of positive chronotropic (heart rate) and inotropic (contractility) agents, also known as sympathomimetics. An example is dobutamine. If heart rate is less than 85%

of predicted maximal heart rate, then another agent that blocks the vagus nerve, atropine, may be given to further increase heart rate.

Recommendations for Exercise Programming

Mode, intensity, frequency, and duration recommendations for exercise training/physical activity can be found in the Angina and Silent Ischemia: Exercise Programming table (see page 44). Comprehensive exercise programming (e.g., cardiac rehabilitation) has been proven to be a vital component in helping people with CAD.

Prior to exercise training, people with angina must be able to:

- define *angina;*
- define possible anginal symptoms;
- identify their own anginal symptoms;
- describe the immediate treatment (this includes understanding the necessity and protocol for taking nitroglycerin in the event of an anginal attack); and

Angina and Silent Ischemia: Exercise Programming

Modes	Goals	Intensity/ Frequency/Duration	Time to Goal
Aerobic • Large muscle activities	• Improve functional capacity • Decrease CAD risk factors • Decrease BP response to submaximal exercise • Decrease myocardial O_2 demand	• HR 10-15 contractions/min below ischemic threshold • 3-7 days/wk • 20-60 min/session • 5-10 min of warm-up and cool-down activities	• 4-6 mo
Strength • Circuit training*	• Improve functional capacity	• Light resistance; 40-50% maximal voluntary contraction (avoid Valsalva) • 2-3 days/wk • 15-20 min/session	• 4-6 mo
Flexibility • Upper and lower body ROM activities	• Decrease risk of injury	• 2-3 days/wk	• 4-6 mo

*Avoid isometric exercises.

Medications	Special Considerations
• See appendixes A, B, and C. • Most cardiac medications can alter hemodynamics during exercise.	• See chapter 4 exercise programming table. • Clients need to be encouraged to stay below their ischemic threshold. • If signs or symptoms change, clients should be referred to their physician. • Clients should always carry nitroglycerin if diagnosed with CAD. • Lower-intensity walking is useful. • Clients with low ejection fraction, poor exercise capacity, or frequent dysrhythmias should be closely monitored. • Home-based cardiac rehabilitation may be appropriate for many low-risk patients. • Prolonged warm-up and cool-down (> 10 min) have an anti-anginal effect. • Upper body exercises may precipitate angina more readily than lower body exercises because of a higher pressor response.

• understand the appropriate upper limits of exercise (including heart rate, ratings of perceived exertion, and angina scales).

A prolonged warm-up and cool-down ($\geq$ 10 min), which includes range-of-motion, stretching, and low-intensity aerobic activities, has been shown to have an anti-anginal effect. A goal for people with angina should be to increase heart rate within 10 to 20 contractions/min of the lower limit of the exercise prescription.

The upper exercise intensity limit should be set at least 10 to 15 contractions/min below the RPP at the original threshold measured during the exercise test. As previously stated, this is the heart rate and blood pressure that corresponds to the silent ischemic (ST-segment depression of $\geq$ 1 mm) or symptomatic ischemic (anginal) threshold. In addition to the ischemic threshold, the upper limit may be based on ventricular dysrhythmia threshold or inadequate blood pressure response threshold. Exercise prescription greater than the ischemic threshold may induce life-threatening ventricular dysrhythmias or increase the risk of thrombus formation from catecholamines. The lower limit of the exercise prescription should be about 20 contractions/min below the upper limit.

The duration of the exercise session should use ischemic preconditioning (intervals), exercise periods of short duration (e.g., 5-10 min/session) separated by short rest periods, 2 to 3 sessions/day. These brief episodes of ischemia protect the heart muscle from further damage of subsequent episodes of ischemia. In addition, exercising in the cold should be avoided because of the increased chance of Prinzmetal's angina.

If there is a change in frequency, type, or severity of anginal symptoms before, during, or after an exercise session, this must be recorded in the person's chart and a physician should be notified. Persons presenting with anginal symptoms should subjectively verbalize them using the following angina scale:

1 = Perceptible but mild
2 = Moderate
3 = Moderately severe
4 = Severe

If a person verbalizes a 2 or greater, decrease exercise intensity until resolved or stop exercise completely. Terminate exercise and use standard nitroglycerin protocol if

a client develops angina during an exercise session. Standard nitroglycerin protocol includes the following:

- discontinue exercise if chest pain develops;
- check pulse, blood pressure, and cardiac rhythm using telemetry monitor;
- if no relief with 1 to 3 min of rest, take one sublingual nitroglycerin tablet;
- obtain a 12-lead ECG (if possible);
- if pain is still not relieved, repeat nitroglycerin under the tongue after 5 min;
- give a third nitroglycerin after another 5 min;
- place person on oxygen at 2 to 4 l/nasal prongs (if possible); and
- notify EMS or a physician to determine further course of action.

CASE STUDY Angina Pectoris

A 54-year-old man had been having substernal chest pressure for several months. At first it occurred only when doing very vigorous activities, but later it was brought on by climbing a flight of stairs. The discomfort occasionally radiated to his left shoulder and was associated with some shortness of breath and nausea. Heart catheterization revealed a 75% mid-right coronary artery stenosis, which was opened to less than 10% stenosis by balloon angioplasty. He was referred to cardiac rehabilitation.

S: "I had one of those balloon jobs."

O: Vitals: BP: 142/75 mmHg   HR: 73 contractions/min   Respiration: 14 breaths/min
Lungs: Clear
Heart sounds: Soft fourth heart sound
Normal peripheral pulses; no edema
Labs:
  ECG: Normal
Graded exercise test (stress test; Bruce protocol):
  1.5 mm of flat ST-segment depression in the inferolateral leads at 6 min
Medications: None

A: Exertional angina caused by CAD

P: 1. Refer to Phase II cardiac rehabilitation.
2. Check fasting lipids; initiate lipid-lowering therapy.
3. Prescribe aspirin.

Exercise Program
Goals:
1. Evaluate/improve anginal threshold
2. Increase functional capacity
3. Educate about managing angina symptoms
4. Reinforce lifestyle changes/medical management

(continued)

CASE STUDY Angina Pectoris (continued)

Mode	Frequency	Duration	Intensity	Progression
Aerobic	2 days/wk	20 min/session	THR 10-15 contractions/min below ischemic threshold	Increase to maintain 10-15 contractions/min below ischemic threshold
Strength (all major muscle groups)	3 days/wk	1 set of ≤ 10 reps	40-50% of 1RM	Increase to 2 sets of 10-12 reps after 12 wk
Flexibility (all major muscle groups)	3 days/wk	20 s/stretch	Maintain stretch below discomfort point	Discomfort point should occur at higher ROM
Neuromuscular				
Functional				
Warm-up/Cool-down	Before and after each session	10-15 min	RPE <10/20	Maintain

Suggested Readings

American Association of Cardiovascular and Pulmonary Rehabilitation. 1999. *Guidelines for cardiac rehabilitation and secondary prevention programs.* 3rd ed. Champaign, IL: Human Kinetics.

American College of Sports Medicine. 2000. *ACSM's guidelines for exercise testing and prescription.* Edited by B.A. Franklin, M.H. Whaley, and E.T. Howley. 6th ed. Philadelphia: Lippincott Williams & Wilkins.

Chaitman, B. 1992. Exercise stress testing. In *Heart disease,* edited by E. Braunwald, 161-79. 4th ed. Philadelphia: W.B. Saunders.

Fardy, P.S., and F.G. Yanowitz. 1995. *Cardiac rehabilitation, adult fitness, and exercise testing.* 3rd ed. Baltimore: Williams & Wilkins.

Lilly, L.S. 1997. Ischemic heart disease. In *Pathophysiology of heart disease: A collaborative project of medical students and faculty,* 128-42. 2nd ed. Baltimore: Lilly.

Opie, L.H. 1998. *The heart: Physiology, from cell to circulation.* 3rd ed. Baltimore: Williams & Wilkins.

Opie, L.H. 1995. *Drugs for the heart.* 4th ed. Philadelphia: W.B. Saunders.

Squires, R.W. 1998. *Exercise prescription for the high-risk cardiac patient.* Champaign, IL: Human Kinetics.

Williams, M.A. 1994. Exercise testing and exercise prescription. In *Exercise testing and training in the elderly cardiac patient.* Champaign, IL: Human Kinetics.

CHAPTER 7

Atrial Fibrillation

J. Edwin Atwood, MD
Palo Alto VA Medical Center
Stanford University

Jonathan N. Myers, PhD, FACSM
Palo Alto VA Medical Center
Stanford University

Overview of the Pathophysiology

Chronic atrial fibrillation (AF) is characterized by chaotic, rapid, and irregular atrial depolarizations. It is one of the most common arrhythmias encountered clinically, and it occurs more frequently with advancing age. Although the pathophysiology of AF is not completely understood, most investigators think it is caused by multiple reentrant circuits within the atria. The irregular ventricular response can impair cardiac pump function, leading to a variety of symptoms attributable to hemodynamic variance. Although AF can often be asymptomatic, its disadvantages are generally thought to include the following:

- increased risk of thromboembolic events;
- rapid ventricular rates when AV node is inadequately suppressed;
- incomplete ventricular filling, causing reduced cardiac output;
- decreased exercise capacity; and
- fatigue.

AF is also associated with chronic heart failure, cardiomyopathy, significant valvular disease, coronary artery disease, and hypertension. Some of these disorders may be underlying causes of AF, and in some cases they may be manifestations of AF.

Effects on the Exercise Response

The most notable hemodynamic feature of the exercise response in clients with AF is a rapid, irregular ventricular response. Heart rate is comparatively high at any level of exercise, in part to compensate for the diminished stroke volume and thus cardiac output in AF. Maximal heart rate tends to be considerably higher in clients with AF compared to that among subjects in normal sinus rhythm. However, there is a marked variability in the maximal heart rate response, as evidenced by standard deviations of 30 contractions/min, even among subjects of similar age. The heart rate response will also be affected by comorbid conditions commonly associated with AF (e.g., coronary artery disease, chronic heart failure) and the use of AV nodal suppressant drugs such as beta blockers, digoxin, and diltiazem.

Exercise tolerance is generally reduced in AF relative to age-matched normal subjects. The degree of this reduction is typically in the order of 20% but is highly dependent on the presence and extent of underlying heart disease. Clients with lone AF (i.e., AF without any underlying disease) achieve peak oxygen consumption values typical of age-matched subjects in normal sinus rhythm.

Because of the variability in the diastolic filling period, the determination of systolic blood pressure can be difficult to assess and is poorly reproducible. This is particularly true at rest when, after long RR intervals, Korotkoff sounds may be heard more distinctly.

Effects of Exercise Training

Although few data are available concerning the effects of exercise training in groups of clients with AF specifically, because the prevalence of AF is comparatively high in men older than 60 years, these clients have been included in many rehabilitation studies. Clients with AF would not be expected to have a training response particularly different from individuals in normal sinus rhythm. The major concern in terms of exercise training in clients with AF is the underlying heart disease, particularly valvular disease, chronic heart failure, and coronary artery disease. The presence of these underlying diseases should be the foremost consideration in exercise programming for individuals with AF.

Management and Medications

Management of AF primarily involves converting the individual to normal sinus rhythm, pharmacologic intervention to maintain sinus rhythm, and when AF is chronic, strategies to control the ventricular rate response and reduce the incidence of stroke. In many clients initially diagnosed with AF, an effort will be made to convert the client back to sinus rhythm electrically, pharmacologically, or both. This procedure has been shown to improve exercise capacity in the order of 15 to 20%, although functional gains probably do not occur until at least one month after successful cardioversion. While the initial success rate of electrical cardioversion is high, many clients will return to AF within 4 to 6 weeks. Conversion and maintenance of normal sinus rhythm is particularly difficult when the duration of AF has been long. Medicines commonly used to control the ventricular rate in AF

include digoxin, beta blockers (e.g., propranolol, sotalol, metoprolol, atenolol), and calcium-channel blockers (e.g., diltiazem, verapamil). Other agents are used to convert AF to sinus rhythm or maintain sinus rhythm once cardioversion is successful (e.g., amiodarone, propoferone).

In terms of stroke prevention, several major trials have demonstrated that antithrombotic therapy in clients with AF reduces the risk of stroke. Treatment with warfarin has consistently demonstrated a 64 to 84% reduction in stroke risk. This risk reduction is independent of the duration of AF. Aspirin has also been demonstrated to be effective in reducing stroke risk, but clinical trials have demonstrated that it is less effective than warfarin. Lastly, successful anticoagulation therapy is dependent upon

Atrial Fibrillation: Exercise Testing

Methods	Measures	Endpoints*	Comments
Aerobic Cycle (ramp protocol 10-15 watts/min; staged protocol 20-30 watts/3 min stage) Treadmill (individualized ramp protocol 8- to 12-min target) Moderately incremented protocol (e.g., Naughton, Balke)	• 12-lead ECG, HR • BP, rate pressure product • RPE (6-20) • Angina scale • Gas analysis (VO₂peak) • Radionuclide testing	• Serious dysrhythmias • >2mm ST-segment depression or elevation • Ischemic threshold • T-wave inversion with significant ST change • SBP > 250 mmHg or DBP > 115 mmHg • +3 or earlier on +1-+4 scale (see page 45)	• Better estimate of capacity
Endurance 6-min walk	• Distance walked	• Rest stops allowed; note stops in record	
Flexibility Goniometry	• Angle of flexion/extension		• If lowered ROM

*Measurements of particular significance; do not always indicate test termination.

Medications	Special Considerations
• See appendixes A, B, and C. • Digoxin/Digitalis: May control ventricular response; diffuse ST effects. • Calcium-channel blockers: May mask ischemia and decrease exercise HR response (e.g., verapamil). • Diltiazem, verapamil: Help control ventricular response; may improve exercise capacity. • Beta blockers: Help control ventricular response; may reduce exercise capacity. Decrease submaximal and maximal HR and BP response; sometimes exercise capacity, especially with nonselective medications.	• Age-predicted maximal HR targets are not valid. • Irregular ventricular response may make BP less precise or more difficult to determine.

regular (e.g., at least monthly) measurements of the international normalized ratio (INR), with careful adjustment to maintain a level between 2.0 and 3.0.

Recommendations for Exercise Testing

Maximal exercise testing can be safely used to objectively characterize the functional capabilities of the client with AF (see the Atrial Fibrillation: Exercise Testing table). The reduction in exercise capacity associated with AF is a direct function of the underlying heart disease. Because underlying heart disease is common, moderately incremented protocols such as the Naughton or ramp are recommended.

Contraindications to exercise testing related to underlying conditions such as stability of chronic heart failure, valvular disease, or complex ventricular arrhythmias should take precedence over AF itself. In the absence of other clinical indications for stopping, clients with AF may be safely taken to fatigue or shortness of breath endpoints. The fact that many clients with AF are taking digoxin, beta blockers, or other antiarrhythmic agents, along with the fact that left bundle branch block and left ventricular hypertrophy are common in AF, complicates the interpretation of ST-segment changes on the exercise electrocardiogram. Age-predicted maximal heart rate targets are particularly useless in AF because of the rapid and highly variable ventricular response. Because of the irregular ventricular response, it has been demonstrated that heart rate is most accurately measured using calipers over at least a 6-s rhythm strip during exercise.

Recommendations for Exercise Programming

As the population ages, the number of individuals with AF referred for exercise rehabilitation will increase. There are two major factors to consider in exercise programming for clients with AF:

- concomitant or underlying heart disease, and
- inherent unreliability of the pulse rate in prescribing exercise intensity.

Because AF is frequently accompanied by ischemic heart disease, chronic heart failure, or valvular heart disease, exercise programming considerations for these conditions should take precedence over AF. In addition, some clients with AF referred to a rehabilitation program

Atrial Fibrillation: Exercise Programming

Modes	Goals	Intensity/ Frequency/Duration	Time to Goal
Aerobic • Large muscle activities • Arm/leg ergometry	• Increase $\dot{V}O_2$peak • Increase ADLs	• RPE 11-16/20 • 50-80% $\dot{V}O_2$peak or HR reserve • 3-7 days/wk • 30-45 min/session	• 3 mo
Strength • Weight machines	• Increase strength	• High reps, low resistance • 3 days/wk	• 2-3 mo
Flexibility • Upper and lower body ROM activities	• Increase flexibility • Reduce risk of injury	• 3-5 days/wk	• 2-4 mo

Medications	Special Considerations
• See exercise testing table.	• Longer sampling of pulse may be needed for reliable HR. • AF has varied effects; some patients will experience fatigue, while others will not. • Ascertain rhythm on a daily basis. • AF is frequently intermittent. • Many clients will be elderly; consider co-morbid conditions such as osteoporosis, CAD, and hypertension.

will have experienced a stroke, in which case the goals of the rehabilitation program change accordingly (see chapter 36). Regardless of the concomitant disease, all clients with AF will require frequent monitoring of the INR. Because of the chronically irregular ventricular rate, exercise intensity should be prescribed based on METs and perceived exertion levels. Frequency, duration, intensity, and progression of exercise are similar to clients in normal sinus rhythm referred to a rehabilitation program and should follow ACSM guidelines.

AF can be intermittent (i.e., the client may be in AF one day and in normal sinus rhythm the next); this will influence not only the client's heart rate response to exercise but perhaps also exercise tolerance and level of fatigue. Limited data have demonstrated that clients with AF can achieve significant functional gains from exercise rehabilitation (see the Atrial Fibrillation: Exercise Programming table on page 49).

CASE STUDY Atrial Fibrillation

A 54-year-old male had a 10-year history of intermittent AF before it became chronic AF. He had a history of post-traumatic stress disorder, depression, herniorrhaphy, and laminectomy, but no history of myocardial infarction, hyperlipidemia, or hypertension. He had a 30 pack-year history of smoking, but had stopped smoking.

S: "I want to be able to play with my grandchildren."

O: Vitals: Height: 6′ 0″ (1.8 m)   Weight: 177.2 lb (80.4 kg)   BMI: 24.8 kg/m²
HR: 86 contractions/min, irregular   BP: 135/96 mmHg, irregular

Middle-aged male in no distress

Cardiovascular: Irregular rhythm; no rubs, gallops, or murmurs

Medications: Warfarin, Metoprolol

INR: 1.88

ECG: Atrial fibrillation with a ventricular response of 86 contractions/min, but otherwise normal; cardiac exam is unremarkable

Echocardiogram: Mildly enlarged left and right atria, normal left ventricle, normal wall thicknesses, and normal ejection fraction (70%); aortic and mitral valves show mild thickening; mild mitral and tricuspid regurgitation; findings are similar to an echocardiogram performed one year earlier.

Graded exercise test (Naughton protocol):
Peak exercise: 5.5 METs (68% of predicted)
Peak RPE: 18/20
Termination from leg fatigue
Chronotropic response to exercise: Normal
Peak HR: 155 contractions/min
Peak BP: 186/94 mmHg
No significant ST changes during exercise or recovery
No report of chest discomfort

A: 1. Chronic AF

2. Low exercise tolerance for age

P: 1. Cardioversion after INR is between 2.0-3.0.

2. Undergo cardiovascular rehabilitation.

Exercise Program
Goals:

1. Improve cardiovascular endurance

2. Monitor ventricular response to exercise

3. Monitor pressor response to exercise

4. Refer to cardiologist for changes in goals 2 and 3

Mode	Frequency	Duration	Intensity	Progression
Aerobic	3 days/wk	20 min/session	THR (50-75% $\dot{V}O_2$peak) RPE 11-16/20	Increase to 40 min @ 60-80% THR after 12 wk
Strength (all major muscle groups)	3 days/wk	1 set of ≤ 10 reps	50-70% of 1RM	Increase to 2 sets of 10-12 reps after 12 wk
Flexibility (all major muscle groups)	3 days/wk	20 s/stretch	Maintain stretch below discomfort point	Discomfort point should occur at higher ROM
Neuromuscular				
Functional				
Warm-up/Cool-down	Before and after each session	10-15 min	RPE <10/20	Maintain

Suggested Readings

Atwood, J.E., and J. Myers. 1997. Exercise hemodynamics of atrial fibrillation. In *Atrial fibrillation: Mechanisms and management*, edited by R.H. Falk and P.J. Podrid. Philadelphia: Lippincott-Raven. 219-39.

Atwood, J.E., J. Myers, M. Sullivan, S. Forbes et al. 1989. The effect of cardioversion on maximal exercise capacity in patients with chronic atrial fibrillation. *American Heart Journal* 118: 913-18.

Atwood, J.E., J. Myers, M. Sullivan, S. Forbes et al. 1988. Maximal exercise testing and gas exchange in patients with chronic atrial fibrillation. *Journal of the American College of Cardiology* 11: 508-13.

Mertens, D.J., and T. Kavanagh. 1996. Exercise training for patients with chronic atrial fibrillation. *Journal of Cardiopulmonary Rehabilitation* 16: 193-96.

Sra, J., A. Dhala, Z. Blanck, S. Deshpande et al. 2000. Atrial fibrillation: Epidemiology, mechanisms, and management. *Current Problems in Cardiology* 25: 405-524.

Ueshima, K., J. Myers, W.F. Graettinger, J.E. Atwood et al. 1993. Exercise and morphologic comparison of chronic atrial fibrillation and normal sinus rhythm. *American Heart Journal* 126: 260-61.

Ueshima, K., J. Myers, C.K. Morris, J.E. Atwood et al. 1993. The effect of cardioversion on exercise capacity in patients with atrial fibrillation. *American Heart Journal* 126: 1021-24.

Vanhees, L., D. Schepers, J. Defoor, S. Brusselle et al. 2000. Exercise performance and training in cardiac patients with atrial fibrillation. *Journal of Cardiopulmonary Rehabilitation* 20: 346-52.

CHAPTER 8

Pacemakers and Implantable Cardioverter Defibrillators

Michael West, MD
Lovelace Health Systems

Scott O. Roberts, PhD, FACSM
California State University, Chico

Overview of the Pathophysiology

Several factors contribute to optimal cardiac function, including atrioventricular synchronization and the responsiveness of heart rate and contractility to neurohormonal control. Loss of the normal sequence of atrial and ventricular filling and contraction can result in deterioration of hemodynamics and significant symptoms at rest and during exercise. Pacing techniques are sometimes used in such persons to improve symptoms and enhance exercise performance. Individuals who cannot increase their heart rate in response to increased metabolic demand usually have sinus node dysfunction and may require cardiac pacing. Other individuals who have worrisome life-threatening ventricular arrhythmias are sometimes candidates for an implantable cardioverter defibrillator (ICD).

Pacing Terminology

Chronotropic incompetence: The inability to augment one's heart rate to an appropriate level with increases in metabolic demand. It is somewhat arbitrarily defined as the inability to increase the heart rate above 100 contractions/min or reach 70% of maximal predicted heart rate despite maximal exertion.

Symptomatic bradycardia: Symptoms directly attributable to a slow heart rate include activity intolerance, transient dizziness, lightheadedness, and complete or near loss of consciousness (syncope).

Rate-adaptive pacemakers: Pacemakers equipped with sensors that allow adaptation of the pacemaker's rate commensurate with increases in demand (i.e., exercise). These units utilize various types of sensors, including those that respond to physiological, mechanical, or electrical signals. This facilitates pacing in a more physiologic manner.

Pacemaker syndrome: Constellation of clinical signs and symptoms that occur as a consequence of the inadequate timing of atrial and ventricular contraction. Most typically results from single-chamber (i.e., ventricular) pacing with loss of atrioventricular (AV) synchrony and retrograde atrial activation. Generally, symptoms result from a reduced cardiac output, negative atrial contribution to stroke volume, or both. Symptoms include lethargy, fatigue, lightheadedness, hypotension, shortness of breath, syncope, neck pulsations, and impaired exercise capacity.

Tiered therapy: ICDs that utilize antitachycardia pacing, shock therapies, and bradycardia safety pacing in a step-wise approach to the treatment of life-threatening ventricular arrhythmias.

Sudden cardiac death syndrome: A clinical scenario during which the person experiences loss of consciousness usually due to a ventricular tachyarrhythmia, usually ventricular tachycardia (VT) and/or ventricular fibrillation (VF). Unless there is prompt restoration to normal rhythm, death ensues. Severe bradycardia and asystole can also account for sudden death in a minority of cases.

Pacemakers

The use of permanent cardiac pacemakers increases survival, decreases symptoms, and improves quality of life. Some commonly accepted indications for pacemaker implantation include:

- sick sinus syndrome with symptomatic bradycardia;
- acquired AV block; and
- persistent advanced AV block after myocardial infarction.

Other less common indications for use of a pacemaker are:

- neurally mediated syncope;
- carotid sinus hypersensitivity; and
- AV block intentionally created by ablative procedures.

A typical pacemaker system consists of two basic components: either 1 or 2 leads and a pulse generator. Leads are insulated and are implanted transvenously into the right atrium, right ventricle, or both. The leads are connected to the pulse generator, which is typically implanted near the clavicle. The two main functions of the leads are sensing and pacing. Sensing involves receiving electrical signals (i.e., P waves and R waves) from the heart. In the absence of such sensed signals, the pacemaker generator will fire, causing the atria or ventricles to contract. Optimally, the pacing system utilizes an atrial and ventricular lead to maintain AV synchrony, which in turn facilitates cardiac output and exercise capacity. Pacemakers are categorized by a standardized code. By convention, the first letter represents the chamber paced, the second is the chamber sensed, and the third connotes the response to a sensed event. The fourth position is utilized to indicate that the pacemaker has rate-response capabilities. For example, VVIR is the abbreviation used when the ventricle (V) is the chamber being paced and sensed. When the pacemaker senses a normal ventricular contraction, the pacemaker is inhibited (I). The R indicates that the pulse generator is rate responsive during exercise.

Another common pacemaker system is dual chamber paced, dual chamber sensed, dual chamber inhibited response (DDDR), which paces and senses both the atrium and ventricle and the response is to either "trigger" or inhibit a pacing stimulus depending on the presence or absence of atrial and/or ventricular rhythm above the programmed rate cutoff. The DDDR pacemaker is widely regarded as the optimal pacing mode in individuals who have normal sinoatrial (SA) node function because it provides AV synchrony and utilizes the client's own sinus rhythm as the sensor-driven heart rate.

Implantable Cardioverter Defibrillators

Persons with coronary artery disease and prior myocardial infarction, congestive heart failure, as well as those with various forms of cardiomyopathy, are at increased risk of sudden cardiac death. Implantable cardioverter defibrillators are utilized to electrically terminate life-threatening ventricular tachyarrhythmias. They consist of two basic parts: the lead system and the cardioverter defibrillator. Currently utilized ICDs have lead systems that are placed transvenously, typically by way of the subclavian vein. The ICD leads track the cardiac rhythm and transmit the information to the pulse generator, which is usually implanted subcutaneously in the pectoral region. When a tachyarrhythmia is detected, preprogrammed therapies are sent back to terminate the arrhythmia. The units can pace-terminate an arrhythmia and/or deliver electric cardioversion/defibrillation shocks. In order to terminate an arrhythmia, the pulse generator must be programmed to recognize specific heart rates. Ventricular tachycardia and fibrillation are typically recognized by their rapid rates. If either is sensed, the pulse generator will deliver the appropriate preprogrammed therapy to the heart through the lead system.

Effects on the Exercise Response

Because of abnormalities in sinus node function, cardiac conduction, and neurohormonal systems, many persons benefit from an improved heart rate response to exercise. Inadequate heart rate responses to exercise, with attendant symptoms, can be markedly improved with current pacemaker technologies.

Persons with ICDs are at risk of receiving inappropriate shocks during exercise. This can occur if the heart rate exceeds the programmed threshold rate for therapy or if the person develops an exercise-induced supraventricular tachycardia. For this reason, people with ICDs should be closely monitored during exercise to ensure that their heart rate does not approach the activation rate for the device.

Effects of Exercise Training

During exercise, cardiac output must increase to support the increased tissue oxygen demand. This increase is

Pacemakers and ICDs: Exercise Testing

Methods	Measures	Endpoints*	Comments
Aerobic Cycle (ramp protocol 17 watts/ min; staged protocol 10-25 watts/3-min stage) Treadmill (1-2 METs/3-min stage)	• 12-lead ECG, HR	• Peak HR must be below activation rate for ICD • Serious dysrhythmias • > 2 mm ST-segment depression or elevation • Ischemic threshold • T-wave inversion with significant ST change	• Peak HR may be blunted. • ECG sensitivity is low for detecting ischemia. • Know HR activation rate for ICD before testing.
	• BP, rate pressure product	• SBP > 250 mmHg or DBP > 115 mmHg • Watch for drop or no increase in SBP with increased work rate	• Peak SBP may be blunted. SBP may decrease or not increase with left ventricular dysfunction.
	• RPE (6-20)		• Better guide of intensity because of possible HR inability to increase with exercise.
	• Radionuclide testing or stress echocardiogram		• May be more useful in assessing ischemic heart disease.

*Measurements of particular significance; do not always indicate test termination.

Medications	Special Considerations
• See chapter 4 exercise testing table.	• Individuals with ICDs are at risk for receiving inappropriate shocks. • HR should not approach the activation rate of the ICD. • Some individuals with pacemakers and ICDs have moderate to severe left ventricular dysfunction. Therefore, appropriate precautions for this population may need to be followed as well (see chapter 10).

accomplished primarily through an increase in the heart rate via sympathetic stimulation and activation of neurochemical and neurohormonal systems. Recent technologic advances have dramatically advanced pacemaker function to the point where pacemakers can nearly mimic normal cardiac function, both at rest and during exercise. It is important that the exercise training upper heart rate limit in DDDR and VVIR pacemakers be set below the person's ischemic threshold. At least a 10% safety margin between exercise heart rate and rate cutoff for the device is advised. An inappropriately delivered shock can be proarrhythmic and itself induce a life-threatening ventricular dysrhythmia. Despite a high level of caution, however, inappropriate shocks are common and have many causes. Therefore, full knowledge of the person's ICD programming is essential before exercise, and close

consultation with the client's electrophysiologist is advised.

Management and Medications

Individuals with pacemakers or ICDs may be taking cardiac medications such as antihypertensives or beta blockers. Persons receiving a pacemaker or ICD may have left ventricular dysfunction, necessitating vasodilator therapy. In addition to the precautions associated with a pacemaker or ICD, precautions for possible side effects during exercise or exercise training should be followed on the basis of the type of medications currently being taken (see appendix B).

Pacemakers and ICDs: Exercise Programming

Modes	Goals	Intensity/Frequency/Duration	Time to Goal
Aerobic • Large muscle activities	• Increase functional capacity and ability to perform ADLs • Increase self-efficacy	• 50-85% VO_2peak or HR reserve • Target HR should be kept below ischemic threshold and ICD activation threshold • 4-7 days/wk • 20-60 min/session	• 4-6 mo
Strength • Circuit training	• Increase ability to perform leisure and occupational activities and ADLs • Increase muscle strength and endurance	• Low to moderate intensity • 2 days/wk • 15-20 min/session • Should be avoided initially after implantation	
Flexibility • Upper and lower body ROM activities	• Maintain ROM	• 2-3 days/wk	

Medications	Special Considerations
• See chapter 4 exercise programming table.	• Upper-extremity ROM may be restricted due to pacemaker and ICD incision. • It is important to know the type and function of pacemaker. • RPE should be used in conjunction with HR to monitor intensity. • Know the ICD activation rate. • Ventricular tachyarrhythmias should be anticipated. • See guidelines for left ventricular dysfunction (chapter 10).

Recommendations for Exercise Testing

Exercise testing can be used as a diagnostic tool as well as a therapeutic tool in the adjustment of rate-responsive pacemakers. Once a permanent pacemaker with rate-responsive pacing capabilities has been implanted, exercise testing is sometimes useful in the evaluation of pacemaker behavior as well as for optimization of the pacemaker activity response. As for all people, those with pacemakers and ICDs require an exercise protocol suited to their age, health/medical status, and present functional capacity. Exercise protocols such as the modified Bruce, Balke, or Naughton protocol can often be helpful in this population. It is important to remember that in persons with a pacemaker, induced heartbeat ST-segment changes may not reflect ischemic changes; thus, other diagnostic tests should be considered. Stress imaging with echocardiography or thallium is often useful in these

circumstances (see the Pacemakers and ICDs: Exercise Testing table).

Recommendations for Exercise Programming

Persons with ICDs and pacemakers can benefit from exercise training. Before an exercise program begins, the upper training heart rate should be established and documented. In addition to improving functional capacity, exercise training can also help to reduce cardiac risk factors (e.g., through cholesterol modification, hypertension reduction) and improve psychosocial outcomes. Activities should be selected so that the intensity can be carefully regulated during exercise. Because some upper body movement may dislodge implanted leads, upper body exercises are not advised initially for people with pacemakers. Before exercise training, full knowledge of the individual's ICD programming is essential, and close consultation with the client's electrophysiologist is advised. The upper exercise training intensity must be set below the person's ischemic threshold and must not approach a heart rate causing activation of the ICD (see the Pacemakers and ICDs: Exercise Programming table on page 55).

CASE STUDY Pacemaker

A 63-year-old female rancher was referred for a 2- to 3-week history of palpitations, which she described as forceful, "squishy" heartbeats. An ECG revealed 2:1 AV block with a right bundle branch block. Carotid sinus massage improved conduction to 1:1, proving that the 2:1 block was distal and likely in need of permanent pacing. She denied the typical symptoms of "symptomatic bradycardia," such as activity intolerance, dyspnea, lightheadedness, or syncope. To better assess for limited aerobic capacity, she was given a regular treadmill test. Her maximal heart rate was 82 contractions/min with persistent 2:1 block throughout the exercise period. Remarkably, she completed more than 8 min of a Bruce protocol. After a dual-chamber pacemaker was implanted, she had a follow-up exercise test in which she exercised for over 14 min. The "squishy" heartbeats resolved with pacing.

S: "My heart's been fluttering."

O: Vitals: Height: 5'6" (1.7 m)   Weight: 140 lb (63.5 kg)   BMI: 21.97 kg/m^2
         RHR: 50 contractions/min   BP: 116/70 mmHg

Graded exercise test (treadmill, Bruce protocol):
  Duration: 8 min 30 s (3.4 mph at 14% grade)
  Max HR: 82 contractions/min with persistent 2:1 block throughout exercise
Medications: Estrogen replacement

A: 1. 2:1 AV block
    2. Very active rancher, tolerating AV block well

P: 1. Undergo dual-chamber permanent pacemaker implantation.
    2. Refer to cardiac rehabilitation.

Exercise Program
Goals:
  1. Improve functional capacity
  2. Educate about managing angina symptoms
  3. Reinforce lifestyle changes/medical management

Mode	Frequency	Duration	Intensity	Progression
Aerobic	3 days/wk	20 min/session	THR (55-70% $\dot{V}O_2$max) RPE 11-14/20	Increase to 40 min @ 60-70% THR after 12 wk
Strength (all major muscle groups)	3 days/wk	1 set of ≤ 10 reps	50-70% of 1RM	Increase to 2 sets of 10-12 reps after 12 wk
Flexibility (mainly back/lower extremity)	3 days/wk	30-60 s/stretch	Below discomfort point	Maintain
Neuromuscular				
Functional				
Warm-up/Cool-down	Before and after each session	10-15 min	RPE <10/20	Maintain

Suggested Readings

ACC/AHA guidelines for pacing and ICDs. 1998. *Journal of the American College of Cardiology* 31 (5): 1175-1209.

Lampman, R.M., and B.P. Knight. 2000. Prescribing exercise training for patients with defibrillators. *American Journal of Physical Medicine and Rehabilitation* 79 (3): 292-97.

Landzberg, J.S., J.O. Franklin, S.K. Mahawar et al. 1990. Benefits of physiologic atrioventricular synchronization for pacing with an exercise rate response. *American Journal of Cardiology* 66 (2): 193-97.

Pashkow, F.J. 1992. Patients with implanted pacemakers or implanted cardioverter defibrillators. In *Rehabilitation of the coronary patient*, edited by N. Wenger and H. Hellerstein, 431-38. 3rd ed. New York: Churchill Livingstone.

Pashkow, F.J., C. Walters, G. Blackburn, and P. McCarthy. 1993. Exercise training with an implantable ventricular assist device. *Journal of the American College of Cardiology* 21 (2): 188A.

Podrid, P.J., and P.R. Kowey, eds. 1995. *Cardiac dysrhythmia: Mechanisms, diagnosis, and management.* Baltimore: Williams & Wilkins.

Sharp, C.T., E.F. Busse, J.J. Burgess, and R.G. Haennel. 1998. Exercise prescription for patients with pacemakers. *Journal of Cardiopulmonary Rehabilitation* 18 (6): 421-31.

Smith, L.K. 1991. Exercise training in patients with impaired left ventricular function. *Medicine and Science in Sports and Exercise* 23 (6): 654-60.

Wilkoff, B.L., and R.E. Miller. 1992. Exercise testing for chronotropic assessment. *Cardiology Clinics* 10 (4): 705-17.

CHAPTER 9

Valvular Heart Disease

Martha Canulette, MSN, RN
Cardiac Rehabilitation Department, New Mexico Presbyterian Healthplex

Adam Gitkin, MS
Cardiac Rehabilitation Department, New Mexico Presbyterian Healthplex

Daniel Friedman, MD, FACSM
New Mexico Presbyterian Heart Group

Overview of the Pathophysiology

The primary causes for disease of the heart valves include rheumatic fever, valves with congenital abnormalities, infection, and aging. The symptoms, limitations, and recommendations with respect to physical activity in clients with valvular heart disease depend on the following:

- heart valve(s) involved (i.e., mitral, aortic, tricuspid, and/or pulmonary);
- condition of the valve (e.g., narrowing, or stenosis; or not closing properly, regurgitation or insufficient);
- severity of the valve lesions; and
- presence of coronary artery disease, myocardial dysfunction, or other organ system disease.

Mitral Stenosis

With mitral stenosis (MS), blood flow is obstructed across the mitral heart valve; thus, emptying of the left atrium is impeded. Resistance is increased across the mitral valve, which decreases ventricular filling. This may lead to a decreased left ventricular stroke volume and cardiac output. MS also causes elevation of the left atrial pressure, which may result in pulmonary hypertension. In addition, the left atrium is chronically overloaded, which may stretch the atrial conduction fibers and lead to atrial fibrillation (a rapid irregular heart rhythm). Particularly, in combination with atrial fibrillation, MS may lead to an atrial thrombus formation and subsequent stroke or other embolic event. The predominant cause of MS is rheu-matic fever (approximately 60% of cases). Other causes of MS include a congenital etiology, lupus, carcinoid, and amyloid disease. Pathologic features of rheumatic MS include thickening and shortening of the chordae tendineae, calcification of the valve leaflets, and fusion of the commissures (the borders where the leaflets meet).

Dyspnea is usually the presenting symptom, occurring as the valve orifice is reduced to 2 to 2.5 cm^2 or less. Severe MS is said to present at 1.0 cm^2. Other symptoms include hemoptysis, chest pain, thromboembolism, infective endocarditis, and hoarseness. Symptoms increase with heart rate, which may limit exercise capacity. Neck veins often demonstrate an elevated pressure and a prominent A wave. On auscultation, a loud S1, an opening snap, and a low-pitched diastolic murmur are present. Echocardiography is helpful in evaluating the left atrial size to assess the presence and severity of MS and mitral regurgitation, and pulmonary hypertension. Transesophageal echocardiography, in particular, helps to define the feasibility of balloon valvuloplasty.

Mitral Regurgitation

Mitral regurgitation (MR) occurs when the leaflets of the mitral valve do not close properly. Annular dilatation is the major cause of MR. Other factors are more frequently involved, including congenital abnormalities, myxomatous degeneration, mitral valve prolapse, chordae tendineae rupture, bacterial destruction, and annular disease. Symptoms of MR depend on the severity and the rate of development of the MR. Mild MR produces no symptoms. Moderately severe MR can lead to increased left atrial and left ventricular volumes. This can manifest itself to pulmonary venous congestion, elevation of pulmonary artery pressures, and dyspnea. A systolic murmur is the most prominent feature during the physical exam. Echocardiography is useful to determine the etiology and severity of MR. It helps to determine whether or not left ventricular dysfunction or pulmonary hypertension has developed. Angiography remains the gold standard for determining the severity of MR.

Mitral Valve Prolapse

Mitral valve prolapse (MVP) is a bowing of the mitral valve leaflets into the left atrium during ventricular systole. It is sometimes accompanied by mitral regurgitation and is most often asymptomatic. However, clients may present with chest pains or palpitations because of associated arrhythmias. A physical examination may identify MVP by the presence of a midsystolic "click" and/or murmur. The click represents the sudden tensing of the involved mitral leaflet or chordae tendineae as the leaflet is forced back toward the left atrium. The murmur represents the regurgitant flow through the incompetent valve.

Aortic Stenosis

Aortic stenosis (AS) is a narrowing of the aortic valve leaflets. It is commonly caused by gradual fibrosis and calcification of the aortic valve in adults. In this type, the valve neither opens nor closes normally. Other causes include congenital aortic stenosis, a bicuspid valve, and rheumatic heart disease. AS is accompanied by dyspnea, angina, and/or syncope. The common time for the symptoms to occur is between ages 60 and 80. On physical examination, carotid upstrokes are diminished, the second heart sound is single and may be soft, and a harsh systolic murmur at the upper left sternal border (often radiating to the neck) is present. Echocardiography can help to determine the severity of AS. It is important to follow people with mild or moderate disease in anticipation of future surgical replacement. Angiography is performed before surgery to determine whether coronary disease is present and CABG is needed. People with symptomatic AS are not candidates for exercise programs. The danger of sudden death is present, particularly during exercise. Clients with mild or moderate AS may have a normal exercise capacity. Angina, dyspnea, and fatigue are common symptoms with exercise.

Aortic Regurgitation

Aortic regurgitation (AR) occurs when the leaflets of the aortic valve do not close properly. It may be caused by disease of the aortic root or valve leaflets. Valvular disease may develop in the setting of rheumatic disease, infective endocarditis, trauma, congenital lesions, or in connective tissue-related diseases including Marfan's syndrome and Ehlers-Danlos syndrome. Aortic root disease occurs in a wide range of conditions that cause dilation of the ascending aorta. Long- standing hypertension (HTN) or aging can cause dilation of the aortic root, resulting in mild AR.

People with significant AR usually present with exertional dyspnea in their 40s or 50s. Mild to moderate AR is tolerated for years. Exaggerated arterial pulses are notes, systolic ejection murmur, and an early diastolic murmur. Echocardiography can both diagnose this lesion and help in following clients to determine the appropriate time for surgical intervention.

Strenuous exercise (e.g., isometric exercises) should be avoided in AR if weakening of the aortic wall (e.g., Marfan's or Ehlers-Danlos) is present. People with mild to moderate AR can pursue normal exercise activities.

Tricuspid Stenosis

Tricuspid stenosis (TS) is a rare condition resulting from narrowing of the tricuspid valve. It is almost always secondary to rheumatic heart disease. Other causes are infection and tumors. People with TS commonly complain of fatigue and swelling in the lower extremity and abdomen regions. Physical examination reveals distended neck veins and significant edema. Lungs are often clear, and the murmur may be difficult to auscultate. Echocardiography is a noninvasive method to determine the presence, cause, and severity of disease. Capacity will depend on the other valves involved. Often people with TS are not candidates for testing or rehabilitation until after valve surgery.

Tricuspid Regurgitation

Tricuspid regurgitation (TR) occurs when the leaflets of the tricuspid valve do not close properly. TR is often caused by dilation of the right ventricle and tricuspid annulus. Most common causes are left-sided myocardial or valvular disease and pulmonary lung disease leading to pulmonary HTN and right ventricle enlargement. Other causes include Ebstein's anomaly, carcinoid syndrome, rheumatic heart disease, and infections. If pulmonary arterial pressure is elevated, fatigue and peripheral edema develop. A holosystolic murmur, increasing with inspiration, is heard at the lower left sternal border. With the use of Doppler echocardiography, the presence and severity of this lesion can be determined and the right ventricle pressure estimated.

Pulmonic Stenosis

Pulmonic stenosis (PS) is a narrowing or tightening of the pulmonary valve. It is most often congenital. Other causes include rheumatic heart disease and carcinoid plaques. Pulmonic regurgitation can be secondarily caused by dilation of the pulmonary artery or valve ring secondary to pulmonary HTN. People with mild PS are usually asymptomatic. People with PS can present with heart failure, exertional dyspnea, syncope, or chest pain, caused by the inability to increase pulmonary blood flow during exercise.

Pulmonic Regurgitation

Pulmonic regurgitation (PR) occurs when the leaflets of the pulmonary valve do not close properly. The major symptoms of PR usually relate to the underlying cause. People with PR often have a harsh, rapidly louder then softer, systolic murmur at the upper left sternal border. In significant PR, an early diastolic murmur in the same region can be heard. Echocardiography can generally determine the presence and possible cause. It can also estimate the significance of each of these lesions.

Effects on the Exercise Response

During submaximal treadmill exercise, ST depression is commonly seen, especially with AS and MS. With MS, ST depression may represent reduced coronary perfusion or pulmonary hypertension. With MVP, ST depression has been seen with normal coronary arteries. These changes can be improved with beta blockers. However, the presence of ST-depression in the exercise ECG has no diagnostic value in people with valvular disease. Exercise capacity measurements provide only a gross assessment of the severity of the hemodynamic limitation associated with valvular heart disease. Exercise testing is contraindicated in persons with critical aortic stenosis because of the risk of dysrhythmia and death. This is probably caused by some combination of carotid hyperactivity, baroreceptor stimulation, left ventricular failure, dysrhythmia, and poor coronary perfusion. If pulmonic stenosis is present, risk of syncope is present.

Effects of Exercise Training

The mechanical function of a valve will not improve with exercise. However, the working capacity of the skeletal muscles (i.e., skeletal muscle efficiency) can be improved with training. This may assist the person with valvular

Valvular Heart Disease: Exercise Testing

Methods	Measures	Endpoints*	Comments
Aerobic Cycle (ramp protocol 17 watts/ min; staged protocol 25-50 watts/3-min stage) Treadmill (1-2 METs/3-min stage)	• 12-lead ECG, HR	• Ischemic threshold • > 2 mm ST-segment depression or elevation • T-wave inversion with significant ST change • Serious dysrhythmias	• May help determine need for surgery
	• BP, rate pressure product	• SBP > 250 mmHg or DBP > 115 mmHg	
	• Resting/stress echocardiogram		• Useful in determining degree of stenosis, regurgitation, left ventricular function • Helpful to determine timing of surgery • ST changes may lose specificity with mitral and aortic valve prolapse in terms of the diagnosis of CAD
	• RPE (Borg 6-20 scale)		

*Measurements of particular significance; do not always indicate test termination.

Medications	Special Considerations
• See appendixes A, B, and C. • Most cardiac medications can alter hemodynamics during exercise and possibly alter the sensitivity of the test (refer to appendixes A, B, and C).	• Severe symptomatic aortic stenosis is an absolute contraindication to exercise testing (see *ACSM's Guidelines for Exercise Testing and Prescription*). • TS, TR, PS, and AS are contraindications to exercise testing. • Clarify symptoms prior to testing. • If exercise test is used to establish appropriate training intensity, medication regimen should be continued at time of test. • Clarify complete testing procedures prior to starting exercise test.

disease in achieving activities of daily living at a given cardiovascular work rate that were previously unattainable. Significant mitral stenosis may cause limitation to exercise because demands of the exercising muscle may be greater than the cardiac output available. People with severe aortic stenosis and people with limited cardiac reserve secondary to aortic insufficiency should avoid vigorous physical activity because there is an increased risk of syncope or sudden death.

Management and Medications

Medications used to manage valvular diseases depend on the valve involved and symptoms. In severe valvular diseases, control of the heart failure is often the goal. Several medications are used to control symptoms, including: diuretics, beta blockers, ACE inhibitors, digoxin, and calcium-channel blockers. To prevent blood clots, anticoagulants such as Coumadin are prescribed. This medication must be monitored regularly with an international normalized ratio (INR) blood test. While on Coumadin, clients should avoid contact sports and carry identification with them. Signs of bleeding need to be reported, such as dark stools or pink or red urine, severe headaches, abdominal pain, severe bruising, vomitus that looks like coffee grounds, and/or heavy bleeding related to nose bleeds, gums, menstruation, or cuts. Prophylactic antibiotics are considered prior to minor surgery in persons with aortic stenosis, mitral valve disease, and valve replacements or repairs to prevent infective endocarditis.

Valvular Heart Disease: Exercise Programming

Modes	Goals	Intensity/Frequency/Duration	Time to Goal
Aerobic •Large muscle activities	•Improve functional capacity •Improve muscle function •Improve ADLs with decreases in symptoms	•3-7 days/wk •20-60 min/session •After surgery: resting HR + 20-30 contractions/min •THR: 40-70% $\dot{V}O_2$max •RPE 11-14/20 •10-15 min of warm-up and cool-down activities	•4-6 mo
Strength •Isotonic/Isokinetic	•Improve muscle function •Increase strength for vocational and avocational activities	•30-50% maximal voluntary contraction (avoid Valsalva) •2-3 days/wk •4-8 exercises (major groups) •12-15 reps (increasing 5-10 lb) •1-2 sets •< 1 h	•4-6 mo
Flexibility •Upper and lower body ROM activities	•Increase ROM •Increase functioning for vocational and avocational activities	•≥ 3 days/wk •To a position of mild discomfort •10-30 s/stretch •Static (slow, controlled)	•4-6 mo

Medications	Special Considerations
•Coumadin: No effect on HR or BP. •Cardiac medications: Most can alter hemodynamics during exercise (see appendixes A, B, and C).	•See precautions for exercise after CABGS if client has had prosthetic valve replacement. •If signs of symptoms change, refer client to physician. •Monitor high-risk clients closely. •Avoid strength training with significant aortic stenosis and pulmonic stenosis.

Once AS symptoms develop, valve replacement is generally necessary. Although balloon valvuloplasty can increase the cross-sectional area of the valve opening, it is not highly effective in this condition. Treatment for people with AR, who are minimally symptomatic with minimally increased or normal cardiac size, can be managed medically. Surgery is indicated when the heart dilates significantly. In MS, surgery is considered when symptoms cannot be controlled medically, particularly when the mitral valve area is less than $1.0\,cm^2$. In general, some heart valves can be repaired, but many require replacement. For people with TS, surgical repair is the treatment of choice and usually done at the time of mitral valve surgery. However, salt restriction and diuretics can help to lessen the volume overload. If pulmonic valve stenosis is severe, it can usually be repaired with a balloon or through surgery.

Clients with highly abnormal values or those post valve surgery must take special precautions to avoid minor infections that could damage the new valve. Before going through any dental work and certain surgical procedures, antibiotics may be taken. With isolated TR, no intervention is generally required. These people usually respond to an improvement or correction of the underlying cause. The edema that develops can be improved with diuretics. Narrowing the tricuspid annulus with a prosthesis, such as a Carpentier ring, can improve regurgitation.

Recommendations for Exercise Testing

A cardiac examination should be performed prior to exercise testing to rule out AS and determine if exercise testing is contraindicated. Examination should include, but not be limited to, findings of murmurs, clicks, gallop rhythms, and other abnormal heart and lung sounds. Although it is not of diagnostic value in valvular heart disease, exercise testing can provide important information about a person's functional capacity. Exercise testing can be utilized to quantify the extent of hemodynamic impairment (chest pain, dyspnea, arrhythmias, and other symptoms) consequent to valvular heart disease. The results can be used for continued follow-up and deter-

mine appropriate time for interventions (see the Valvular Heart Disease: Exercise Testing table on page 60).

Severe AS is an absolute contraindication to exercise. Severe TS, TR, and PS are also contraindications to exercise. Indications for terminating exercise testing include:

- ECG changes (>2 mm ST-segment depression or elevation, T-wave inversion with significant ST change, and serious dysrhythmias); and

- abnormal changes in blood pressure (SBP > 250 mmHg or DBP > 115 mmHg).

Recommendations for Exercise Programming

Before an exercise program begins, the upper training rate and description of any symptoms should be documented from a diagnostic exercise test. The extent of the stenosis and/or regurgitation also needs to be established. No limitations are indicated in people with mild disease. People with significant PS or severe AS should refrain from vigorous physical activity due to the risk of syncope. With mitral valve disease, MS, MR, and MVP, physical activity is limited by individual symptoms. For people who are unable to undergo surgery of the heart valves, the primary goal is to improve the working capacity of the skeletal muscles. The mechanical function of the valve will not improve with exercise. In many people, long-term systematic increases in physical activity can improve with submaximal working capacity. Signs of heart failure need to be documented and reported to the physician because of possible progression of left ventricular or valvular dysfunction.

With respect to exercise programming, frequency should include 3 to 7 days a week with duration increasing to 20 to 60 min/session. For deconditioned people with valve disease, intermittent exercise of 5 to 15 min/session may be used. Exercise intensity shortly post surgery should use resting heart rate and then add 20 to 30 contractions/min, with a long-term goal of increasing to 40 to 70% of aerobic capacity (see the Valvular Heart Disease: Exercise Programming table on page 61).

CASE STUDY Valvular Heart Disease

A 50-year-old obese white male complained of occasionally having dyspnea on exertion. He had been hypertensive for approximately 10 years and had been inconsistent in taking medication. He had no other history of cardiac disease.

S: "Sometimes I can't catch my breath after I walk."

O: Vitals: HR: 80 contractions/min   BP: 138/85 mmHg

Obese male

Systolic ejection murmur in the 2nd intercostal space with a loud S4

ECG: Left ventricular hypertrophy

Echocardiogram: Thickened aortic valve leaflets, mild hypertrophy of left ventricle; valve area approximately 1.2 cm^2

A: 1. Mild to moderate AS

P: 1. Utilize calcium-channel blockers and ACE inhibitors for medical afterload reduction.

   2. Conduct serial echocardiograms every 6 to 12 months, depending on symptoms and function.

   3. Consider surgical replacement if he develops syncope, angina, or heart failure.

Exercise Program

Goals:

   1. Maintain function

   2. Observe for symptoms of worsening stenosis

Mode	Frequency	Duration	Intensity	Progression
Aerobic	3 days/wk	20 min Rest for symptoms	THR (<60% $\dot{V}O_2$max) RPE <14/20	Very slow, ≤ 60 min over several mo
Strength	Contraindicated			
Flexibility (all major muscle groups)	3 days/wk	20-60 s/stretch	Maintain stretch below discomfort point	
Neuromuscular				
Functional				
Warm-up/Cool-down	Before and after each sesson	10-15 min	RPE <10/20	

Suggested Readings

American Association of Cardiovascular and Pulmonary Rehabilitation. 1999. *Guidelines for cardiac rehabilitation and secondary prevention programs.* 3rd ed. Champaign, IL: Human Kinetics.

American College of Sports Medicine. 2000. *ACSM's guidelines for exercise testing and prescription.* Edited by B.A. Franklin, M.H Whaley, and E.T. Howley. 6th ed. Philadelphia: Lippincott Williams & Wilkins.

Atwood, J.E., S. Kawanisi, J. Myers, and V.F. Reoelicher. 1988. Exercise testing in patients with aortic stenosis. *Chest* 93: 1083-87.

Braunwald, E. 1992. Valvular heart disease: In *Heart disease,* edited by E. Braunwald. 4th ed. Philadelphia: Saunders.

Broustet, J.P., H. Douard, and B. Mora. 1987. Exercise testing in dysrhythmias of idiopathic mitral valve prolapse. *European Heart Journal* 8 (supplement D): 37-42.

Fardy, P.S., and F.G. Yanowitz. 1995. *Cardiac rehabilitation, adult fitness, and exercise testing.* 3rd ed. Baltimore: Williams & Wilkins.

Fletcher, G.F., V.F. Balady, L.H. Hartley, W.L. Haskell, and M.L. Pollock. 1995. Exercise standards: A statement for healthcare professionals from the American Heart Association. *Circulation* 91 (2): 580-615.

Lilly, L.S. 1997. Valvular heart disease. 2nd ed. Baltimore: Lilly.

Opie, L.H. 1995. *Drugs for the heart.* 4th ed. Philadelphia: W.B. Saunders.

Skinner, J.S. 1993. *Exercise testing and exercise prescriptions for special cases: Theoretical basis and clinical application.* 2nd ed. Media, PA: Lea & Febiger.

Squires, R.W. 1998. *Exercise prescription for the high-risk cardiac patient.* Champaign, IL: Human Kinetics.

Williams, M.A. 1994. *Exercise testing and training in the elderly cardiac patient.* Champaign, IL: Human Kinetics.

CHAPTER 10

Chronic Heart Failure

Jonathan N. Myers, PhD, FACSM
Palo Alto VA Medical Center
Stanford University

Peter H. Brubaker, PhD, FACSM
Wake Forest University

Overview of the Pathophysiology

Chronic heart failure (CHF) is characterized by the inability of the heart to adequately deliver oxygen to the metabolizing tissues. The underlying pathophysiology in individuals with CHF is either depressed systolic function, abnormal diastolic function, or their combination. The former condition occurs from either loss of muscle (i.e., myocardial infarction) or loss of contractility. The latter condition is characterized by increased resistance to ventricular filling, and resultant increased ventricular pressure, higher than normal filling pressures, and reduced ventricular compliance. While diastolic dysfunction was once thought to be an infrequent cause, recent studies indicate that it may account for as much as 40% of all CHF. Several central hemodynamic changes are associated with CHF:

- decreased cardiac output during exercise, or in severe cases at rest;
- elevated left ventricular filling pressures;
- compensatory ventricular volume overload; and
- elevated pulmonary and central venous pressures.

In addition to these abnormalities in central hemodynamics, CHF is associated with secondary organ changes, including major derangements in skeletal muscle metabolism, impaired vasodilation, and renal insufficiency leading to sodium and water retention. These changes underlie the hallmark signs and symptoms of CHF—namely, fatigue, dyspnea, and reduced exercise tolerance.

Effects on the Exercise Response

A number of central, peripheral, and ventilatory abnormalities influence the single exercise responses among persons with CHF:

- central factors, including systolic function, pulmonary hemodynamics, diastolic dysfunction, and neurohumoral mechanisms;
- peripheral factors, including blood flow abnormalities, vasodilatory capacity, and skeletal muscle biochemistry; and
- ventilatory factors, including pulmonary pressure, physiologic dead space, ventilation-perfusion mismatch, respiratory control, and breathing patterns.

Independent of etiology (systolic vs. diastolic dysfunction), the major pathophysiological feature of the client with CHF is a reduction in cardiac output relative to the demands of the work. The resultant compensatory responses lead to the "syndrome" of CHF and a number of characteristic responses to exercise. Poor cardiac output underlies a mismatching of ventilation to perfusion in the lung, causing an elevation in physiologic dead space and leading to shortness of breath. Interestingly, although dyspnea on exertion is a hallmark of CHF, most individuals (roughly two-thirds) are limited by leg fatigue during exercise testing. Early fatigue is related to the heart's inability to supply adequate blood flow and oxygen to the working muscles. Lactate accumulates in the blood at low work rates relative to those for healthy individuals. This contributes to the hyperventilation response to exercise and early fatigue.

Abnormal neurohumoral mechanisms contribute to reduced cardiac performance during exercise in persons with CHF. Catecholamine levels are usually elevated among these persons, and abnormalities in beta receptor density likely contribute to reduced contractile function. This occurs because beta-adrenergic receptors play an important inotropic regulatory role in the myocardium, and these receptors are less sensitive to endogenous and exogenous beta-agonist stimulation in the presence of CHF. Altered baroreceptor reflexes have been observed in animals with heart failure and may also contribute to diminished chronotropic responses or to reduced systolic pressure during exercise, the latter perhaps contributing to peripheral perfusion abnormalities.

There are significant peripheral abnormalities that also influence the response to exercise in persons with CHF. These include not only reductions in blood flow but also abnormal redistribution of blood, reduced vasodilatory capacity, endothelial dysfunction, and abnormal skeletal muscle biochemistry. Abnormalities in skeletal muscle metabolism include reduced mitochondrial enzyme activities and histological changes (reduced type I aerobic fibers and increased type II fibers). The cumulative effect of these skeletal muscle abnormalities is reduced exercise tolerance as a result of greater glyco-lysis, reduced oxidative phosphorylation, and greater metabolic acidosis.

Effects of Exercise Training

Before the mid-1980s, persons with CHF were generally discouraged from participating in formal programs of exercise training. This was due to concerns over safety and questions about whether or not exercise training caused harm to a weak heart. In the last decade, however, numerous studies have documented the safety and benefits of exercise training in persons with heart failure. These studies suggest that improvements in exercise capacity after training result more from peripheral adaptations (e.g., improvements in skeletal muscle metabolism, endothelial function, vasodilatory capacity, and distribution of cardiac output) than from cardiac changes (e.g., central hemodynamics including volumes, ejection fraction, and pulmonary pressures at rest and during exercise).

Chronic Heart Failure: Exercise Testing

Methods	Measures	Endpoints*	Comments
Aerobic Cycle (ramp protocol 10-15 watts/min; staged protocol 10-50 watts/3-min stage)	• 12-lead ECG, HR • BP, rate pressure product • RPE, dyspnea scales • Respired gas analysis	• Serious dysrhythmias • T-wave inversion with significant ST change • Hypotensive response • Perceived shortness of breath and fatigue • $\dot{V}O_2$peak and ventilatory threshold	
Treadmill (Naughton)			• Peak performance is often < 5 METs, so a low-level ramp or Naughton protocol is preferred.
Endurance 6-min walk	• Distance	• Note stops for rest (time/distance)	• Useful throughout training program.
Functional Lifestyle-specific tests	• Performance related to ADLs		

*Measurements of particular significance; do not always indicate test termination.

Medications	Special Considerations
• Digoxin: Diffuse ST effects. May increase performance. • Diuretics: May induce ectopy. May lower BP. • Vasodilators: May increase HR, lower BP, and increase performance. • ACE inhibitors: Lower BP. May improve performance. • Antiarrhythmics: May increase HR but have little or no effect on performance.	• Ventilation/perfusion inequalities cause increased dead space and hyperventilation/dyspnea. • Increased risk of dysrhythmias.

There has been some controversy regarding the possibility that exercise training in clients with heart failure could cause abnormal ventricular remodeling and infarct expansion, particularly for exercise performed early after a heart attack. This concern arose because a group of individuals who had ventricular asynergy were initially found to have worsening asynergy, myocardial expansion, and decreased ejection fraction after training. Recent reports, including studies using high-intensity training and assessment of the myocardium using Doppler 2-D echocardiography and magnetic resonance imaging (MRI), have allayed these concerns. Some clients with reduced ventricular function after a myocardial infarction will continue to deteriorate despite intensive intervention, and studies demonstrate that exercise training does not lead to further myocardial damage. Generally, studies have demonstrated that exercise training neither harms nor results in significant benefit to the heart muscle in CHF clients. Recent exercise training studies in older individuals with isolated diastolic dysfunction have demonstrated similar improvements in functional capacity. These appear to be caused by peripheral adaptations because no changes in left ventricular function or volumes have been observed.

Management and Medications

Initial management of CHF involves identifying the underlying cause. For example, a stenotic valve may need to be replaced, hypertension or myocardial ischemia controlled, or alcohol use discontinued. In some persons, these measures alone may restore cardiac function to normal. A major manifestation of CHF in clients with systolic dysfunction is increased ventricular volume and pressure; therefore, the second goal is to reduce these manifestations pharmacologically. Therapy generally reduces symptoms; often, however, a period of time in therapy is required before exercise capacity improves. Since excessive salt and water retention is a hallmark of CHF, most clients will need to use a diuretic. Afterload reduction by angiotensin converting enzyme (ACE) inhibition, ACE-II receptor blockers, or

Chronic Heart Failure: Exercise Programming

Modes	Goals	Intensity/Frequency/Duration	Time to Goal
Aerobic • Large muscle activities	• Increase $\dot{V}O_2$peak and ventilatory threshold • Increase peak work and endurance	• RPE 11-16/20 • 40-70% $\dot{V}O_2$peak or HR reserve • 3-7 days/wk • 20-40 min/session	• 3 mo
Strength • Circuit training	• Reduce atrophy	• High reps, low resistance	• 3 mo
Flexibility • Upper and lower body ROM activities	• Maintain ROM	• 2-3 days/wk	• 4-6 mo
Functional • Activity-specific exercise	• Increase ADLs • Return to work • Improve quality of life and maintain independence	• 2-3 days/wk	• 3 mo

Medications	Special Considerations
• Beta blockers: Attenuate HR by ~ 10-30 contractions/min. Long-term effects may be beneficial. • ACE inhibitors and diuretics: Combining with a vasodilator may increase performance but cause postexertional hypotension.	• See chapter 4 exercise programming table. • Tolerance of exercise intensity will most likely be lower in CHF patients. • Some patients have prolonged fatigue after exercise. • Weight gain and/or increased dyspnea may indicate decompensated heart failure.

other arterial vasodilators tends to reduce left ventricular end-diastolic pressures and improve stroke volume and cardiac output, and this reduces symptoms. ACE inhibition may lower mortality, while digoxin or other inotropic agents increase myocardial contractility.

In recent years, beta-blocking agents have gained acceptance as an effective treatment option for clients with CHF, and studies have demonstrated that these agents improve symptoms and reduce mortality. Beta blockers act by inhibiting sympathetic activation, and their beneficial effects are related to the prevention of the deleterious effects of chronically increased adrenergic stimulation on the failing heart. In terms of pharmacologic management, the primary difference between clients with systolic and diastolic dysfunction is that the latter do not require positive inotropes. In addition, the use of calcium-channel blockers has been shown to improve ventricular relaxation, increase end diastolic volume, and increase functional capacity in clients with diastolic dysfunction.

Recommendations for Exercise Testing

Exercise testing can be a valuable tool to objectively characterize the severity of CHF and to evaluate the efficacy of therapeutic interventions. In general, the standard exercise electrocardiogram offers little insight into the nature of the person's symptoms. It is frequently more appropriate to characterize the cardiopulmonary (ventilatory gas exchange) response to exercise, quantify exercise tolerance, and identify the pathophysiological abnormalities responsible for the limitation in exercise capacity. Exercise capacity measured by gas exchange techniques accurately quantifies functional limitations, identifies ventilatory abnormalities, and helps to optimize risk stratification in persons with CHF. The normal central and peripheral responses to the exercise test may not be present in these persons. For example, relative to what is seen in healthy individuals, cardiac output is reduced, blood is redistributed abnormally, and peripheral vascular resistance is high. Heightened ventilation is a characteristic feature of the exercise response in CHF. Exercise can cause a drop in ejection fraction, stroke volume, or both, and exertional hypotension may occur. Although exercise testing in these individuals has the potential for a higher rate of complications, limited data on the safety of exercise testing in CHF suggests it is similar to that observed among persons with coronary artery disease (see the Chronic Heart Failure: Exercise Testing table on page 65).

The following considerations relate to exercise testing with this population:

- symptoms are frequently observed under 5 METs, so lower level, moderately incremented, individualized protocols are recommended (Naughton or ramp);

- symptoms indicative of unstable or decompensated CHF are a contraindication;

- respiratory gas exchange measurements increase precision, optimize risk stratification, and permit assessment of breathing efficiency and patterns; these are particularly useful in clients with CHF;

- 6-min walk tests are an effective supplement to the graded exercise test;

- exertional hypotension, clinically significant dysrhythmias, and chronotropic incompetence may occur in CHF; and

- test endpoints should focus on symptoms, hemodynamic responses, and standard clinical indications for stopping (and not target heart rate).

Recommendations for Exercise Programming

Because of the improvements in therapeutic and surgical techniques, persons with CHF compose one of the fastest-growing cardiac rehabilitation populations. Formal exercise training programs are effective in lessening symptoms and improving exercise capacity. An improvement in the ability to sustain low-level activities can mean that a person can live independently and continue to work instead of being disabled. For these reasons, exercise programs may significantly enhance the quality of these individuals' lives (see the Chronic Heart Failure: Exercise Programming table).

However, the potential complications and outcomes differ from those of the standard cardiac rehabilitation client. For example, many clients with CHF will deteriorate irrespective of exercise or medical therapy. In these persons, the exercise regimen needs to be reassessed. Persons with CHF are at higher risk of sudden death, and they frequently experience psychosocial and vocational problems brought on by their disease. Some may experience prolonged fatigue after a single exercise session. Careful consideration should be given to absolute contraindications (particularly obstruction to left ventricular outflow, decompensated CHF, or unstable dysrhythmias). Relative contraindications to exercise are the same for persons with CHF as for persons with normal left ventricular function. These considerations necessitate that programs be designed carefully and that the staff be trained to recognize specific needs of this population as well as specific precautions that should be taken.

- Status can change quickly, and clients should be reevaluated frequently for signs of decompensation, rapid changes in weight or blood pressure, worse-than-usual dyspnea or angina on exertion, or increases in dysrhythmias.
- Warm-up and cool-down sessions should be prolonged.
- Some clients may tolerate only limited work rates and may necessitate lower intensity/longer-duration exercise sessions.
- Perceived exertion and dyspnea scales should take precedence over heart rate and work rate targets.

- Isometric exercise should be avoided.
- ECG monitoring is required for persons with a history of ventricular tachycardia, cardiac arrest (sudden death), or exertional hypotension.
- Consider ancillary study data (e.g., exercise echocardiogram, radionuclide studies, hemodynamic studies, ventilatory gas analysis) when developing the exercise program. In general, do not exceed a work rate that produces wall motion abnormalities, a drop in ejection fraction, a pulmonary wedge pressure greater than 20 mmHg, or the ventilatory threshold.

CASE STUDY Chronic Heart Failure

A 70-year-old male complained of increasing difficulty sustaining recreational activities and household chores. The client had a 10-year history of reduced left ventricular function from ischemic heart disease and had bypass surgery performed five years ago. He was not smoking, but had a 40 pack-year history of smoking. Other risk factors included a sedentary lifestyle, history of high blood pressure (controlled pharmacologically), and slightly excessive weight. He carried nitroglycerin for chest pain and an albuterol inhaler for bronchitis, but he rarely used either one.

S: "I get fatigued when I'm doing things."

O: Vitals: HR: 55 contractions/min   BP: 130/65 mmHg

Elderly male, grossly normal appearance

ECG: Sinus bradycardia

Echocardiogram:

  LVEF: 30%, mild ventricular hypertrophy, posterior wall dyskinesis, inferior wall akinesis, mild mitral valve thickening and moderate regurgitation, mild tricuspid valve regurgitation

Spirometry:

  FVC: 2.84 l (60.6% of expected)

  FEV_1: 70.4% of normal (low)

Graded exercise test:

  Peak exercise: 4.6 METs (estimated)

  $\dot{V}O_2$peak: 15.3 ml · kg^{-1} · min^{-1} (measured, 62% of age-predicted)

  Terminated due to shortness of breath @ RPE 17/20

  No chest discomfort

  Peak HR: 95 contractions/min

  Peak BP: 160/70 mmHg

  ECG: No significant ST changes during exercise or recovery; occasional PVCs

Medications: Lisinopril, Hydrochlorothiazide, Atenolol, Naproxen

A: 1. CHF, NYHA class III

  2. Coronary artery disease, s/p CABG

  3. Mild COPD

P: 1. Introduce home-based exercise.

  2. Increase physical activity level.

  3. Reevaluate in 6 months.

Exercise Program

Goals:

1. Improve functional capacity.
2. Monitor for symptoms of worsening CHF.
3. Assist with lifestyle changes to decrease cardiovascular risk.

Mode	Frequency	Duration	Intensity	Progression
Aerobic	Daily	20 min/session as tolerated	THR (40-70% $\dot{V}O_2$max) RPE 10-16/20	As tolerated
Strength (all major muscle groups)	2-3 days/wk	1 set of 5-10 reps	50-70% of 1RM	Limit to 2 sets of 10-12 reps
Flexibility (all major muscle groups)	2-3 days/wk	20-60 s/stretch	Maintain stretch below discomfort point	
Neuromuscular				
Functional				
Warm-up/Cool-down	Before and after each sesson	10-15 min	RPE <11/20	

Suggested Readings

Brubaker, P.H. 1999. Clinical considerations and exercise responses of patients with primary left ventricular diastolic dysfunction. *Journal of Clinical Exercise Physiology* 1: 5-12.

Dubach, P., J. Myers, G. Dziekan, U. Goebbels, W. Reinhart, P. Vogt, R. Ratti, P. Muller, R. Miettunen, and P. Buser. 1997. Effect of exercise training on myocardial remodeling in patients with reduced left ventricular function after myocardial infarction: Application of magnetic resonance imaging. *Circulation* 95: 2060-67.

Hambrecht, R., E. Fiehn, J, Yu, J. Niebauer, C. Weigl, L. Hilbrich, V. Adams, U. Riede, and G. Schuler. 1997. Effects of exercise endurance training on mitochondrial ultrastructure and fiber type distribution in skeletal muscle of patients with stable chronic heart failure. *Journal of the American College of Cardiology* 29: 1067-73.

Hambrecht, R., S. Gielen, A. Linke, E. Fiehn, J. Yu, C. Walther, N. Schoene, and G. Schuler. 2000. Effects of exercise training on left ventricular function and peripheral resistance in patients with chronic heart failure: A randomized trial. *Journal of the American Medical Association* 283: 3095-3101.

Harrington, D., and A.J.S. Coats. 1997. Mechanisms of exercise intolerance in congestive heart failure. *Current Opinion in Cardiology* 12: 224-32.

Keteyian, S.J., C.A. Brawner, and J.R. Schairer. 1997. Exercise testing and training of patients with heart failure due to left ventricular systolic dysfunction. *Journal of Cardiopulmonary Rehabilitation* 17: 19-28.

Myers, J., G. Dziekan, U. Goebbels, and P. Dubach. 1999. Influence of high-intensity exercise training on the ventilatory response to exercise in patients with reduced ventricular function. *Medicine and Science in Sports and Exercise* 31: 929-37.

Myers, J., L. Gullestad, R. Vagelos, D. Do, D. Bellin, H. Ross, and M.B. Fowler. 1998. Clinical, hemodynamic, and cardiopulmonary exercise test determinants of survival in patients referred for evaluation of heart failure. *Annals of Internal Medicine* 129: 286-93.

Piepoli, M.F., M. Flather, and A.J.S. Coats. 1998. Overview of studies of exercise testing in chronic heart failure: The need for a prospective randomized multicenter European trial. *European Heart Journal* 19: 830-41.

Sullivan, M.J., H.J. Green, and F.R. Cobb. 1991. Altered skeletal muscle metabolic response to exercise in chronic heart failure: Relation to skeletal muscle aerobic enzyme activity. *Circulation* 84: 1597-1607.

Sullivan, M.J., and M.H. Hawthorne. 1995. Exercise intolerance in patients with chronic heart failure. *Progress in Cardiovascular Disesases* 38: 1-22.

Management and Medications

Controlling immune system rejection of the donor heart while avoiding the adverse side effects of immunosuppressive therapy (infections, hyperlipidemia, hypertension, obesity, osteoporosis, renal dysfunction, and diabetes) is a main issue soon after transplantation. One year after surgery, the likelihood for acute rejection lessens, but there is increased probability of developing accelerated atherosclerosis (i.e., concentric fibrointimal hyperplasia) that affects the epicardial and intramural coronary arteries and veins of the donor heart. By five years after transplantation, malignancy is the second most common cause of mortality after accelerated atherosclerosis.

Acute graft rejection is common among all transplant individuals, especially within the first year, and is characterized by perivascular infiltration of killer T lymphocytes into the myocardium, including possible cellular necrosis. The severity of acute rejection is generally classified as mild-early, moderate, or severe. Treatment for acute graft rejection includes medication (e.g., corticosteroids, antilymphocyte therapy) and in rare cases retransplantation.

Two approaches are used to lessen the occurrence of acute rejection. First, since rejection is silent, endomyocardial biopsy (by catheters) is performed both to detect preclinical cellular involvement and to assess the efficacy of therapy. Second, immunosuppressive agents (e.g., prednisone, cyclosporine, azathioprine, mycophenolate, tacrolimus) are used to prophylactically suppress killer T lymphocyte function. Doing so, however, renders individuals more susceptible to certain infections and cancers. Also, although confirmatory evidence is still lacking, a possible cyclosporine-induced calf discomfort is experienced in approximately 15% of the individuals during walking. Otherwise, the immunosuppressive medications mentioned do not necessarily affect exercise testing or training.

Recommendations for Exercise Testing

Considerations that relate to assessing exercise safety and the various components of fitness among individuals with cardiac transplant are as follows (also see the Cardiac Transplant: Exercise Testing table on page 71):

- To assess cardiorespiratory fitness, conduct a continuous incremental test using a treadmill or stationary cycle ergometer. Arm ergometry testing can be used to assess the safety and ability of these individuals to perform arm work.

- Exercise protocols can be either ramp or steady state (3 min/stage). With the use of cycle ergometry, work rates should be increased by 10 to 15 watts/min or 25 to 30 watts/stage for ramp or steady-state protocols, respectively.

- Steady-state exercise tests conducted with the use of a treadmill should increase work rates by 2 METs per stage.

- Because of the delayed and blunted response of heart rate to exercise, ratings of perceived exertion as well as oxygen consumption should be assessed. These assessments are helpful when quantifying functional capacity, developing an appropriate exercise prescription, and determining whether a peak effort was attained. $\dot{V}O_2$peak in untrained cardiac transplant individuals is generally between 10 and 22 ml $\cdot$ kg^{-1} $\cdot$ min^{-1}. If measured before and after a training regimen, ventilatory threshold can also serve as a marker for change in submaximal cardiorespiratory endurance.

- To assess recovery following a session of maximal or submaximal exercise, observation of systolic blood pressure is a better indicator than heart rate alone.

- Although not mandatory, determination of oxygen consumption at the ventilatory threshold, typically assessed using the V-slope method, can help set initial work rates for exercise training.

Although isolated cases of chest pain associated with accelerated graft atherosclerosis have been observed, for the most part decentralization of the myocardium eliminates anginal symptoms. Exercise electrocardiography is also inadequate with respect to assessing ischemia, as evidenced by its low sensitivity (i.e., < 25%) for detecting true disease in these individuals. Thus, radionuclide testing may be more useful for assessing ischemic heart disease.

Following an adequate warm-up, assessment of skeletal muscle strength can be accomplished using a 1RM method. In most clients, 1RM is reached within 3 to 5 trials. Be sure to allow at least 2 min recovery between trials.

Although the restoration and maintenance of range of motion is important for all adults, among people with cardiac transplant, there are no unique joint or muscle issues. As a result, specific testing beyond that needed to assess progress achieved during a training program is not needed. A general flexibility assessment such as the sit-and-reach test is adequate.

Recommendations for Exercise Programming

As in most other people with chronic disease, progressive exercise training in individuals with cardiac transplant is

Cardiac Transplant: Exercise Programming

Modes	Goals	Intensity/Frequency/Duration	Time to Goal
Aerobic • Large muscle activities	• Increase self-efficacy • Increase cardiorespiratory fitness • Improve risk factors (e.g., body mass, insulin sensitivity, BP)	• RPE 11-14/20 • 50-75% $\dot{V}O_2$peak • 3-5 days/wk • 15-60 min/session or accumulated throughout the day	• > 6 mo
Strength • All major muscle groups	• Increase ability to perform leisure, occupational activities and ADLs • Increase muscle strength/endurance • Delay/reverse harmful effects of long-term corticosteroid therapy	• Low to moderate intensity • 1-2 sets of 10-15 reps • 2-4 days/wk	• > 8 wk
Flexibility • Upper and lower body ROM activities	• Improve upper body ROM following sternotomy	• 2-3 days/wk	• > 4 wk

Medications	Special Considerations
• See exercise testing table.	• Corticosteroids: Possible bone/joint-related disorders because of demineralization effects. • Cyclosporine: Increase in resting and submaximal BP. • Start slow! Severe deconditioning is common, especially if prolonged bed rest was required prior to surgery. Intermittent exercise or short periods throughout the day may be needed until longer, continuous exercise can be tolerated. • ROM and stretching exercises are important for upper body due to sternotomy; however, these exercises should be limited for up to 6-8 wk after surgery. • RPE should be primary method of monitoring exercise intensity.

an effective means to reestablish self-efficacy and improve both cardiorespiratory fitness and muscle endurance. Less established, however, is whether the modification of cardiovascular risk factors through exercise alters the progression of accelerated graft atherosclerosis, which is the major factor limiting long-term survival in these individuals.

The current recommended methods to guide exercise intensity in persons with cardiac transplant are ratings of perceived exertion, fixed distance/fixed speed, percentage of $\dot{V}O_2$peak, and ventilatory threshold. When incorporated into training studies involving persons with cardiac transplant, these methods have resulted in increases in $\dot{V}O_2$peak of 15 to 40%. The minimal threshold of intensity (i.e., 40, 50, or 60% of $\dot{V}O_2$peak) needed to significantly improve $\dot{V}O_2$peak is not known.

The use of heart rate alone to guide exercise intensity is not appropriate. In fact, it is not uncommon to find persons with cardiac transplant achieving an exercise heart rate that not only exceeds 85% of measured peak heart rate but is equal to or greater than peak heart rate. Instead, a rating of perceived exertion between 11 and 14 should be used to guide exercise intensity. Also, these persons should perform an aerobic activity 4 to 5 times per week while progressively increasing the duration from 15 to 60 min (see the Cardiac Transplant: Exercise Programming table).

Since a leg-strength deficit contributes, in part, to the reduced $\dot{V}O_2$peak observed in these individuals, most may benefit from two sessions per week of progressive resistance training that involves the legs, lower back, arms, and shoulders. Such a program will also help negate or reverse the glucocorticoid-induced myopathy and bone loss that occurs in these clients after surgery. One to two sets of 10-15 repetitions is generally sufficient to accomplish these goals.

CASE STUDY Cardiac Transplant

A 62-year-old female underwent heart transplantation because of ischemic heart failure. Prior to surgery, she did not participate in any regular physical activity. She had a long history of obesity, non-insulin dependent diabetes, and hypertension, and was referred to cardiac rehabilitation for a reconditioning program and cardiovascular risk reduction.

S: "I just had a heart transplant."

O: Vitals: HR: 60 contractions/min   BP: 180/110 mmHg   Weight: 207 lb (93.92 kg)

Height: 5'2" (1.57 m)   BMI: 38.1 kg/m^2

Obese female post heart transplant

Graded exercise test:
  Peak exercise: 4.3 METs
  $\dot{V}O_2$peak: 15.1 ml $\cdot$ kg^{-1} $\cdot$ min^{-1}
  Peak HR: 99 contractions/min
  Peak BP: 179/90 mmHg
  Peak RPP: 17,028 mmHg/min
  No ECG changes or ischemia indications
  Test terminated due to fatigue

Echocardiogram: Normal left ventricular ejection fraction (60%), mild mitral and tricuspid regurgitation

Estimated PA pressure: 34 mmHg

Total cholesterol: 286 mg/dl
  HDL: 52 mg/dl
  LDL: 160 mg/dl
  Trig: 368 mg/dl

Medications: Cyclosporine, Mycophenolate mofetil, Prednisone, Ganciclovir, Isosorbide dinitrate, Pravastatin, Furosemide, Lisinopril, Clonodine, Trimethoprim, Glyburide, Aspirin, Magnesium

A: 1. Status post cardiac transplant
2. Exercise intolerance
3. Hypertension, poorly controlled
4. Hypercholesterolemia
5. Type 2 diabetes
6. Obesity

P: 1. Introduce an aerobic conditioning program.
2. Introduce diabetic/weight loss dietary counseling.
3. Follow resting BP and pressor response to exercise.

Exercise Program
Goals:
1. Increased functional capacity
2. Weight loss
3. Improved diabetes control
4. Better lipid profile

Mode	Frequency	Duration	Intensity	Progression
Aerobic	3 days/wk	5-10 min/session	RPE 11-14/20	Increase to 30-45 min over 1 mo
Strength				10-12 reps after 12 wk
Flexibility all (major muscle groups)	3 days/wk	20 s/stretch	Maintain stretch below discomfort point	Discomfort point should occur at higher ROM; progress as tolerated
Neuromuscular				
Functional				
Warm-up/Cool-down	Before and after each sesson	5-10 min	RPE <10/20	

Follow-Up

After 12 sessions of cardiac rehabilitation, she had increased her training work rate from 1.7 to 4.1 METs and enrolled in a maintenance cardiac rehabilitation program.

Suggested Readings

Albrecht, A.E., D. Lillis, M.D. Pease, P. Harrison, B.J. Morgan, J.E. Schairer, and W.H. Boganhagen. 1993. Heart rate and catecholamine responses during exercise and recovery in cardiac transplant recipients. *Journal of Cardiopulmonary Rehabilitation* 13: 182-87.

Badenhop, D.T. 1995. The therapeutic role of exercise in patients with orthotopic heart transplant. *Medicine and Science in Sports and Exercise* 27 (7): 975-85.

Braith, R.W., and D.G. Edwards. 2000. Exercise following heart transplantation. *Sports Medicine* 30 (3): 171-92.

Costanzo, M.R. 2000. Management of the cardiac transplant patient. *Harrison's Online*. [Online]. Available: **www.harrisonsonline.com**.

Ehrman, J.K., S.J. Keteyian, A.B. Levine, K.L. Rhoads, L.R. Elder, T.B. Levine, and P.D. Stein. 1993. Exercise stress tests after cardiac transplantation. *American Journal of Cardiology* 71: 1372-73.

Kavanagh, T. 1992. Exercise and therapy of the cardiac transplant patient. In *Exercise and the heart in health and disease*, edited by R.J. Shepard and H.S. Miller Jr., 257-82. New York: Marcel Dekker.

Keteyian, S.J., C.R.C. Marks, A.B. Levine, F. Fedel, T. Kataoka, and T.B. Levine. 1994. Cardiovascular responses of cardiac transplant patients to arm and leg exercise. *European Journal of Applied Physiology* 68: 441-44.

Keteyian, S.J., C.R.C. Marks, A.B. Levine, T. Kataoka, F. Fedel, and T.B. Levine. 1994. Cardiovascular responses to submaximal arm and leg exercise in cardiac transplant patients. *Medicine and Science in Sports and Exercise* 26 (4): 420-24.

Kobashigaws, J.A., D.A. Leaf, N. Lee, M.P. Gleeson, H.H. Liu, M.A. Hamilton, J.D. Moriguchi, N. Kawata, K. Einhorn, E. Herlihy, and H. Laks. 1999. A controlled trial of exercise rehabilitation after heart transplantation. *New England Journal of Medicine* 34 (4): 272-77.

Squires, R.W. 1991. Rehabilitation after cardiac transplantation: 1980 to 1990. *Journal of Cardiopulmonary Rehabilitation* 11: 84-92.

Young, J.B., W.L. Winters, R. Bouge, and B.F. Uretsky. 1993. Task force 4: Function of the heart transplant recipient. *Journal of the American College of Cardiology* 22: 31-41.

CHAPTER 12

Hypertension

Neil F. Gordon, MD, PhD, MPH, FACSM
The Heart and Lung Group

Overview of the Pathophysiology

Hypertension is a major public health problem in most Western industrialized countries. It is estimated that in the United States, as many as 50 million individuals have an elevated blood pressure (BP) or are taking antihypertensive medication. In these persons, the risk for nonfatal and fatal cardiovascular disease (especially coronary artery disease and stroke), renal disease, and all-cause mortality increases progressively with higher levels of both systolic and diastolic BP. At any level of high BP, risks of cardiovascular disease are increased several-fold for persons with target-organ disease. Cardiovascular risks are also related to the presence of other risk factors.

Table 12.1 shows how adult BP is classified in the 1997 report of the Joint National Committee on Prevention, Detection, Evaluation, and Treatment of High Blood Pressure. Among hypertensive adults between the ages of 18 and 65 who are seen in typical clinical practice, 95% have no identifiable cause. Their hypertension is defined as either primary, essential, or idiopathic. Although their

cardiac output may be high initially, hypertension usually persists in these clients because of an increased peripheral resistance.

Effects on the Exercise Response

A single session of dynamic exercise usually evokes a normal rise in systolic BP from baseline levels in unmedicated persons with hypertension, although the response may be exaggerated or diminished in certain individuals. However, because of an elevated baseline level, the absolute level of systolic BP attained during dynamic exercise is usually higher in persons with hypertension. In addition, their diastolic BP may not change, or may even slightly rise, during dynamic exercise, probably as a result of an impaired vasodilatory response.

Recent studies have documented a 10 to 20 mmHg reduction in systolic BP during the initial 1 to 3 hours following 30 to 45 min of moderate-intensity dynamic exercise in persons with hypertension. This response, which may persist for up to 9 hours, appears to be mediated by a transient decrease in stroke volume rather than peripheral vasodilation.

Untreated hypertension may be accompanied by some limitation in exercise tolerance. The use of certain antihy-

Table 12.1 Classification of Blood Pressure for Adults Aged 18 Years and Older*

Category	Systolic BP (mmHg)	Diastolic BP (mmHg)
Optimal	< 120	80
Normal	< 130	< 85
High-normal	130-139	85-89
Hypertension**		
Stage 1	140-159	90-99
Stage 2	160-179	100-109
Stage 3	180	110

*Not taking antihypertensive drugs and not acutely ill. When systolic and diastolic BP fall into different categories, the higher category should be selected to classify the individual's BP status.

**Based on the average of 2 or more readings taken at each of 2 or more visits after an initial screening.

Reprinted from the Joint National Committee on Prevention, Detection, Evaluation, and Treatment of High Blood Pressure. 1997. The sixth report of the Joint National Committee on Prevention, Detection, Evaluation, and Treatment of High Blood Pressure (JNC VI). *Archives of Internal Medicine* 157: 2413-46.

pertensive drugs may further impair exercise performance. However, exercise tolerance may be enhanced by control of hypertension with lifestyle modification and, if warranted, well-tolerated antihypertensive medications.

Effects of Exercise Training

Existing evidence indicates that endurance exercise training reduces the magnitude of rise in BP that can be expected over time in persons at increased risk for developing hypertension. Longitudinal studies further show that endurance training may elicit an average reduction of about 10 mmHg in both systolic and diastolic BP in persons with stage I or II hypertension. Both the Joint National Committee and ACSM (1993) advocate regular aerobic exercise as a preventive strategy to reduce the incidence of high BP and indicate that exercise training can be effectively used as definitive or adjunctive therapy for hypertension.

The mechanisms by which exercise training lowers BP are unclear. Possibilities include:

- decrease in plasma norepinephrine levels;
- increase in circulating vasodilator substances;
- amelioration of hyperinsulinemia; and
- alteration in renal function.

Physically active persons with hypertension and those with higher levels of cardiorespiratory fitness have been shown to have markedly lower mortality rates than sedentary and less-fit persons.

The cardiovascular responses to a single session of resistance exercise differ from those for endurance exercise in several fundamental ways. In particular, heavy-resistance exercise elicits a pressor response that involves only moderate increases in heart rate and cardiac output, relative to those seen with dynamic exercise, but a greater elevation in systolic and diastolic BP. With the exception of circuit weight training, chronic strength or resistive training has not consistently been shown to lower resting BP.

Management and Medications

According to the Joint National Committee, the goal of treating persons with hypertension is to prevent morbidity and mortality associated with high BP and to control BP by the least intrusive means possible. To accomplish this, BP should be lowered and maintained below 140/90 mmHg while other modifiable cardiovascular risk factors are controlled concurrently.

For hypertension control or overall cardiovascular risk reduction, or both, it is recommended that people make the following lifestyle modifications:

- lose weight, if overweight;
- limit alcohol intake to no more than 1 oz/day (3 cl/day) of ethanol (24 oz [71 cl/day] of beer, 10 oz [30 cl/day] of wine, or 2 oz [6 cl/day] of 100-proof whiskey) for men or 0.5 oz/day (1.5 cl/day) for women and lighter people;
- increase aerobic physical activity (30-45 min most days of the week);
- reduce sodium intake to no more than 2.4 g/day;
- maintain adequate dietary potassium, calcium, and magnesium intake; and
- stop smoking and reduce intake of dietary saturated fat and cholesterol for overall cardiovascular health.

The decision to initiate drug therapy requires consideration of several factors:

- severity of BP elevation;
- presence or absence of clinical cardiovascular disease or target-organ disease; and
- presence or absence of other medical conditions and cardiovascular disease risk factors.

Beta blockers and, to a lesser degree, the calcium antagonists diltiazem and verapamil reduce the heart rate response to submaximal and maximal exercise. In contrast, dihydropyridine-derivative calcium antagonists and direct vasodilators may increase the heart rate response to submaximal exercise.

With the exception of beta blockers, most antihypertensive agents do not substantially alter the systolic BP response to a single session of dynamic exercise. However, they do lower the resting BP and therefore the absolute level attained. Beta blockers have been shown to attenuate the magnitude of rise in systolic BP from the baseline level as well as to reduce the resting BP. Unfortunately, the usefulness of beta blockers, especially nonselective agents, is often considerably limited by a concomitant impairment of exercise tolerance in persons without myocardial ischemia, by a possible blunting of exercise training-induced lowering of BP and triglycerides, and by increases in high-density lipoprotein cholesterol.

Antihypertensive agents that reduce total peripheral resistance by vasodilation may predispose to postexercise hypotension. This potential adverse effect can usually be prevented by avoidance of abrupt cessation of exercise and use of a longer cool-down period. Diuretics may result in serum potassium derangements and thereby accentuate the risk for exercise-induced dysrhythmias.

Recommendations for Exercise Testing

Standard exercise testing methods and protocols may be used for persons with hypertension. Individuals with an additional coronary risk factor, and those who are male and older than 45 years or female and older than 55 years, should perform an exercise test with ECG monitoring before starting a vigorous exercise program. Irrespective of the intensity of exercise training, persons with symptoms of cardiovascular disease or with known cardiovascular disease should perform an exercise test with ECG monitoring before commencing an exercise program. When exercise testing is performed for the purpose of exercise prescription, the individual should be taking his or her usual antihypertensive medications. A resting systolic BP over 200 mmHg or diastolic BP under 115 mmHg is considered a relative contraindication to exercise testing. Attainment of a systolic BP over 250 mmHg or diastolic BP under 115 mmHg is an indication for exercise test termination (see the Hypertension: Exercise Testing table).

Recommendations for Exercise Programming

It is recommended that people with more marked elevations in BP (> 180/110 mmHg) add endurance training to their treatment regimen only after initiating drug therapy. The mode (large muscle, aerobic activities), frequency (3-7 days/wk), duration (30-60 min), and intensity of exercise (40-70% of maximal oxygen consumption [$\dot{V}O_2$max]) recommended for persons with hypertension are similar to those for healthy adults (see the Hypertension: Exercise Programming table). Interestingly, exercise training at somewhat lower intensities (40-70% of $\dot{V}O_2$max) appears to lower BP as much as, if not more than, exercise at higher intensities. The latter is especially important in certain specific populations of persons with hypertension, such as those who are elderly or who have chronic diseases in addition to hypertension.

Strength or resistive training is not recommended as the only form of exercise training for persons with hypertension because, with the exception of circuit weight training, it has not consistently been shown to lower BP. Thus, resistive exercise training is recommended when

Hypertension: Exercise Testing

Methods	Measures	Endpoints*	Comments
Aerobic Cycle (ramp protocol 17 watts/ min; staged protocol 25-50 watts/3min stage) Treadmill (1-2 METs/3-min stage)	•12-lead ECG, HR	•Serious dysrhythmias •>2 mm ST-segment depression or elevation •Ischemic threshold •T-wave inversion with significant ST change	•Medications should be taken at usual time relative to the exercise session.
	•BP, rate pressure product	•SBP > 250 mmHg or DBP > 115 mmHg •Headache or other significant symptoms	
	•Respired gas analysis •RPE (6-20)	•$\dot{V}O_2$max ventilatory threshold	
Strength Free weights, machines	•1RM or maximal voluntary contraction		•Observe for exaggerated pressor response (SBP > 250 mmHg or DBP > 115 mmHg).

*Measurements of particular significance; do not always indicate test termination.

Medications

•See chapter 4 testing table.
•Beta blockers: Cause low chronotropic response of ~ 30 contractions/min.

Hypertension: Exercise Programming

Modes	Goals	Intensity/Frequency/Duration	Time to Goal
Aerobic • Large muscle activities	• Increase $\dot{V}O_2$max and ventilatory threshold • Increase peak work and endurance • Increase caloric expenditure • Control BP	• 50-80% peak HR • 40-70% $\dot{V}O_2$max or maximal HR reserve • RPE 11-14/20 • 3-7 days/wk • 30-60 min/session • 700-2000 kcal/wk	• 4-6 mo
Strength • Circuit training	• Increase strength	• High reps, low resistance	• 4-6 mo

Medications	Special Considerations
• Beta blockers: Attenuate HR by ~ 30 contractions/min • Alpha$_1$ blockers, alpha$_2$ blockers, calcium-channel blockers, and vasodilators: May cause postexertional hypotension	• See chapter 4 programming table. • Do not exercise if resting systolic BP > 200 mmHg or diastolic BP > 115 mmHg. • Exercise when pressor response is well controlled by medications. • Exercise at 40-70% $\dot{V}O_2$max appears to lower resting BP as much as, if not more than, exercise at higher intensities. • 700 kcal/wk should be the initial goal; 2000 kcal/wk should be the long-term goal.

done as one component of a well-rounded exercise program, but not when done independently. Resistive training using low resistances and high repetitions should be prescribed.

CASE STUDY Hypertension

A 59-year-old male was interested in starting an exercise program. He had no health complaints but did have hypertension and hyperlipidemia. He also was overweight. He had been sedentary for many years, did not smoke cigarettes, and had a family history of premature atherosclerosis.

S: "I think I should start an exercise program."

O: Vitals: Height: 6'0" (1.83 m)   Weight: 210 lb (95.2 kg)   BMI: 29.4 kg/m^2
          HR: 58 contractions/min   BP: 144/92 mmHg

Moderately obese male; no distress

No vascular changes on funduscopic exam; peripheral pulses nondelayed; no bruits

Normal heart sounds, nondisplaced ventricular apical impulse

Graded exercise test (Bruce protocol):
  Terminated at 6 min because of leg fatigue
  Peak RPE: 18/20
  Peak HR: 136 contractions/min
  Peak BP: 186/90 mmHg
  ECG: no significant ST changes; occasional PVCs
  No chest discomfort reported

Medications: Atenolol, Simvastatin

(continued)

CASE STUDY Hypertension (continued)

A: 1. Hypertension
2. Hyperlipidemia
3. Obesity
4. Sedentary lifestyle/deconditioning

P: Initiate an aerobic exercise program

Exercise Program
Goals:

1. Improved blood pressure and pressor response to exercise
2. Weight loss
3. Cholesterol control

Mode	Frequency	Duration	Intensity	Progression
Aerobic (treadmill, stationary cycling)	3 days/wk	15-min/session	40-70% of HRR (89-113 contractions/min) RPE 11-14/20	Build to 5 days/wk Add ~5 min/wk until 30-45 min/session*
Strength Resistance (all major muscle groups)	2-3 days/wk	1 set of 10-15 reps	RPE 13/20	Arms: Add 2-5 lb/wk (0.9-2.3 kg/wk) Legs: Add 5-10 lb/wk (2.3-4.5 kg/wk) Aim for ~ RPE 15 after 4-6 wk
Flexibility (all major muscle groups)	3 days/wk	20 s/stretch	Maintain stretch below discomfort point	Discomfort point should occur at higher ROM; progress as tolerated
Neuromuscular				
Functional				
Warm-up/Cool-down	Before and after each session	10-15 min	RPE <11/20	

*He was told that the time interval between taking his atenolol and exercise training could alter his cardiovascular response to exercise and, thus, to attempt to exercise at the same time each day.

Suggested Readings

American College of Sports Medicine. 2000. *ACSM's guidelines for exercise testing and prescription,* edited by B.A. Franklin, M.H Whaley, and E.T. Howley. 6th ed. Philadelphia: Lippincott Williams & Wilkins.

American College of Sports Medicine. 1993. Position stand: Physical activity, physical fitness, and hypertension. *Medicine and Science in Sports and Exercise* 25: i-x.

Blair, S.N., H.W. Kohl, C.E. Barlow, and L.W. Gibbons. 1991. Physical fitness and all-cause mortality in hypertensive men. *Annals of Medicine* 23: 307-12.

Fletcher, G.F., G. Balady, V.F. Froelicher, L.H. Hartley, W.L. Haskell, and M.L. Pollock. 1995. Exercise standards: A statement for health care professionals from the American Heart Association. *Circulation* 91: 580-615.

Gordon, N.F., C.B. Scott, W.J. Wilkinson, J.J. Duncan, and S.N. Blair. 1990. Exercise and mild essential hypertension: Recommendations for adults. *Sports Medicine* 10: 390-404.

Hagberg, J.M. 1990. Exercise, fitness, and hypertension. In *Exercise, fitness, and health*, edited by C. Bouchard, R.J. Shephard, T. Stephens, J.R. Sutton, and B.D. McPherson, 455-66. Champaign, IL: Human Kinetics.

Joint National Committee on Prevention, Detection, Evaluation, and Treatment of High Blood Pressure. 1997. The sixth report of the Joint National Committee on Prevention, Detection, Evaluation, and Treatment of High Blood Pressure (JNC VI). *Archives of Internal Medicine* 157: 2413-46.

Kaplan, N.M., R.B. Deveraux, and H.S. Miller Jr. 1994. Task force 4: Systemic hypertension. *Medicine and Science in Sports and Exercise* 26: S268-70.

Paffenbarger, R.S., Jr., R.T. Hyde, A.L. Wing, and C.-C. Hsieh. 1986. Physical activity, all-cause mortality, and longevity of college alumni. *New England Journal of Medicine* 314: 605-13.

CHAPTER 13

Peripheral Arterial Disease

Christopher J. Womack, PhD, FACSM
Michigan State University

Andrew W. Gardner, PhD
Baltimore VA Medical Center

Overview of the Pathophysiology

Peripheral arterial disease (PAD) results from stenoses and occlusions of the arteries of the lower extremities, causing a reduction in blood flow beyond the obstructions. The severity of PAD may be classified into the following categories according to recent guidelines:

- Grade 0 = asymptomatic
- Grade 1 = intermittent claudication
- Grade 2 = ischemic rest pain
- Grade 3 = minor or major tissue loss from the foot

Effects on the Exercise Response

The primary effect of PAD on a single exercise session is the development of claudication pain in the leg musculature during exercise because of insufficient blood flow. Ankle systolic blood pressure is measured to noninvasively assess the peripheral circulation and is expressed relative to the brachial systolic pressure, termed the ankle/brachial systolic pressure index (ABI). Ankle systolic pressure and ABI are obtained while the client is supine at rest and following exercise.

The time and/or distance to onset and to maximal claudication pain during walking are used as criteria for assessing the functional severity of disease. Ankle systolic pressure and ABI are reduced following exercise because blood flow is shunted into the proximal leg musculature at the expense of the periphery and distal areas of the leg.

Effects of Exercise Training

The clinical status of intermittent claudication in clients with PAD is improved through physical conditioning. Proposed mechanisms for an increase in exercise tolerance include the following adaptations:

- increase in leg blood flow;
- more favorable redistribution of blood flow;
- improved hemorheological and fibrinolytic properties of blood (e.g., reduced viscosity);
- greater reliance upon aerobic metabolism because of a higher concentration of oxidative enzymes;
- less reliance upon anaerobic metabolism;
- an improvement in the efficiency of walking economy and oxygen uptake kinetics; and
- increased free-living daily energy expenditure.

Management and Medications

Common medications for intermittent claudication include the following:

- pentoxifylline (Trental);
- cilostazol (Pletal);
- dipyridamole (Persantine);
- warfarin (Coumadin); and
- aspirin.

Either clients should not take these medications until the exercise test procedures have been completed, or the time of day at which the medications were taken should be recorded and kept consistent upon repeated tests. Clients will commonly take medications for related forms of cardiovascular disease and/or related risk factors (e.g., hypertension, dyslipidemia, diabetes). In terms of exercise programming, little information is available on the interaction between exercise training and medication therapy for the treatment of intermittent claudication.

Recommendations for Exercise Testing

The primary objectives of a treadmill test for clients with PAD are to:

- obtain reliable measures of claudication pain times;
- obtain reliable measures of ankle pressure following exercise; and
- assess whether coronary artery disease is present.

(See the Peripheral Arterial Disease: Exercise Testing table.)

The procedures for treadmill testing clients with PAD are as follows:

- Ankle and brachial systolic blood pressures are measured and ABI is calculated after the client has been in a supine position for 15 min.

- Blood pressure is measured in both arms and in the posterior tibial and dorsalis pedis arteries of both legs (via Doppler). The artery yielding the higher systolic pressure in each leg is used for the measurement of ankle systolic pressure, and the higher pressure between the two arms is used to calculate ABI.

- An exercise test with gradual increments in percent grade is then performed. Small increments in grade allow claudication times of clients to be stratified according to disease severity. A highly reliable protocol

Peripheral Arterial Disease: Exercise Testing

Methods	Measures	Endpoints*	Comments
Aerobic Treadmill (1-2 METs/stage; preferred)	• 12-lead ECG HR	• Serious dysrhythmias • >2 mm ST-segment depression or elevation • Ischemic threshold • T-wave inversion with significant ST change	• Cycle protocols can underestimate the severity of PAD.
	• BP	• SBP > 250 mmHg or DBP > 115 mmHg	
	• 4-point claudication scale		• Record time of pain onset and maximal pain.
Endurance Constant work rate	• Time to maximal pain	• Maximal pain	• Record time of pain onset and maximal pain.
Neuromuscular Gait analysis	• Speed • Step rate • Step length		• May change with disease progression.
Functional 6-min walk (majority of patients)	• Distance	• Time to maximal pain • Maximal pain	• Record time of pain onset and maximal pain.

*Measurements of particular significance; do not always indicate test termination.

Medications	Special Considerations
• Pentoxyphylline, dipyridamole, aspirin, and warfarin: May improve time to claudication. • Beta blockers: May decrease time to claudication.	• High risk for CAD (refer to chapters 4 and 6). • High prevalence of smoking/COPD (refer to chapter 15). • Diabetic neuropathy can mimic claudication. • Skin ulcers common in persons with pain at rest (grade 2). • Consider leg pain not of vascular origin.

Peripheral Arterial Disease: Exercise Programming

Modes	Goals	Intensity/ Frequency/Duration	Time to Goal
Aerobic • Large muscle activities (walking highly preferred)	• Improve pain response; perform longer in time trials or grade achieved on GXT	• 40-70% $\dot{V}O_2$peak HR reserve • Intermittent walk to 3 (out of 4) on claudication scale (monitor HR) • 3 days/wk • 20-40 min/session	• 4-6 mo • Decrease CAD risk factors • Increase duration before intensity
Neuromuscular • Walking	• Improve gait		
Functional • Walking	• Increase ADLs, work potential, and quality of life		

Medications	Special Considerations
• Pentoxyphylline, cilostazol, dipyridamole, aspirin, and warfarin: May improve time to claudication. • Beta blockers: May decrease time to claudication.	• Improvement may unmask angina pectoris. • Aggressive lifestyle and lipid management necessary. • May need repeat TM testing to judge increases in program. • Quality of life questionnaire (e.g., Short Form 36) may be useful. • Watch for changes in co-morbidity. • Refer to chapters 4 and 6 for clients with CAD. • Cold weather may worsen symptoms; need a longer warm-up.

uses a constant speed of 2 mph (3.2K/h) and an increase in grade of 2% every 2 min beginning at 0% grade.

• A validated pain scale ranging from 0 to 4 (0 = no pain, 1 = onset of pain, 2 = moderate pain, 3 = intense pain, and 4 = maximal pain) is used to assist clients in identifying progression of claudication pain during the test to maximal pain (a score of 4). The time elapsed from the start of exercise to each pain score is recorded. Holding on to the handrails is discouraged, except for brief moments to maintain balance, because it alters metabolic demands, resulting in changes in physiological responses that cause variability in claudication times. Heart rate and brachial blood pressure are recorded during the last minute of each 2-min exercise stage.

• The client recovers in a supine position for 15 min. The time elapsed from the start of recovery to the relief of claudication pain (a score of 0) is recorded. Ankle and brachial blood pressures are recorded throughout the recovery period.

• Use of indirect calorimetry during treadmill testing can alter the client's perception of claudication pain. Repeated tests should be consistent as to whether indirect calorimetry is used.

Recommendations for Exercise Programming

Exercise programs for clients with PAD should be designed with a goal of improving claudication pain symptoms and reducing cardiovascular risk factors (see the Peripheral Arterial Disease: Exercise Programming table). Most persons should do interval walking or stair climbing three times a week, at an intensity that causes pain of a 3 score on a 4-point scale. The onset of claudication should occur in approximately 5 min; full recovery is allowed between intervals. This type of program may start with 20 min of exercise per session at 40% of heart rate reserve, and gradually progress to 40 min at 70% of heart rate reserve, over a period of about 6 months. Non-weight-bearing tasks (e.g., cycling) may be used for warming up and cooling down. There are circumstances in which it is inappropriate for clients with PAD to exercise.

• Exercise training should not be performed until medical clearance, based on a physical exam, blood screening, and graded exercise test has been completed.

- Exercise should not be performed when there are concomitant comorbidities that may limit exercise tolerance.

CASE STUDY Peripheral Arterial Disease

A 75-year-old man complained of cramps in his right leg during walking across a small room or up a flight of stairs. The pain was always on the right, brought on by activity and relieved by rest. He did not get nocturnal cramps or cramps when sitting still. He smoked cigarettes but did not have high blood pressure. He was sent to the exercise laboratory for an evaluation of intermittent claudication. After the evaluation, he wished to enroll in an exercise program.

S: "I get cramps in my right leg when I walk."

O: Vitals: Height: 5'8" (1.73 m)   Weight: 154 lb (69.85 kg)   BMI: 23.3 kg/m²
RHR: 80 contractions/min   BP: 110/70 mmHg

Elderly male, smelling of cigarettes

Bilateral inguinal hernias

Cervical laminectomy scar

Abdominal scar (bowel resection)

Ankle/brachial systolic pressure index: 0.66

Graded exercise test: Continuous treadmill at 2.0 mph, 0.0% grade increasing 2% every 2 min:
 Time to onset of claudication pain: 306 s
 Time to maximal claudication pain: 503 s
 Free-living daily energy expenditure as measured by accelerometer: 53 kcal/day
 6-minute walk distance: 760 ft (231.6 m)

Blood lipids: not available

Medications: None

A: 1. Peripheral arterial disease with intermittent claudication
2. Low functional capacity caused by early onset claudication

P: 1. Initiate a walking program.
2. Refer to atherosclerosis clinic.
3. Recommend smoking cessation.
4. Consider platelet inhibition medications.

Exercise Program
Goal:
1. Increased time to claudication onset and maximal pain
2. Increased free-living energy expenditure
3. Increased functional capacity

Mode	Frequency	Duration	Intensity	Progression
Aerobic (walking)	3-7 days/wk	15 min/session	60% of $\dot{V}O_2$peak Elicit 3/4 pain of claudication	Increase to 45 min @ 70% over a period of 6 mo; increase nominally every 3-4 weeks
Strength			10-12 reps after12 wk	
Flexibility (all major muscle groups)	3 days/wk	20 s/stretch	Maintain stretch below discomfort point	Discomfort point should occur at higher ROM; progress as tolerated
Neuromuscular				
Functional				
Warm-up/Cool-down	Before and after each sesson	5-10 min; longer in cold weather	RPE <10/20	

Follow-Up

The 6-month rehabilitation program increased the time to onset of claudication pain by 4 min, and time to maximal claudication pain by 7 min. His free-living daily activity increased from 53 kcal/day to 373 kcal/day. One year after completing the formal rehabilitation program, he maintained a 1.5-min improvement in time to onset of claudication, a 2-min improvement in time to maximal claudication, and an increase of 100 kcal/day free-living physical activity.

Suggested Readings

Adhoc Committee on Reporting Standards. 1986. Suggested standards for reports dealing with lower extremity ischemia. *Journal of Vascular Surgery* 4: 80-94.

Gardner, A.W., J.S. Skinner, B.W. Cantwell, and L.K. Smith. 1991. Progressive vs. single-stage treadmill tests for evaluation of claudication. *Medicine and Science in Sports and Exercise* 23: 402-8.

Gardner, A.W., J.S. Skinner, and L.K. Smith. 1991. Effects of handrail support on claudication and hemodynamic responses to single-stage and progressive treadmill protocols in peripheral vascular occlusive disease. *American Journal of Cardiology* 68: 99-105.

Regensteiner, J.G., and W.R. Hiatt. 1995. Exercise rehabilitation for patients with peripheral arterial disease. *Exercise and Sport Sciences Reviews* 23:1-24.

Skinner, J.S., and D.E. Strandness Jr. 1967. Exercise and intermittent claudication: I. Effect of repetition and intensity of exercise. *Circulation* 36: 23-29.

Womack, C.J., D.J. Sieminski, L.I. Katzel, A. Yataco, and A.W. Gardner. 1997. Improved walking economy in patients with peripheral arterial occlusive disease. *Medicine and Science in Sports and Exercise* 29: 1286-90.

Yao, S.T., T.N. Needham, C. Gourmoos, and W.T. Irvine. 1972. A comparative study of strain-gauge plethysmography and Doppler ultrasound in the assessment of occlusive arterial disease of the lower extremities. *Surgery* 71: 4-9.

CHAPTER 14

Aneurysms

Geoffrey E. Moore, MD, FACSM
McGill University

Peter H. Brubaker, PhD, FACSM
Wake Forest University

Overview of the Pathophysiology

Many diseases can cause a dilated enlargement (aneurysm) of arteries. Aneurysms can be caused by congenital or acquired diseases, are usually asymptomatic, and are often not discovered until they rupture or cause symptoms due to localized pressure on an adjacent tissue. Most aneurysms are diseases of aging, but some occur during childhood and adolescence. With regard to exercise, the main risks for persons with an aneurysm are progressive enlargement of the aneurysm, tearing of the arterial wall (dissection), and sudden rupture of the artery. These risks apply to any aneurysm, regardless of location in the body.

The most common site for aneurysms is in the brain, where sac-like bulges in the wall of a cerebral artery (berry aneurysm) occur in perhaps 2 to 5% of the population. Most berry aneurysms cause no symptoms or illness during the person's entire life. When a berry aneurysm enlarges, however, it takes up space within the skull; this can squeeze on that area of the brain and cause neurologic problems. A rupture (cerebral hemorrhage) can cause severe disability or death, or it may cause mild, reversible damage and be treatable by medicines, surgery, or both. Unfortunately, except for some associations with polycystic kidney disease and coarctation of the aorta, there is generally no way of knowing who has a berry aneurysm until it ruptures.

The aorta is the next most common artery site of aneurysms. The enlargement usually occurs in a well-defined location, although some regions of this long artery are more susceptible than others. The aortic root (just where the vessel leaves the heart) is one such region. The abdominal aorta (in the region of the branches to the kidneys) is the most common site, affecting about 3% of older adults, particularly men over the age of 60. Other regions of the aorta can enlarge at different ages depending on the disease process.

High blood pressure greatly increases the risk of aneurysm rupture, and aneurysm enlargement is usually without symptoms. Most aneurysms are acquired, such as abdominal aortic aneurysms associated with hypertension, atherosclerosis, and other chronic diseases. High blood pressure and cigarette smoking are the most common coincidental medical problems in older adults with abdominal aortic aneurysms. Other causes of aneurysms include inflammation (aortitis), infection (syphilis), and injury to the aorta (especially deceleration injuries as in automobile accidents). Aneurysms can be acquired from iatrogenic causes, mainly as a complication of surgical attempts to angioplasty a vessel with atherosclerosis. The most common site for this complication is probably the coronary arteries, since these vessels most frequently undergo this procedure.

The main congenital cause of aortic aneurysms is Marfan's syndrome, which is usually discovered because persons with this disease are often tall and lanky, have deformity of the chest such as scoliosis (curvature of the spine) and pectus excavatum (inward-shaped or funnel chest), overly flexible joints, and dislocation of the eye lens, or because a close relative is affected. Marfan's syndrome is caused by a genetic defect in the microfibrils forming the elastic fibers of large arteries as well as in similar microfibrils that give strength and structure to some connective tissues. Marfan's syndrome causes the aortic root to dilate immediately above the aortic valve. As dilatation progresses, the aortic valve begins to leak (aortic regurgitation), and the risk of dissection increases.

Effects on the Exercise Response

Early in the course of aneurysmal disease, when the dilation is minimal, there is usually no effect on the exercise response. Even in persons with existing aneurysms, there is likely to be little change in the exercise response other than a delay and blunting in pulse pressure. Indeed, it is more likely that exercise will affect an aneurysm than the aneurysm will alter the exercise response.

Biomechanical modeling of flow through an aortic aneurysm suggests that exercise may be detrimental in the progression of the disease. Pulsatile flow through an aneurysm creates vortices and turbulence within the aneurysm that markedly increase wall stress. This may contribute to endothelial damage and stimulation of the inflammatory phase of atherogenesis. This situation is most notable for markedly enlarged aneurysms and is exaggerated during exercise.

Exercise has, in rare circumstances, been associated with aneurysm dissection or rupture. This complication has been reported for cerebral, aortic, renal, and coronary arteries, and any artery is theoretically at risk. In most case reports of such incidents, it was not known whether the aneurysm was present prior to the onset of symptoms. One study of abdominal aortic aneurysms suggests that the risk of dissection or rupture caused by exercise is about 1%. Because this was a retrospective survey of a selected population, however, the true risk is not known. Athletes with Marfan's syndrome have died while playing sports, including the volleyball Olympic gold medalist Flo Hyman. Such high-profile events have increased the awareness of Marfan's syndrome among team physicians but, more importantly, point out the need for caution when managing the exercise program of a client with aneurysmal disease.

Effects of Exercise Training

To the extent that exercise increases blood pressure, exercise increases the tension on the wall of an aneurysm and so increases the risk of dissection or rupture for an already weakened aneurysm. The wall tension of a vessel increases with the square of the radius, so the increased blood pressure associated with exercise is markedly increased in the dilated section of the vessel. Also, the progression of enlargement, or worsening, of the aneurysm is likely to be increased by exercise. These complications may be attributable to an increase in heart rate as well as blood pressure because rapid heart rates cause more pulsations acting on the weakened wall in a given period of time. Thus, exercise training is relatively contraindicated in persons with aneurysmal disease.

Aneurysms: Exercise Testing

Methods	Measures	Endpoints	Comments
Aerobic Not recommended			• Raises HR/BP too high.
Strength Not recommended			• Raises HR/BP too high.
Endurance Time trial, 6-min walk	• Distance	• Time	• Assess low-level exercise endurance.
Flexibility Goniometry Sit and reach			
Functional Balance		• Assess need for occupational/physical therapy	

Medications	Special Considerations
• Beta-adrenergic blockade: Limits chronotropic response.	• Elevated HR and BP (double product) potentially harmful. • HR should never go > 100 contractions/min. • Risk of dissection. • In Marfan's syndrome: joint contractures, hypermobility, scoliosis, hyperlordosis, kyphosis, protusio acetabulae.

Management and Medications

Does all this mean that people with aneurysms should not exercise? In the ideal situation, a risk profile should be generated for each individual. This approach has at least three limitations. First, there has been little scientific work, in humans or animals, on the actual risk of a given degree of dilatation. Second, many people with aneurysms are asymptomatic (or even undiagnosed) and may want to exercise. Third, exercise offers benefits that people with aneurysms should not be denied, as long as the risks are not too high.

For people diagnosed with an aneurysm, the key step in medical management is to follow the progress of the enlarged area. This might involve echocardiography, abdominal ultrasound, magnetic resonance imaging, or (less and less commonly) angiography. The next most important step is lowering blood pressure to the low-normal range. A beta-adrenergic blocking drug, like atenolol or propranolol, is ideally suited to blood pressure management because it will also reduce the strength of arterial pulses. Even people with a low-normal baseline blood pressure should be treated with a beta blocker if there is not a contraindication to this medicine. Finally, when the vessel wall reaches about double the diameter it would ordinarily be, strong consider-ation should be given to surgical repair. Some people, such as those with a strong family history of dissection, should have surgery even sooner.

Recommendations for Exercise Testing

In general, people with known aneurysms of any type should not undergo maximal exercise testing. Limited retrospective data suggest that the risk of complication is low for diagnostic exercise stress testing prior to surgery. Submaximal stress tests can be used to optimize therapeutic control of heart rate and blood pressure. In particular, it is important to avoid raising the heart rate–blood pressure product (HR × systolic BP), which is a measure of stress on the arteries. Stress tests can help adjust medications so that pulse rate does not rise above 100 contractions/min (adults).

There are no good exercise data on the likelihood that an increase in rate-pressure product will cause an aneurysm to rupture, but it is thought that the larger the aneurysm, the greater the likelihood of exercise to cause a rupture. Maximal strength testing should similarly be avoided since resistance exercise can markedly increase blood pressure (see the Aneurysms: Exercise Testing table on page 87).

Aneurysms: Exercise Programming

Modes	Goals	Intensity/ Frequency/Duration	Time to Goal
Aerobic • Large muscle activities (walking, swimming)	• Increase peak work, endurance, and time to exhaustion	• Do not exceed HR of 100 contractions/min • 30 min • 3-4 days/wk • Emphasize duration over intensity	• 4-6 mo
Flexibility • Stretching	• Maintain/increase ROM		
Neuromuscular • Gait/Balance training	• Improve gait (for joint disorders)		
Functional • Activity specific	• Maintain ADLs		

Special Considerations

• See exercise testing table in this chapter and in chapters 4 and 5.
• Avoid overstretching in persons with Marfan's syndrome, who are typically hypermobile.
• Do not elevate HR > 100 contractions/min in order to keep double-product low.

Recommendations for Exercise Programming

The recommended modes of exercise are limited. In general, contact sports and competition should be avoided. Sports that have low cardiovascular demand, such as bowling, are recommended by the American College of Cardiology (1994) for clients with aneurysmal disease. The larger the diameter of the aneurysm relative to the normal diameter of the vessel, the more exercise should be restricted. In any case, any aerobic isotonic activity should be performed at a moderate to low intensity.

For individuals taking beta-adrenergic blocking drugs, the heart rate is not a good guide of intensity unless the peak heart rate has been ascertained by way of a graded exercise test. If peak heart rate is unknown, perceived exertion scales should be used. Resistance exercise should also be performed at moderate to low intensity. In persons with Marfan's syndrome, flexibility training (e.g., some yoga positions) should not be done by persons with joint involvement because it may risk joint dislocation. Some yoga activities may be useful, however, for blood pressure control (see the Aneurysms: Exercise Programming table).

Special Considerations

One management difficulty with aneurysmal disease is in advising persons who want to exercise. In particular, what about people who want to engage in sports? Indeed, some people with Marfan's syndrome may be particularly suited to sport because of their stature and flexibility. Unfortunately, the very sports for which these individuals are predisposed to have talent involve body contact and extreme elevation of the rate-pressure product, most notably basketball. Furthermore, high doses of beta-blocking medications are likely to decrease aerobic performance needed for an intense fast-break style of play. The psychological characteristics that lead to athletic success may present problems with adherence to recommendations of limiting this activity and may warrant the involvement of an expert in sport psychology.

CASE STUDY Abdominal Aortic Aneurysm

A 74-year-old male with a history of myocardial infarction (MI) (21 years prior), hypertension, hyperlipidemia, gout, renal insufficiency, and ventricular ectopy presented to cardiac rehabilitation three weeks after a second MI and redo coronary artery bypass grafting and mitral valve repair. A preoperative physical examination uncovered a tender abdomen and a soft abdominal bruit, and a sonogram revealed a distal aortic aneurysm of 3.7 cm diameter.

S: "They sent me to cardiac rehabilitation."

O: Vitals: HR: 68 contractions/min   BP: 130/76 mmHg   Weight: 174 lb (78.9 kg)
           Height: 5'11" (1.8 m)   BMI: 24.4 kg/m^2

Mechanical heart valve; abdominal bruit; femoral pulses intact and nondelayed

Graded exercise test: modified Bruce protocol
  5.6 METs
  Peak HR: 119 contractions/min
  Peak BP: 170/110 mmHg
  No ischemia; frequent PVCs, couplets, triplets

Medications: Atenolol, Norvasc, Allopurinol, Indomethacin, ASA

A: 1. Low exercise tolerance secondary to
    • extensive atherosclerosis/recent cardiac surgery
    • deconditioning
    • gouty arthritis

    2. Abdominal aortic aneurysm (no vascular compromise)

    3. Brisk pressor response to exercise

P: 1. Initiate an exercise (walking) program.

    2. Initiate aggressive HR and BP control.

    3. Monitor BP during exercise program.

(continued)

CASE STUDY Abdominal Aortic Aneurysm (continued)

Exercise Program
Goals:

1. Maintain functional capacity
2. Monitor cardiovascular (especially pressor) response to exercise

Special considerations: Avoid exaggerated blood pressure response. If observed, increase blood pressure medications.

Mode	Frequency	Duration	Intensity	Progression
Aerobic	3-7 days/wk	5 to 10-min intervals	THR (50-65% $\dot{V}O_2$max) RPE $\leq$ 11/20	Advance to 15-20 min/ session in 3-4 wk
Strength				
Flexibility				Stretching contra-indicated in Marfan's syndrome
Neuromuscular				
Functional				
Warm-up/Cool-down	Before and after each sesson	5-10 min	RPE <10/20	

Follow-Up

He successfully completed Phase II cardiac rehabilitation and entered into a center-based "maintenance" exercise program. The aneurysm was periodically assessed by sonograms and after 2 1/2 years it had enlarged to a diameter of 4.8 cm. The aneurysm was repaired in elective surgery. After 3 weeks of convalescence, he reentered cardiac rehabilitation where an exercise test revealed a functional capacity of 4.1 METs. Peak heart rate and blood pressure were 115 contractions/min and 172/60 mmHg, respectively. He resumed exercise training with a target heart rate of 78 to 97 contractions/min.

Suggested Readings

Best, P.A., A.J. Tajik, R.J. Gibbons, and P.A. Pellikka. 1998. The safety of treadmill exercise stress testing in patients with abdominal aortic aneurysms. *Annals of International Medicine* 139 (8): 628-31.

Braverman, A.C. 1998. Exercise and the Marfan syndrome. *Medicine and Science in Sports and Exercise* 30 (10 supplement): S387-95.

Cheitlin, M.D., P.S. Douglas, and W.M. Parmley. 1994. Task force 2: Acquired valvular heart disease. 26th Bethesda Conference: Recommendations for determining eligibility for competition in athletes with cardiovascular abnormalities. *Journal of the American College of Cardiology* 24 (4): 874-80.

Egelhoff, C.J., R.S. Budwig, D.F. Elger, T.A. Khraishi, and K.H. Johansen. 1999. Model studies of the flow in abdominal aortic aneurysms during resting and exercise conditions. *Journal of Biomechanics* 32: 1319-29.

Ellis, C.J., G.A. Haywood, and J.L. Monro. 1994. Spontaneous coronary artery dissection in a young woman resulting from an intense gymnasium "work-out." *International Journal of Cardiology* 47: 193-94.

Graham, T.P., Jr., J.T. Bricker, F.W. James, and W.B. Strong. 1994. Task force 1: Congenital heart disease. 26th Bethesda Conference: Recommendations for determining eligibility for competition in athletes with cardiovascular abnormalities. *Journal of the American College of Cardiology* 24 (4): 867-73.

Provenzale, J.M., D.P Barboriak, and J.M. Taveras. 1995. Exercise-related dissection of cranio-cervical arteries: CT, MR, and angiographic findings. *Journal of Computer-Assisted Tomography* 19 (2): 268-76.

Pyeritz, R.E., and U. Francke. 1993. Conference report: The second international symposium on the Marfan syndrome. *American Journal of Medical Genetics* 47: 127-35.

Sherrid, M.V., J. Mieres, A. Mogtader, N. Menezes, and G. Steinberg. 1995. Onset during exercise of spontaneous coronary artery dissection and sudden death. *Chest* 108 (1): 284-87.

Thomas, M.C., R.J. Walker, and S. Packer. 1999. Running repairs: Renal artery dissection following extreme exertion. *Nephrology, Dialysis, Transplantation* 14: 1258-59.

SECTION III

Pulmonary Diseases

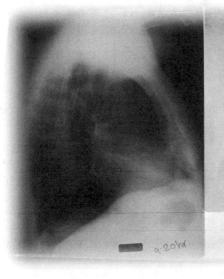

Christopher B. Cooper,
MD, FACSM

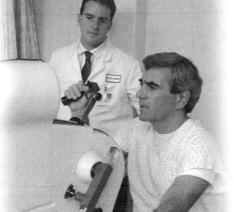

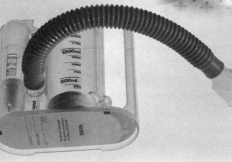

CHAPTER 15

Chronic Obstructive Pulmonary Disease

Christopher B. Cooper, MD, FACSM
UCLA School of Medicine

Overview of the Pathophysiology

Chronic obstructive pulmonary disease (COPD) imposes multiple pathophysiological problems, not only through obvious ventilatory and gas exchange impairments but also through complex interactions with the cardiovascular and muscular systems. To appreciate the nature of these impairments, it is instructive to divide the pathophysiology into a number of categories.

Ventilatory Impairments

• Increased airway resistance as seen in obstructive pulmonary diseases such as chronic bronchitis and asthma. Airflow obstruction is compromised mainly during expiration because the airways tend to become smaller as lung volume decreases. While smoking-related chronic bronchitis is slowly progressive, asthma can be intermittent and of varying severity. In the special case of exercise-induced bronchoconstriction, pulmonary function can be normal between attacks.

• Reduced compliance as seen in restrictive pulmonary diseases—for example, reduced lung compliance as seen in pulmonary fibrosis or reduced chest wall compliance as seen in kyphoscoliosis.

• Increased work of breathing, which occurs in both obstructive and restrictive diseases.

• Ventilatory muscle weakness due to either hyperinflation or neuromuscular weakness. Hyperinflation occurs with expiratory airflow obstruction placing the inspiratory muscles at a mechanical disadvantage. Neuromuscular weakness of the respiratory muscles also causes a restrictive ventilatory defect as seen in poliomyelitis or muscular dystrophy.

• Ventilatory inefficiency due to increased dead space and an inappropriately high ratio between physiological dead space and tidal volume (VD/VT).

• Ventilatory muscle fatigue resulting from increased work of breathing, ventilatory muscle weakness, ventilatory inefficiency, or a combination of these factors.

• Ventilatory failure with inadequate alveolar ventilation, hypoxemia, and hypercarbia. This condition arises in the later stages of many COPDs.

Abnormalities of Gas Exchange

• Destruction of the alveolar-capillary membrane is seen in emphysema and pulmonary fibrosis. Because of diffusion impairment, both conditions can result in hypoxemia during exercise or even at rest in advanced disease.

• Ventilation-perfusion inequality as seen particularly in COPD and recurrent pulmonary emboli. These conditions can also result in hypoxemia, which usually worsens during exercise.

Cardiovascular Impairments

• Cardiovascular deconditioning, which is an inevitable consequence of reduced physical activity in COPD. Individuals may experience an accumulation of lactic acid at low work rates.

• Reduced pulmonary vascular conductance is seen in chronic hypoxemia and pulmonary vascular disease, such as thromboembolism and emphysema. As a result of increased pulmonary vascular resistance, the right ventricle is unable to respond adequately to the demand for increased cardiac output during exercise.

Muscular Impairments

• Peripheral muscle deconditioning, which is an inevitable consequence of reduced physical activity in COPD.

• Muscle wasting and weakness are also present due to inactivity and malnutrition.

Symptomatic Limitations

• Breathlessness (dyspnea) is a frightening symptom with a complex etiology. Dyspnea results from a summation of neurological inputs from pulmonary receptors, chemoreceptors, and mechanoreceptors in the chest wall and limbs. Some individuals have dyspnea that is disproportional to their ventilatory limitations.

Psychological Disturbances

• Chronic anxiety afflicts many individuals with COPD because of the frightening nature of their symptoms.

• Depression sometimes follows from limited ability to pursue normal daily activities with resulting social isolation, feelings of helplessness, and despair.

Effects on the Exercise Response

Some, but not all, people with COPD have true ventilatory limitation whereby the ventilatory requirement at maximum exercise equals the ventilatory capacity that can be measured over 12 or 15 s (maximal voluntary ventilation) or calculated from spirometry. Individuals with obstructive disease have impeded expiration requiring a longer time for adequate lung emptying. In these persons, increased breathing frequency during exercise tends to lead to hyperinflation and smaller tidal volumes, circumstances that worsen breathing efficiency by increasing VD/VT. Individuals with restrictive diseases characteristically have limited inspiratory capacity (e.g., tidal volume constraint) but usually have unimpeded or even accelerated expiration. These persons characteristically exhibit rapid respiratory rates (e.g., > 50 breaths/min) at maximum exercise.

In the absence of true ventilatory limitation, exercise can be limited by cardiovascular factors such as deconditioning, impaired left ventricular function due to hypoxemia, or reduced pulmonary blood flow secondary to chronic hypoxemia. Peripheral muscle deconditioning can lead to lactic acid accumulation at low work rates, increased CO_2 output from bicarbonate buffering, and consequently an increased ventilatory requirement (which compounds the situation).

Impairment of gas exchange occurs in emphysema because of destruction of the alveolar-capillary membrane and in pulmonary fibrosis because of loss of functioning lung units. Both conditions might cause hypoxemia during exercise, particularly when increases in pulmonary blood flow increase shunting through areas of incomplete gas exchange. Chronic hypoxemia also causes erythrocytosis, and the resulting increase in blood viscosity can further compromise the circulation during exercise. In smokers, increases in carboxyhemoglobin, which does not carry oxygen, will impair blood oxygen transport. Finally, in some individuals, symptoms (predominantly dyspnea) and psychological factors might limit exercise capacity independently.

Effects of Exercise Training

Regular participation in physical activity can manifest beneficial changes in persons with COPD. These changes include the following:

• cardiovascular reconditioning;

• desensitization to dyspnea;

• improved ventilatory efficiency;

• increased muscle strength;

• improved flexibility;

• improved body composition;

• better balance; and

• enhanced body image.

The accomplishment of these changes requires careful attention to medications to obtain optimal respiratory mechanics and may require use of oxygen therapy to maintain adequate oxygenation during exercise.

Management and Medications

Because individuals with COPD have some degree of physical deconditioning, exercise training is a crucial aspect of clinical management and rehabilitation. The specific goals of management are the following:

• optimization of respiratory system mechanics by careful attention to bronchodilator therapy, inhaler dosage, and technique;

• correction of hypoxemia whether it occurs at rest, during exercise, or during sleep;

• desensitization to dyspnea, fear, and other potentially limiting symptoms;

• breathing retraining to improve ventilatory efficiency;

• energy conservation by improved coordination, balance, and mechanical efficiency during activities of daily living; and

• exercise training to correct physical deconditioning, reduce lactic acidosis, and reduce ventilatory requirement during exercise.

All but the last goal are directed toward enabling an individual to perform exercise at higher intensity, thus increasing the potential for obtaining a reconditioning effect from exercise training.

Individuals with COPD are often taking several medications that could have implications for exercise testing and training. Furthermore, COPD often coexists with cardiovascular diseases such as coronary artery disease,

Chronic Obstructive Pulmonary Disease: Exercise Testing

Methods	Measures	Endpoints*	Comments
Aerobic Cycle (preferred) (ramp protocol 10, 15, or 20 watts/min; staged protocol 25-50 watts/3-min stage) Treadmill (1-2 METs/stage)	• 12-lead ECG, HR	• Serious dysrhythmias • >2mm ST-segment depression or elevation • Ischemic threshold • T-wave inversion with significant ST change	• Clients with COPD often have coexistent CAD.
	• BP	• SBP > 250 mmHg or DBP > 115 mmHg	
	• RPE, dyspnea scales (0-10) • Pulse oximetry/arterial PaO_2 • Respired gas analysis	 • Maximum ventilations • $\dot{V}O_2$peak • Lactate/ventilatory threshold	• Breathing pattern analysis may also be helpful.
	• Blood lactate		• Lactic acidosis may contribute to exercise limitation in some patients.
Endurance 6-min walk	• Distance	• Note rest stop distance/ time, dyspnea index, vitals	• Useful for measurement of improvement throughout conditioning program.
Strength Isokinetic/Isotonic	• Peak torque • Maximum number of reps • 1RM		
Flexibility Sit and reach	• Hip, hamstring, and lower back flexibility		
Neuromuscular Gait analysis Balance			• Body mechanics, coordination, and work efficiency are often impaired.
Functional Sit to stand Stair climbing Lifting	• Time to 10 reps		

*Measurements of particular significance; do not always indicate test termination.

Medications	Special Considerations
All of the following medications, despite potential effects, may improve exercise capacity through bronchodilation, relief of congestive heart failure, and psychotropic effects. • Methylxanthines: May cause tachycardia, cardiac dysrhythmias, and increased dyspnea.	• High risk for CAD. Worsening hypoxia during exertion may induce angina and/or dysrhythmias. • Monitoring of 12-lead ECG, BP, and oxygen saturation is essential.

Medications *(continued)*	Special Considerations *(continued)*
• Sympathomimetic bronchodilators: May cause tachycardia. • Loop and thiazide diuretics: May cause hypokalemia leading to dysrhythmias and muscle weakness. • Antidepressants: May cause tachycardia at rest and during exercise.	• Spirometry, especially maximal voluntary ventilation, is helpful in defining ventilatory limitations. • Exercise testing in mid to late morning or afternoon is desirable. Pulmonary patients often have worse symptoms in the early morning. • Medications should be taken as usual to obtain best exercise performance, especially when using test results for exercise prescription purposes. • Clients may become more dyspneic when lifting objects. Specific evaluation and training may be necessary.

hypertension, and peripheral arterial disease. The potential effects of medications for these conditions are described in chapters 4, 5, 6, 11, and 12.

• Sympathomimetic agonists (e.g., albuterol, metaproterenol, and salmeterol) are selective beta$_2$-adrenoceptor agonists intended to produce bronchodilation. However, they also reduce peripheral vascular resistance and tend to cause tachycardia, palpitations, and tremulousness. Nonselective sympathomimetic drugs (e.g., epinephrine and isoprenaline) should not be used because of unwanted effects on the cardiovascular system.

• Methylxanthines (e.g., theophylline and aminophylline) have potent bronchodilator action but also cause tachycardia, cardiac dysrhythmias, and central nervous system stimulation with increased respiratory drive and the risk of seizures.

• Thiazide diuretics (e.g., hydrochlorothiazide) and loop diuretics (e.g., furosemide) are prescribed to control fluid retention in cor pulmonale. Intravascular volume depletion might cause hypotension during exercise. Hypokalemia might predispose clients to cardiac dysrhythmias and muscle weakness.

• Glucocorticoids (e.g., prednisone) are prescribed for COPD and idiopathic pulmonary fibrosis with the hopes of reducing inflammation and improving pulmonary function. Many individuals with COPD end up on long-term glucocorticoid therapy. Important side effects that influence exercise include skin atrophy and fragility, osteoporosis, muscle atrophy, and myopathy (including the ventilatory muscles).

• Antidepressants (e.g., tricyclics), like many psychotropic drugs, cause resting and exercise tachycardia.

Recommendations for Exercise Testing

Exercise testing is extremely valuable in persons with COPD to distinguish between several possible causes of limited exercise capacity as described in this chapter's section on pathophysiology. It is also essential to identify coexistent exercise-induced hypoxemia, hypertension, cardiac dysrhythmias, or myocardial ischemia.

Maximal exercise testing is safe with appropriate monitoring and gives the best definition of the limitations, including psychological problems and symptoms. The cycle ergometer offers the best means of controlling external work rate, measuring gas exchange, and blood sampling. A typical protocol might include 3 min of unloaded pedaling followed by a ramp increase in work rate of 5, 10, 15, or 20 watts/min, depending on the degree of impairment. The aim should be to obtain between 8 and 10 min of exercise data. A constant work rate protocol on a cycle ergometer can be used repetitively to allow accurate comparison of physiological responses and to show improvements after therapeutic interventions including exercise training.

Treadmill exercise testing is helpful for the oxygen-dependent person and can be repeated with different oxygen systems and flows to determine the best means of correcting hypoxemia (see the Chronic Obstructive Pulmonary Disease: Exercise Testing table).

Recommendations for Exercise Programming

Exercise is to be encouraged in persons with COPD. The exercise prescription should be individualized and flexible to account for fluctuations in clinical status. Any significant change in the medical condition of the person requires reassessment of the goals and risks of the exercise program.

Exercise rehabilitation should involve several different professionals. Respiratory therapists evaluate, teach, and ensure effective use of bronchodilator medications and oxygen therapy. Physical therapists and exercise professionals evaluate exercise endurance, muscle strength, flexibility, and body composition. They

Chronic Obstructive Pulmonary Disease: Exercise Programming

Modes	Goals	Intensity/Frequency/Duration	Time to Goal
Aerobic • Large muscle activities (walking, cycling, swimming)	• Increase $\dot{V}O_2$peak • Increase lactate threshold and ventilatory threshold • Become less sensitive to dyspnea • Develop more efficient breathing patterns • Facilitate improvement in ADLs	• RPE 11-13/20 (comfortable, pace and endurance) • Monitor dyspnea • 1-2 sessions, 3-7 days/wk • 30 min/session (shorter intermittent exercise sessions may be necessary initially) • Emphasize progression of duration > intensity	• 2-3 mo to ensure compliance
Strength • Free weights • Isokinetic/Isotonic machines	• Increase maximal number of reps • Increase isokinetic torque/work • Increase lean body mass	• Low resistance, high reps • 2-3 days/wk	• 2-3 mo
Flexibility • Stretching • Tai chi	• Increase ROM	• 3 days/wk	
Neuromuscular • Walking, balance exercises • Breathing exercises	• Improve gait, balance • Improve breathing efficiency	• Daily	

Medications	Special Considerations
• Corticosteroids: May contribute to psychological disturbances. • See exercise testing table.	• RPE and dyspnea are the preferred methods of monitoring intensity. Many patients are unable to achieve a peak HR but still show physiological improvement. • CAD, peripheral artery disease, and musculoskeletal problems (e.g., arthritis, osteoporosis) are common in patients with COPD. • Muscular myopathy (including respiratory muscles) may be present due to corticosteroids and disuse atrophy. • Patients usually respond best to exercise in mid to late morning. • Avoid extremes in temperature and humidity. • Supplemental O_2 flow rate should be adjusted to $SaO_2 > 90\%$. • Anxiety, depression, and/or fear are common due to dyspnea and physical disability.

determine and adjust the exercise prescription and demonstrate and supervise techniques for improving flexibility, balance, and muscle strength. Occupational therapists evaluate activities of daily living and quality of life. They teach energy conservation and improved body mechanics aimed at reducing the oxygen requirement for specific activities. All therapists teach improved breathing efficiency using methods such as pursed lips and diaphragm breathing, which slow the respiratory rate.

The recommended mode of exercise training can be walking, cycling, swimming, or conditioning exercises based on energy centering and balance, such as tai chi (see the Chronic Obstructive Pulmonary Disease: Exercise Programming table). The mode of exercise selected should be one that is enjoyable and directly improves ability to perform usual daily activities. In addition to the accepted specificity of training effect in terms of muscle performance, there is some evidence that desensitization to dyspnea is task specific.

Oxygen should be administered during exercise to individuals who have had a fall in arterial oxygen tension to less than 55 mmHg or in oxyhemoglobin desaturation to less than 88%. Prevention of exercise-induced hypoxemia is likely not only to improve exercise capacity but also to enhance the effects of exercise training. The goal of oxygen therapy during exercise is to maintain an oxyhemoglobin saturation above 90%.

Modifications to the duration and frequency of exercise might be necessary. Commonly the person with chronic respiratory disease is unable to sustain 20 or 30 min of exercise, and interval exercise consisting of 5- or 10-min sessions might be necessary until adaptations have occurred that allow reduction of rest intervals and gradual increases in work intervals.

An intensive six-week exercise program with group interaction is helpful to begin the process of physical reconditioning. However, the importance of maintaining a higher level of physical activity cannot be overemphasized. The individual with COPD is at particular risk of relapsing into a state of inactivity and physical deconditioning. Membership in a health and fitness facility is worth considering.

CASE STUDY Chronic Obstructive Pulmonary Disease

A 60-year-old male was known to have COPD with emphysema. He was diagnosed 4 years ago. He had a 75 pack-year smoking history but had not smoked in 3 years. His exercise capacity varied considerably from day to day, but he generally was able to walk about half a city block and climb 15 steps at home, although he had some difficulty climbing stairs. In a motor vehicle accident 20 years ago, he sustained 5 fractures to his left lower leg and was left with a residual varus deformity of his foot. Consequently, he often walked with a cane. He used supplemental oxygen overnight at a flow rate of 2 l/min.

S: "I need help getting around."

O: Vitals: HR: 80 contractions/min BP: 140/90 mmHg Weight: 176 lb (80 kg)
Height: 5'11" (1.8 m) BMI: 24.7 kg/m²

Male, moderately dyspneic at rest, using pursed-lip breathing and accessory respiratory muscles with thoracoabdominal paradox

Chest hyperinflated and hyperresonant to percussion; breath sounds considerably diminished throughout

Heart sounds regular but indistinct; no right ventricular heave, no increased jugular venous pressure or peripheral edema

Truncal obesity; mild degree of muscle wasting affecting all limbs; left foot has a 45° varus deformity

Chest X ray: Bilateral emphysematous changes prominent in the upper lobes

Pulmonary function tests:
FVC: 45% of predicted
FEV_1: 16% of predicted with 13% improvement after bronchodilator
FEV_1/FVC: 35%
DL_{CO}: 52% of predicted

Arterial blood gas:
pH: 7.43
Pco_2: 41 mmHg
Po_2: 75 mmHg (breathing room air)

Graded exercise test (treadmill):
Speed: 0.8 mph, 0% grade
Duration: 10 min
RPE: 16/20
Breathlessness: 92/100 (visual analog scale)
Arterial Po_2 decreased to 59 mmHg

Medications: Albuterol MDI, Ipratropium MDI, Prednisone (intermittent courses)

(continued)

CASE STUDY   Chronic Obstructive Pulmonary Disease (continued)

A:
1. Severe COPD with emphysema secondary to tobacco smoking
2. Left leg deformity
3. Hypoxemia during low-intensity exercise
4. Moderate deconditioning with marked symptomatic limitation during exercise
5. Excess fat weight with loss of lean body mass

P:
1. Increase Ipratropium MDI to 4 puffs qid, and albuterol MDI to 2 puffs qid.
2. Consider Combivent MDI to improve compliance, and avoid systemic corticosteroids.
3. Prescribe portable O_2 with a flow rate of 1 l/min during exercise.
4. Initiate a multidisciplinary pulmonary rehabilitation program.

Exercise Program
Goal:

Improve functional capacity to increase and maintain ADLs

Mode	Frequency	Duration	Intensity	Progression
Aerobic	3 days/wk	30 min/session	THR (110 contractions/ min) RPE 11/20	Progress as tolerated over 6-wk program to 13/20 RPE
Strength (upper and lower extremities)	2 days/wk	2 sets of 12 reps	To fatigue	Add resistance until 12 reps achieves fatigue
Flexibility	3 days/wk	Hold 20-60 s/ stretch	Below discomfort threshold	Progress as ROM allows
Neuromuscular (walk drills, balance drills, breathing exercises)	Daily	5 min each	As tolerated	Maintain skill level
Functional (O.T.)	If needed for ADL tasks	Match to ADL tasks/needs	As tolerated	As tolerated
Warm-up/Cool-down	Before and after each session	10 min	RPE <10/20	Maintain

Suggested Readings

Casaburi, R., A. Patessio, F. Ioli, S. Zanaboni, C.F. Donner, and K. Wasserman. 1991. Reductions in exercise lactic acidosis and ventilation as a result of exercise training in patients with obstructive lung disease. *American Review of Respiratory Diseases* 143: 9-18.

Cochrane, L.M., and C.J. Clark. 1990. Benefits and problems of a physical training program for asthmatic patients. *Thorax* 45: 345-51.

Cooper, C.B. 1995. Determining the role of exercise in patients with chronic pulmonary disease. *Medicine and Science in Sports and Exercise* 27: 147-57.

Cooper, C.B. 1993. Long-term oxygen therapy. In *Principles and practice of pulmonary rehabilitation*, edited by R. Casaburi and T.L. Petty, 183-203. Philadelphia: W.B. Saunders.

Criner, G.J., and B.R. Celli. 1988. Effect of unsupported arm exercise on ventilatory muscle recruitment in patients with severe chronic airflow obstruction. *American Review of Respiratory Diseases* 138: 856-61.

Davidson, A.C., R. Leach, R.J.D. George, and D.M. Geddes. 1988. Supplemental oxygen and exercise ability in chronic obstructive airways disease. *Thorax* 43: 965-71.

Mahler, D.A. 1992. The measurement of dyspnea during exercise in patients with lung disease. *Chest* 101 (supplement 5): 2425-75.

Ries, A.L. 1990. Position paper of the American Association of Cardiovascular and Pulmonary Rehabilitation: Scientific basis of pulmonary rehabilitation. *Journal of Cardiopulmonary Rehabilitation* 10: 418-41.

CHAPTER 16

Chronic Restrictive Pulmonary Disease

Connie C.W. Hsia, MD
University of Texas Southwestern

Overview of the Pathophysiology

Restrictive pulmonary disease encompasses diverse disorders characterized by a diminished lung volume. These disorders are caused by various pathological processes involving the chest wall, respiratory muscles, nerves, pleura, and the pulmonary parenchyma, and exhibit common pathophysiological features as follows:

Etiologies

- extrapulmonary causes;
- neuromuscular disorders: muscle disorders (muscular dystrophy, myositis), phrenic nerve paralysis, neuritis, neuromuscular junction (myasthenia gravis, botulism, Eaton-Lambert syndrome), spinal cord disorders, and trauma (amyotrophic lateral sclerosis, Guillain-Barré syndrome);
- chest wall disorders: kyphoscoliosis, ankylosing; spondylitis, thoracoplasty, obesity;
- pleural disorders: fibrosis, effusion;
- pulmonary parenchymal causes;
- malignancy;
- pulmonary edema;
- major lung resection;
- radiation exposure;
- infectious agents;
- inhaled particles;
- immunologic diseases;
- drugs; and
- loss of functioning lung units.

In parenchymal lung diseases, alveolar units are destroyed or replaced by fibrous tissue. In diseases involving the pleura, chest wall, and neuromuscular system, the lung is intrinsically normal but unable to expand normally with respiration. Eventually alveolar units collapse and secondary inflammation and fibrosis develop. The common end result is a loss of alveolar surface area, leading to impaired oxygen diffusion.

Diffusion impairment is evidenced by a decline in arterial oxygen saturation, widened alveolar-arterial oxygen tension gradient, and reduced rate of gas uptake from alveolar air to capillary red cells. The latter is commonly measured as diffusing capacity for carbon monoxide (DL_{CO}).

Abnormal Mechanical Ventilatory Function

Airflow rates are reduced in proportion to the reduction in lung volume. The ratio of forced expiratory volume in 1 s to forced vital capacity (FEV_1/FVC) is normal or elevated. Ventilatory muscle strength, endurance, and mechanical efficiency are reduced especially in neuromuscular and skeletal diseases of the thorax, evidenced from reductions in maximal respiratory muscle power and maximal ventilatory capacities.

Compliance of the lung or thorax is reduced. A more negative airway pressure is required to inflate the lung with each breath; hence, respiratory muscles must work harder (i.e., the work of breathing is elevated). Dead space is increased, so minute ventilation must be higher to maintain a given level of alveolar ventilation, further increasing the work of breathing. A greater fraction of total body metabolic energy must be diverted to respiratory muscles to sustain a given level of ventilation, leaving a smaller fraction available for working limb muscles during exercise. This leads to greater lactic acid production from limb muscles, further stimulating ventilation and increasing the work of breathing.

Secondary Hemodynamic and Cardiac Dysfunction

Any pathologic process that obliterates the pulmonary vascular bed increases pulmonary vascular resistance and right ventricular afterload, resulting in a higher pulmonary artery pressure (secondary pulmonary hypertension), right heart strain, and a lower stroke volume during exercise.

Because the lungs surround the heart, forming a potential cavity called the cardiac fossa, a stiff lung reduces the compliance of the cardiac fossa and can potentially restrict diastolic ventricular filling, especially during exercise.

Cardiovascular deconditioning inevitably develops with progressive pulmonary disease and contributes to disproportional disability out of keeping with the impairment in lung function.

Effects on the Exercise Response

The client with chronic restrictive pulmonary disease will experience the following altered exercise responses:

• Reduced exercise tolerance and exertional dyspnea are common manifestations. The breathing pattern consists of rapid shallow breaths. Minute ventilation increases mainly via an increased respiratory rate rather than tidal volume.

• Reduced DL_{CO} and alveolar-arterial oxygen tension gradient measured during exercise are more sensitive indicators of diffusion impairment than measurements at rest.

• Normally DL_{CO} increases by 40 to 100% with increasing cardiac output from rest to exercise, primarily the result of the opening or distention of pulmonary capillaries that increases the surface area for gas exchange. The ability to increase DL_{CO} is essential for maintaining a normal arterial oxygen saturation during exercise. Diffuse parenchymal disease such as interstitial pulmonary fibrosis is characterized by an inability to augment DL_{CO} during exercise, associated with a marked decline in arterial oxygen saturation. In contrast, clients after major lung resection who have normal remaining lung units typically show a low lung volume; however, DL_{CO} increases normally with exercise and arterial oxygen saturation is better maintained.

• In early extrapulmonary disease, DL_{CO} is typically reduced because of a small alveolar volume (V_A), while the ratio of DL_{CO} to V_A (DL_{CO}/V_A) is normal at rest and exercise. In advanced stages, however, pulmonary fibrosis often develops and DL_{CO}/V_A also becomes impaired. In parenchymal lung disease, DL_{CO}, V_A, and DL_{CO}/V_A are all reduced.

Effects of Exercise Training

Exercise training can potentially have multiple benefits in chronic restrictive pulmonary disease, including the following:

• improved submaximal exercise endurance;

• improved maximal oxygen consumption variably, depending on existent fitness level;

• improved ventilatory endurance, efficiency, and ventilation-perfusion matching;

• improved cardiovascular conditioning;

• increased maximal DL_{CO} secondarily if maximal cardiac output increases;

• improved oxygen extraction, endurance, and efficiency of skeletal muscles;

• reduced blood flow requirement of respiratory muscles, secondarily increasing blood flow available to working limb muscles;

• reduced lactic acidosis and minimized stimulation of ventilation during exercise; and

• desensitization to the perception of dyspnea and fear of exertion.

Physical training in the client with chronic restrictive lung disease significantly enhances the feeling of well-being, even if large increases of maximal oxygen consumption do not occur. Training ensures that clients are not disproportionately debilitated more than expected from the pulmonary dysfunction and that all steps of oxygen transport are matched within the constraints imposed by the primary disorder. Training optimizes the efficiency of oxygen transport, a critical issue because clients can ill afford any metabolic energy wastage. Careful attention to long-term physical conditioning allows clients to realize the maximum benefit from concurrent specific therapy aimed at correcting the underlying disorder.

Management and Medications

Treatment of the underlying disorder often includes the following. Restrictive lung disorders are often chronic and progressive; treatment is often empirical.

Corticosteroids are prescribed for a wide variety of inflammatory disorders with the intention of reducing inflammation, retarding disease progression, and protecting lung function. Chronic drug therapy can lead to multiple complications, including obesity, skin changes, systemic hypertension, hyperglycemia, loss of bone density leading to pathological fractures, muscle atrophy, gastrointestinal ulcers, immunosuppression, and emotional disability. Steroid-induced respiratory muscle atrophy can aggravate ventilatory insufficiency in severe lung disease.

Immunosuppressive agents (e.g., methotrexate, cyclophosphamide, penicillamine, chlorambucil) are sometimes used to treat systemic immunological disorders. These agents can depress blood leukocyte count and predispose to opportunistic infections; some can directly

Chronic Restrictive Pulmonary Disease: Exercise Testing

Methods	Measures	Endpoints*	Comments
Aerobic Cycle (preferred) (ramp protocol 10, 15, or 20 watts/min; staged protocol 15-30 watts/3-min stage) Treadmill (1-2 METs/stage)	• 12-lead ECG, HR • BP • RPE, dyspnea scales (0-10) • Expired gas analysis • Pulse oximetry/arterial PaO_2 • Blood lactate	• Serious dysrhythmias • >2mm ST-segment depression or elevation • Ischemic threshold • T-wave inversion with significant ST change • SBP > 250 mmHg or DBP > 115 mmHg • Maximum ventilations • $\dot{V}O_2$peak • Lactate/ventilatory threshold	• Patients often have coexistent CAD. • Breathing pattern analysis may be helpful.
Endurance 6-min walk	• Distance	• Note time, distance, dyspnea index/vitals at rest stops	• Useful in assessing improvement during conditioning program.
Strength Isokinetic/Isotonic	• Peak torque • Number of reps • 1RM		
Flexibility Sit and reach	• Hip, hamstring, and lower back flexibility		
Neuromuscular Gait analysis			• Body mechanics, coordination, balance, and work efficiency are often impaired.
Functional Sit to stand Stair climbing Lifting	• Individualized ADLs		

*Measurements of particular significance; do not always indicate test termination.

Special Considerations

- Worsening hypoxia during exertion may induce angina and/or dysrhythmias.
- Monitoring 12-lead ECG, BP, and oxygen saturation is essential.
- Spirometry and maximal voluntary ventilation are helpful in defining ventilatory limitations.
- Exercise testing during late morning or early afternoon is preferable.
- Medications should be taken as usual to obtain the best exercise performance.

Chronic Restrictive Pulmonary Disease: Exercise Programming

Modes	Goals	Intensity/ Frequency/Duration	Time to Goal
Aerobic • Large muscle activities (walking, cycling, swimming)	• Increase $\dot{V}O_2$peak work, and endurance • Increase lactate and ventilatory threshold • Desensitize to dyspnea • Develop efficient breathing patterns • Improve ADLs	• RPE 11-13/20 (comfortable, pace and endurance) • Monitor dyspnea • 1-2 sessions/day • 3-7 days/wk • 30 min/session (shorter intermittent sessions initially) • Emphasize progression of duration > intensity	• 2-3 mo
Strength • Free weights • Isokinetic/isotonic machines	• Increase number of reps • Increase isokinetic torque/ work • Increase lean body mass	• Low resistance, high reps • 2-3 days/wk	• 2-3 mo
Flexibility • Stretching • Tai chi	• Increase ROM	• 1-3 days/wk	
Neuromuscular • Walking, balance exercises • Breathing exercises	• Improve gait, balance, and breathing efficiency	• Daily	

Medications	Special Considerations
• Corticosteroids: May cause psychological disturbances. • Methotrexate: May cause low white cell count, anemia, liver dysfunction. Predisposed to infections. Prolonged use may worsen pulmonary fibrosis. Regular clinical and laboratory monitoring by a physician is mandatory.	• RPE and dyspnea are the preferred methods of monitoring intensity. Patients who are unable to achieve a training HR can still show physiological improvement. • Coexistent CAD, peripheral artery disease, and musculoskeletal problems (e.g., arthritis, osteoporosis) are common. • Muscular dysfunction (including respiratory muscles) may be present. • Clients usually respond to exercise best in mid to late morning. • Avoid extremes in temperatures and humidity. • Supplemental O_2 flow rate should be adjusted to $SaO_2 > 90\%$. • Anxiety, depression, and/or fear are common due to dyspnea and physical disability.

cause pulmonary inflammation and fibrosis or aggravate existing fibrosis.

• Correct hypoxemia with supplemental oxygen therapy as necessary.

• General health maintenance: Optimize body weight, blood pressure, and nutrition. Control exposure to tobacco and environmental irritants. Vaccinate regularly against respiratory pathogens.

Recommendations for Exercise Testing

The goals of exercise testing include the following:

• define disability due to pulmonary dysfunction;

• detect coexistent factors that aggravate disability; and

- monitor progression of impairment and response to therapy.

Either a cycle ergometer or a treadmill can be used. Following a resistance-free warm-up period, work rate should be incremented in small steps in accordance with the severity of impairment. Electrocardiogram and transcutaneous oxygen saturation should be monitored. Supplemental oxygen may be needed during testing to maintain the oxyhemoglobin saturation above 90%. Clients unaccustomed to exercise, particularly on the cycle ergometer, should be coached in the pedaling techniques and allowed several practice runs until they are comfortable with the procedure. Meticulous attention to technical details such as proper seating, mouthpiece fitting, breathing techniques, and verbal reinforcement during testing will greatly reduce subject anxiety and enhance the quality of the measurements (see the Chronic Restrictive Pulmonary Disease: Exercise Testing table).

Recommendations for Exercise Programming

Evaluation and recommendation from the nutrition therapist, physical therapist, and occupational therapist are very helpful in understanding the client's home environment and occupational and lifestyle constraints before formulating an individualized exercise program. Simple maneuvers should be implemented first, such as learning efficient breathing techniques and improving ergonomics during daily activities to enhance metabolic energy conservation. Long-term exercise training cannot be sustained unless it is both practical and enjoyable. Maintaining subject motivation for exercise requires creativity and clear communication between therapist and client.

Walking is probably the easiest mode of exercise for most clients; it requires no special equipment, can be done at the individual's own pace, and is readily integrated into other activities of daily living. Similarly, arm and leg exercises can often be integrated with other sedentary activities such as watching television or reading (see the Chronic Restrictive Pulmonary Disease: Exercise Programming table on page 102).

In sedentary individuals, an initial period of intense training (20-30 min/day, 5 days/wk for 6-8 wk) is helpful in establishing a baseline level of fitness. Subsequently, sustained training can be continued three times a week. For clients with poor exercise endurance, a training session can be divided into several shorter segments with rest periods in between.

Regular follow-up assessment of exercise and pulmonary function should provide objective feedback of any improvement or retardation of impairment, which helps to sustain the individuals's motivation for continued training.

CASE STUDY Chronic Restrictive Pulmonary Disease

Seven years ago, a 45-year-old African-American female complained of episodic fever with sweats, fatigue, and a rash. She was found to have skin nodules and enlarged liver, spleen, and lymph nodes in the chest. Biopsies of these tissues revealed the diagnosis of sarcoidosis, a multisystem granulomatous inflammatory disease. Initially she had no respiratory complaints, but over the years she gradually developed worsening shortness of breath on exertion to where she could only walk 0.5 mi (0.8K) on a flat surface and climb a single flight of stairs without stopping. Her lung volumes and expiratory flow rate (FEV_1) have been decreasing steadily over the years, but diffusing capacity (DL_{CO}) has markedly decreased. Although she continued to work full time as an insurance clerk, she was easily fatigued. She had been treated with oral prednisone continuously since her diagnosis, and as a result suffered from the side effects of obesity, hypertension, and hyperglycemia.

S: "I can't get around very well."

O: Obese woman at rest, in no acute distress

Multiple flesh-colored skin nodules on face and legs
Bilaterally enlarged parotid glands and cervical lymph nodes
Lung sounds: Clear
Cardiovascular exam normal, no peripheral edema
Enlarged spleen and liver
Labs:
Blood counts and electrolytes: Normal
Liver enzymes: Mildly elevated
Angiotensin-converting enzyme and gamma globulins: Grossly elevated

(continued)

CASE STUDY Chronic Restrictive Pulmonary Disease *(continued)*

Chest X rays: Reticular interstitial infiltrates in both lungs

Spirometry:
FVC: 3.0 l
FEV_1: 3.0 l
DL_{CO}: 12 ml · min^{-1} · mmHg^{-1}

A: 1. Active sarcoidosis involving lung, skin, liver, lymph nodes, and spleen
2. Progressive deterioration of lung function

P: 1. Start low-dose methotrexate and reduce prednisone.
2. Conduct exercise tests to measure aerobic capacity, ventilatory response, and arterial O_2 saturation.
3. Initiate a weight-loss diet.
4. Start a regular exercise program.

Exercise Program
Goals:

1. Aid in weight loss
2. Maintain long-term physical fitness

Mode	Frequency	Duration	Intensity	Progression
Aerobic	5 days/wk	20-30 min/ session	THR (110 contractions/ min) RPE 11/20	Progress as tolerated over 6- to 8-wk program to 13/20 RPE
Strength (upper and lower extremities)	2 days/wk	2 sets of 12 reps	To fatigue	Add resistance until 12 reps achieves fatigue
Flexibility	3 days/wk	Hold 20-60 s/ stretch	Maintain each stretch below discomfort threshold	Progress as ROM allows
Neuromuscular (walk drills, balance drills, breathing exercises)	Daily	5 min	As tolerated	Maintain skill level
Functional (O.T.)	Daily	Match to ADL tasks/needs	As tolerated	As tolerated
Warm-up/Cool-down	Before and after each session	10 min	RPE <10/20	

Suggested Readings

American Thoracic Society. 1987. Single breath carbon monoxide diffusing capacity (transfer factor): Recommendations for a standard technique. *American Review of Respiratory Disease* 136: 1299-1307.

Hsia, C.C. 1999. Cardiopulmonary limitations to exercise in restrictive lung disease. *Medicine and Science in Sports and Exercise* 31 (1 supplement): S28-32.

Hsia, C.C.W., D.G. McBrayer, and M. Ramanathan. 1995. Reference values of pulmonary diffusing capacity during exercise by a rebreathing technique. *American Journal of Respiratory and Critical Care Medicine* 152: 658-65.

Hughes, J.M.B., D.N.A. Lockwood, H.A. Jones, and R.J. Clark. 1991. DL_{CO}/Q and diffusion limitation at rest and on exercise in patients with interstitial fibrosis. *Respiration Physiology* 83: 155-66.

Reynolds, H.Y., and R.B. George, eds. 1995. Interstitial lung disease: Occupational and environmental lung diseases, diseases of the pleura. In *Pulmonary and critical care medicine*, edited by R.C. Bone. Vol. 2, parts M, N, O. St. Louis: Mosby.

West, J.B. 1998. *Pulmonary pathophysiology*. 5th ed. Baltimore: Lippincott Williams & Wilkins.

CHAPTER 17

Asthma

Christopher J. Clark, MD
Hairmyers Hospital

Overview of the Pathophysiology

Bronchial asthma is a syndrome characterized by reversible obstruction to airflow and increased bronchial responsiveness to a variety of stimuli, both allergic and environmental. In persons with asthma, there are three issues influencing exercise performance and athletic competition:

- variability between individuals in severity;
- variability within individuals (exacerbations or attacks, and recovery); and
- interactions between physiological and psychological response to exercise.

There is wide variability between individuals in disease severity, ranging from very mild asthma to severe disease. Some mild cases are only symptomatic when provoked by stimuli such as allergens or exercise. In contrast, severe disease is characterized by largely irreversible airflow obstruction, despite optimal medication. Mild asthma allows participation in athletic competition at the highest level, whereas severe asthma can markedly impair physical function.

Asthma has significant variability in disease severity within each individual, with intermittent exacerbations and remissions. This background liability of airway obstruction influences ability to exercise. Thus, for an individual with asthma, exercise program planning must take into account and respond to fluctuations of asthma severity.

Asthma is a chronic illness often arising during early childhood. Thus, many longstanding misconceptions about the effect of exercise on the illness may exist. In someone with asthma, exercise is not only limited by the disease but also can act as a direct stimulus to exacerbate the disease. As a consequence, some persons with asthma develop an aversion to exercise, although this varies depending on psychosocial variables such as prior attitudes toward exercise, education, social circumstances, and the individual personality.

In considering exercise, the asthmatic population can be grouped into three categories:

- exercise-induced asthma without other symptoms;
- mild asthma (ventilatory limitation does not restrain submaximal exercise); and
- moderate-severe asthma (ventilatory limitation restrains submaximal exercise).

Exercise-induced asthma (EIA) is a syndrome characterized by transient airway obstruction usually occurring 5 to 15 min following physical exertion. Symptoms consist of wheezing, coughing, shortness of breath, chest discomfort, or a combination of these, lasting up to 30 min following exercise cessation. There is some continuing debate as to whether a small subgroup of clients with EIA also have a late reaction (i.e., a further episode of airway obstruction 4-6 h later). The mechanism of EIA is not fully known, but it may be respiratory heat loss, increased osmolality caused by respiratory water loss, or associated vascular events. Increasing minute ventilation during exercise is a potent stimulus to EIA.

If exercise is prolonged, asthma may develop during physical exertion. The physical exertion required to produce symptoms is usually equivalent to an intensity of 75% predicted maximal heart rate. In clients with severe asthma, however, very mild exertion can provoke severe airflow obstruction. Though exercise may provoke an asthmatic episode, exercise should be incorporated in the management plan.

Effects on the Exercise Response

When EIA is well-controlled, there is no effect on the exercise response. In an individual with EIA, during submaximal exercise that is insufficient to induce the asthmatic response, the exercise response is essentially unaffected. During exercise that does induce the asthmatic response, the exercise response is proportional to the ventilatory limitation imposed by the restriction in airflow. In most cases, the symptoms of breathlessness are sufficient to cause the person to stop exercising. In any event, the induction of an asthma exacerbation signifies a need for more intensive medical management to prevent asthma attacks.

Effects of Exercise Training

The situation of adaptability to training is similar to that of the single exercise session response. When EIA is well controlled, asthma has no effect on the adaptations to exercise training. Therefore, one would expect to see good improvements in fitness when adhering to a standard exercise program to improve fitness. In an individual who has submaximal exercise limited by EIA, the exercise intensity is usually insufficient to increase fitness but may increase endurance.

Management and Medications

The most important treatment is the use of a beta-selective sympathomimetic agonist before exercise (ap-

proximately 10 min). The more recently introduced long-acting beta agonists (e.g., salmeterol) extend the period of protection, but the length of time that the drug remains active after a single dose decreases. Thus, it is suggested than long-acting beta agonists might be reserved as a preference for clients who are physically active for more than 30 to 60 min/day. Also, the long-acting beta agonist may be useful for someone in whom objective measures of airflow obstruction demonstrate a late reaction. Protection for some persons with EIA might be provided by leukotriene-receptor antagonists. These medications have some practical advantages, including a protective effect lasting over 24 hours, a single daily dose administration by mouth, and no major adverse effects.

A variety of other agents have variable benefit against EIA. In persons with asthma at rest who also show manifestations of EIA, prophylactic medication such as inhaled steroids should be used in combination with beta agonists. Inhaled steroids reduce susceptibility to EIA when given over 1 to 4 weeks of treatment.

Asthma: Exercise Testing

Methods	Measures	Endpoints	Comments
For individuals undergoing a diagnostic test: Cycle Treadmill (constant load test)	• 12-lead ECG, HR • BP • RPE, dyspnea scale (0-10) • Spirometry before and 8 min after exercise	• 8 min @ ≥ 75% max HR • Decreased FEV_1 of 15% • Decreased peak flow of 20%	• Provide adequate warm-up. • No inhalers or oral bronchodilators.

Medications	Special Considerations
All of the following medications, despite potential side effects, may improve exercise capacity through bronchodilation, relief of congestive heart failure, and psychotropic effects: • Methylxanthines: May cause tachycardia, cardiac dysrhythmias, and increased dyspnea. • Sympathomimetic bronchodilators: May cause tachycardia. • Loop and thiazide diuretics: May cause hypokalemia leading to dysrhythmias and muscle weakness.	• Walking/jogging may be more asthmogenic. • High risk for CAD. Worsening hypoxia during exertion may include angina and/or dysrhythmias. • Monitoring of 12-lead ECG, BP, and oxygen saturation is essential. • Spirometry, especially maximal voluntary ventilation, is helpful in defining ventilatory limitations. • Testing in mid to late morning or afternoon is desirable. Chronic asthma patients often have worse symptoms in the early morning. • Medications should be taken as usual to obtain best exercise performance, especially when using test results for exercise prescription purposes. • Clients may be come more dyspneic when lifting objects. Specific evaluation and training may be necessary. • Several min of warm-up and cool-down may help reduce the likelihood of EIA.

Asthma: Exercise Programming

Modes	Goals	Intensity/ Frequency/Duration	Time to Goal
Aerobic • Large muscle activities	• Increase $\dot{V}O_2$ peak (e.g., walking, cycling, swimming) • Increase lactate threshold and ventilatory threshold • Become less sensitive to dyspnea • Develop more efficient breathing patterns • Facilitate improvement in ADLs	• RPE 11-13/20 (comfortable, pace and endurance) • Monitor dyspnea • 1-2 sessions, 3-7 days/wk • 30 min/session (shorter intermittent sessions may be necessary initially) • Emphasize progression of duration > intensity	• 2-3 mo
Strength • Free weights • Isotonic/Isokinetic machines	• Increase maximal number of reps • Increase isokinetic torque/ work • Increase lean body mass	• Low resistance, high reps • 2-3 days/wk	• 2-3 mo
Flexibility • Stretching	• Increase ROM	• 3 sessions/wk	
Neuromuscular • Walking • Balance exercises • Breathing exercises	• Improve gait, balance • Improve breathing efficiency	• Daily	

*For individuals with EIA controlled by medications, or those with mild asthma (FEV_1 = 60-80% predicted), use ACSM recommendations for normal sedentary persons.

*For individuals with moderate asthma (FEV_1 = 40-60% predicted), use this table.

*For individuals with severe asthma (FEV_1 < 40% predicted), see chapter 15.

Medications	Special Considerations
• Corticosteroids: May contribute to psychological disturbances. • See exercise testing table.	• RPE and dyspnea are the preferred methods of monitoring intensity. Many patients are unable to achieve a high target HR but still show physiological improvement. • CAD, peripheral artery disease, and musculoskeletal problems (e.g., arthritis, osteoporosis) are common in older patients with chronic asthma. • Muscular myopathy (including respiratory muscles) may be present due to corticosteroids and disuse atrophy. • Patients usually respond best to exercise in mid to late morning. • Avoid extremes in temperature and humidity. • Supplemental O_2 flow rate should be adjusted to SaO_2 > 90%. • Anxiety, depression, and/or fear are common due to dyspnea and physical disability. • Several min of warm-up and cool-down may reduce the likelihood of EIA.

It should also be noted that any related condition such as sinusitis, nasal polyps, and so on should be treated to optimize exercise capability.

Recommendations for Exercise Testing

In a person with well-controlled asthma, standard exercise tests can be used to assess physical fitness and the response to exercise. In someone with asthma that is not diagnosed or not in control, exercise testing can be used to make the diagnosis or assess the quality of control.

A common misconception is that EIA is distinct from other forms of asthma. In reality, many asthmatics suffer from EIA when formally given a challenge test. Testing for EIA can be erroneous unless several criteria are fulfilled:

- intensity (75% predicted maximum heart rate or greater);
- duration (8 min exercise at that intensity, following a warm-up period); and
- measurement of airflow obstruction 6 to 8 min after cessation of exercise.

The delay in measuring airflow allows for the development of an immediate (type I) hypersensitivity response. EIA is defined as:

- a fall in either FEV_1 of 15% from baseline, or
- a fall in peak flow of 20% from baseline.

Some individuals experience breathlessness during and after exercise despite medical treatment. Such persons require documentation of pre- to post-exercise changes in peak flow, plus a progressive incremental exercise test to determine the specific cause of exercise limitation. Remember, this type of study is not steady state and, thus, is not a substitute for the formal exercise challenge test specifically required for the diagnosis of EIA (see the Asthma: Exercise Testing table on page 106).

Recommendations for Exercise Programming

The exercise professional must identify realistic outcome targets for the program, which may include improvement of one or all of the following (see the Asthma: Exercise Programming table on page 107):

- fitness as judged by usual physiological criteria;

- exercise tolerance without necessarily improving physiological fitness; and
- musculoskeletal conditioning (i.e., daily kinetic function and activities of daily living).

Improved Fitness

Improving fitness requires participation in a standard aerobic training program, similar to that for previously sedentary normal subjects, where intensity, frequency, duration, and longevity of program are prescribed according to ACSM recommendations for healthy sedentary persons. In practice, persons with EIA only, or with mild asthma (American Thoracic Society criteria: FEV_1 = 60-80% of predicted), can usually participate in and complete such programs. There should be a six-week introductory period during which the client learns to self-monitor exercise intensity.

We also recommend use of the Borg scale to assess the intensity of breathlessness associated with physical activity. Familiarization with this scale can ameliorate the fear of difficulty in breathing, especially when combined with optimal premedication and measurement of peak flow. If peak flow measurements indicate that EIA is not fully controlled, changes in medication should be considered before undertaking an extensive exercise program. The importance of this preparatory process cannot be underestimated.

Improved Exercise Tolerance

Achieving improved exercise tolerance allows more flexibility in terms of the prescribed exercise intensity, and is most appropriate for persons with moderate to severe asthma. Nevertheless, the objective should be to encourage clients to exercise at a work rate that represents a relatively high proportion of their maximal exercise tolerance (e.g., 60% of maximal work rate). Frequency, duration, and length of exercise training program are similar to ACSM recommendations for increased fitness in healthy sedentary persons.

For those individuals with some restriction in exercise tolerance caused by ventilatory limitation, use of the Borg scale for breathlessness allows a comfortable target level of exercise intensity. As a general rule, those with moderate airflow obstruction (American Thoracic Society criteria: FEV_1 = 40-60% of predicted) should be considered the prime target population, with the option of moving to higher-intensity programs if they achieve more rigid control of their asthma. Programs should involve aerobic exercise (e.g., brisk walking, jogging, step-ups, rowing) using an exercise intensity determined as "maximal tolerable" for required session duration.

Musculoskeletal Conditioning

This approach is best considered:

- for the most severe asthmatic individuals (ATS criteria $FEV_1 < 40\%$ predicted);

- as an introduction to exercise for previously very sedentary individuals; and

- during recovery from exacerbations that prevent participation in the usual program.

Musculoskeletal conditioning uses a series of circuit training exercises of the various limb muscle groups, either unloaded with relatively high frequency exercises to build endurance and flexibility or loaded to build strength as an addition to endurance training. Both forms improve exercise performance in persons with chronic airflow obstruction and provide a range of performance requirements to address the needs of all but the most severe asthmatics.

CASE STUDY Asthma

A 20-year-old female college student had a history of asthma from 8 years of age. She had episodic attacks of "wheezy bronchitis," which responded to inhaled bronchodilator therapy, and the frequency and severity of these asthma attacks were successfully suppressed with regular use of sodium cromoglycate. She had been able to perform to a high athletic standard and earned a position on the U.K. international ice skating squad at age 17.

Recently, she complained of a deterioration in her asthma despite escalating therapy. She needed more of an inhaled short-acting beta-2 agonist (albuterol), despite maintenance on an inhaled corticosteroid (beclomethasone 400 g bid) and the recent introductions of a long-acting inhaled beta-2 agonist (salmeterol) as well as a leukotriene antagonist (montelukast). Her skating performance had deteriorated because of fatigue and breathlessness both during and after performance. She was unsure whether her asthma was causing her decrease in exercise tolerance or if this was a case of detraining for reasons unknown, and she was quite anxious both to maintain her competitive sporting activity and to keep her asthma under control.

S: "I think my asthma is hurting my spot on the national team."

O: Young woman at rest, in no respiratory distress

Breath sounds normal, with no rhonchi or wheezes

Chest X ray: Normal lung fields with no evidence of hyperinflation

Spirometry:
  FVC, FEV_1, and FEV_1/FVC: Normal
  Residual volume: 120% of predicted (mild air trapping)
  $D_{L_{CO}}$: Normal
  Diurnal peak flow: < 20% variability (night and morning)

Graded exercise test:
  FEV_1 measured after 6-8 min of exercise at ~75% predicted maximum HR
  60% decrease in FEV_1
  Repeated on medications (including inhaled albuterol 10 min beforehand)
  15% decrease in FEV_1

Maximal graded exercise test:
  Maximal HR: 200 contractions/min (100% of predicted)
  Maximal minute ventilation: 50 l/min (45% of predicted)
  $\dot{V}O_2$max: 26 ml · kg^{-1} · min^{-1} (65% of predicted)

Dynamic kinanometry:
  Normal isokinetic quadriceps strength and endurance

A: 1. Severe EIA

2. Low aerobic exercise tolerance

3. Normal quadriceps strength

(continued)

CASE STUDY Asthma *(continued)*

P:
1. Advise that high level aerobic activities may be limited by asthma.
2. Initiate a self-management program based on peak flow measurement.
3. Switch to noncompetitive sporting activities.

Exercise Program
Goal:

Maintain normal ADLs

Mode	Frequency	Duration	Intensity	Progression
Aerobic	3-7 days/wk	30-45 min/ session	RPE 11-14/20	Maintain current level
Strength (all major muscle groups)	2-3 days/wk	1-2 sets of 8-12 reps	To fatigue	Maintain current level
Flexibility (all major muscle groups)	3-7 days/wk	20-60 s/stretch	Maintain stretch below discomfort point	Maintain current level
Neuromuscular				
Functional				
Warm-up/Cool-down	Before and after each session	10-15 min	RPE <10/20	

Suggested Readings

American Thoracic Society. 1981. Evaluation of impairment/ disability secondary to respiratory disease. *American Review of Respiratory Diseases* 124: 663-66.

Anderson, S.D. 1988. Exercise-induced asthma. In *Allergy: Principles and practice*, edited by E. Middleton, C. Reed, E. Ellis et al. St. Louis: C.V. Mosby.

Clark, C.J., and L.M. Cochrane. 1999. Physical activity and asthma. *Current Opinion in Pulmonary Medicine* 5: 68-75.

Clark, C.J., L. Cochrane, and E. Mackay. 1966. Low-intensity peripheral muscle conditioning improves exercise tolerance and breathlessness in COPD. *European Respiratory Journal* 9: 2590-96.

Morton, A.R. 1995. Asthma. In *Science and medicine in sport*, edited by J. Bloomfield, P.A. Fricker, and K.D. Fitch. 2nd ed. Carlton, South Victoria (Australia): Blackwell Science.

Morton, A.R., and K.D. Fitch. 1993. Asthma. In *Exercise testing and exercise prescription for special cases*, edited by J.S. Skinner. 2nd ed. Philadelphia: Lea & Febiger.

Morton, A.R., and K.D. Fitch. 1990. Exercise-induced bronchial obstruction. In *Current therapy in sports medicine 2*, edited by J.S. Torg, R.P. Welsh, and R.J. Shephard. Toronto: B.C. Decker.

Tan, R.A., and S.L. Spector. 1998. Exercise-induced asthma (review). *Sports Medicine* 25: 1-6.

CHAPTER 18

Cystic Fibrosis

Patricia A. Nixon, PhD, FACSM
Wake Forest University

Overview of the Pathophysiology

Cystic fibrosis (CF) is the most common inherited life-shortening disease in white populations, occurring in 1 in 3,300 live births. The genetic defect causes abnormal epithelial transport of chloride ions, excessive sodium ion resorption, and subsequent extracellular dehydration that results in abnormally salty sweat and thick mucus that clogs ducts, tubes, and tubules. The two organs most adversely affected by the mucus blockage are the pancreas and the lungs. In the pancreas, mucus prevents digestive enzymes from reaching the small intestine to digest fats and proteins, leading to malnutrition and poor growth. In the lungs, the thick mucus blocks the airways and leads to infection, inflammation, and eventually fibrosis and irreversible loss of pulmonary function. The pulmonary involvement accounts for over 90% of the mortality.

Effects on the Exercise Response

Many healthier persons with CF have normal aerobic fitness and normal cardiorespiratory responses to a single session of exercise. However, as the disease progresses and pulmonary function deteriorates, exercise tolerance diminishes. During exercise, individuals must use greater minute ventilation to compensate for airway obstruction and increased dead space. Consequently, the ratio of peak minute ventilation to maximal voluntary ventilation ($\dot{V}_E$/MVV) often exceeds the normal range of 60 to 70%, limiting mechanical ventilatory reserve. Most persons with mild to moderate lung disease are able to maintain adequate gas exchange, although those with more severe lung disease may exhibit oxyhemoglobin desaturation and carbon dioxide retention during exercise.

The likelihood that oxyhemoglobin desaturation will fall below 90% during exercise increases in persons with a forced expiratory volume for 1 s (FEV_1) of less than 50% of the predicted value. Peak heart rate may reach age-predicted maximal levels in healthier persons. However, ventilatory factors may prevent the cardiovascular system from being maximally stressed in persons with worse lung disease, resulting in peak heart rates that are below age-predicted maximal values. In addition, exercise capacity may be limited by peripheral factors associated with deconditioning and malnutrition. Furthermore, in people with very severe lung disease, $\dot{V}_E$/MVV and heart rate at peak exercise may be well below normal, suggesting that other factors such as chest pain, sensations of dyspnea, excessive coughing, or other peripheral factors may limit exercise. During submaximal exercise, oxygen consumption, minute ventilation, and heart rate may be disproportionately high, possibly as a result of physical deconditioning, increased work of breathing, hypoxemia, or any combination of these factors.

Effects of Exercise Training

To date, only one randomized controlled trial has examined the effects of long-term aerobic exercise intervention in persons with CF. Existing research suggests that individuals with CF may derive the following benefits from aerobic exercise training:

- increase in physical work capacity and peak oxygen consumption;
- increase in ventilatory muscle endurance;
- improvement in cardiopulmonary efficiency for a given submaximal work rate;
- greater mucus clearance; and
- temporary increase or delayed deterioration in some indices of pulmonary function.

Higher levels of aerobic fitness have been associated with better quality of well-being and with eight-year survival. However, it is not known whether quality of well-being and survival probability can be improved via exercise training. Individuals may also benefit from upper body weight training through an increase in muscle strength as well as a decrease in air trapping in the lungs. Interventions aimed at improving nutritional status may also improve exercise capacity.

Management and Medications

Standard treatment for individuals with CF now includes:

- oral pancreatic enzyme supplements to enhance digestion of dietary fats and proteins and improve nutritional status;
- chest physical therapy to facilitate mucus clearance from the airways;
- bronchodilator therapy to open airways; and
- antibiotic therapy to fight pulmonary infection.

With the exception of supplemental oxygen, the effects of the following medications on exercise tolerance and responses to exercise have not been studied specifically in persons with CF. Consequently, the following effects are speculative.

- Pancreatic enzyme supplements may indirectly improve exercise capacity by improving nutrition and growth.
- Inhaled bronchodilator (albuterol, ipratropium) therapy may improve exercise tolerance and gas exchange and may reduce exercise-induced bronchospasm, but can also cause tachycardia and cough.
- Oral bronchodilator (theophylline) therapy can cause tachycardia, ventricular dysrhythmia, and tachypnea.
- Anti-inflammatory agents may improve exercise tolerance by reducing airway inflammation and bronchial hyperreactivity.
- Sodium cromolyn and Nedocromil (inhaled) in chronic and acute administration may improve exercise tolerance by diminishing or preventing bronchoconstriction, particularly exercise-induced bronchoconstriction.
- Corticosteroids (inhaled) used on a long-term basis may improve exercise tolerance by reducing bronchial hyperreactivity but may cause effects similar to those of oral corticosteroids if systemically absorbed.
- Corticosteroids (oral) used on a long-term basis may improve exercise tolerance by reducing bronchial hyperreactivity but can cause weight gain, retard growth, and result in below-normal exercise capacity for age. Prolonged use of oral steroids may result in skeletal muscle (including ventilatory muscle) weakness and myopathy that may reduce exercise capacity, as well as elevated blood pressure at rest and during exercise.
- Mucolytic therapy reduces the viscosity of mucus.
- Recombinant human DNase effects on exercise tolerance are not known.

- Insulin may improve exercise tolerance in individuals with diabetes.
- Supplemental oxygen improves oxyhemoglobin saturation at rest and during exercise, and improves cardiopulmonary efficiency (i.e., lower heart rate and minute ventilation) during submaximal and maximal exercise, but may not increase peak oxygen consumption or physical work capacity.

Optimal exercise test results may be obtained if persons undergo testing after chest physiotherapy and bronchodilator therapy. It should be noted, however, that some have a negative or adverse response to bronchodilator therapy and consequently should not include it as part of their treatment.

Recommendations for Exercise Testing

The primary objectives for exercise testing persons with CF are to:

- assess disease severity;
- assess physical work capacity and aerobic fitness;
- observe cardiorespiratory and metabolic responses to exercise;
- observe oxyhemoglobin saturation during exercise;
- provide a basis for prescribing exercise within safe limits; and
- assess changes in fitness and cardiorespiratory responses to exercise that occur with disease progression or medical intervention (e.g., pharmacologic and/or exercise).

Physical work capacity and aerobic fitness are ideally evaluated by a progressive maximal exercise test (see the Cystic Fibrosis: Exercise Testing table). Peak heart rate cannot be estimated from age-predicted equations and therefore must be obtained from a maximal exercise test. Pediatric clients should be tested using a standard pediatric protocol that has established normative data for comparison (e.g., Godfrey protocol). Exercise testing equipment may need to be modified to accommodate children and smaller individuals.

Oxyhemoglobin saturation should be monitored particularly in clients with an FEV_1 less than 50% of the predicted value. If oxyhemoglobin desaturation occurs with the maximal test, a steady-state submaximal test or 6-min walk test should be done because it is not uncommon for greater desaturation to occur with sustained submaximal exercise. If the purpose of the exercise test is

Cystic Fibrosis: Exercise Testing

Methods	Measures	Endpoints	Comments
Aerobic Cycle (preferred) (ramp protocol 10-15 watts/min; staged protocol 25 watts/3 min stage) Treadmill (1 METs/stage)	• HR, BP • Physical work capacity • Respired gas analysis • Oximetry (SaO_2) • ECG • Spirometry • $\dot{V}O_2$peak; $\dot{V}_E$peak/MVV	• Volitional fatigue • End-tidal CO_2 • SaO_2 < 80% may occur	• Increased risk of SaO_2 < 91% or end-tidal CO_2 if FEV_1 < 50% of predicted. • Peak HR may be age-predicted; corticosteroids often increase BP. • ECG usually normal, but may show cor pulmonale in end-stage CF.
Endurance 6-min walk		• Distance covered, HR, SaO_2	• Most useful in persons with very limited exercise tolerance and in persons who exhibit oxyhemoglobin desaturation with exercise.
Anaerobic Wingate protocol	• Peak power output		• May reflect nutritional status.

Medications	Special Considerations
• Beta agonists have a bronchodilator effect in most persons but may cause tachycardia. • Inhaled and oral corticosteroids reduce airway inflammation and bronchospasm; oral steroids may cause truncal obesity, myopathy, diabetes, and hypertension. • Cromolyn diminishes or prevents exercise-induced brochospasm. • Theophylline has a bronchodilator effect but may cause tachycardia, ventricular ectopy, and tachypnea. • Ipratropium has a bronchodilatory effect but may cause tachycardia. • Supplemental oxygen may prevent desaturation, attenuate HR and $\dot{V}_E$, and cause relative hypoventilation.	• May need to adapt equipment to small persons. • Use supplemental O_2 in persons with hypoxemia if exercise tests are being used for exercise programming. • Premedication with bronchodilator therapy may provide optimal results.

to provide a basis for prescribing exercise, persons who exhibit oxyhemoglobin desaturation at rest or during exercise should be tested while breathing supplemental oxygen. To terminate the test because of marked oxyhemoglobin desaturation (for instance, < 80%) may be overly cautious, since no irreversible or harmful effects of short-term hypoxemia have been reported in this population. Submaximal steady-state exercise testing or self-paced walk tests (e.g., 6-min) may be useful for examining cardiorespiratory responses and oxyhemoglobin desaturation with exercise or changes in response to intervention, particularly in severely ill persons for whom a maximal exercise test may be unduly stressful and provide limited information. Exercise may induce excessive coughing in some individuals, causing them to terminate exercise. However, the majority of persons, despite

their obstructive lung disease, report leg fatigue as the reason for terminating exercise, particularly on the cycle ergometer.

Recommendations for Exercise Programming

The primary aim of exercise training is to improve aerobic fitness. The majority of individuals with CF should be able to engage in continuous aerobic exercise for 20 to 30 min at a moderate intensity (i.e., at 60 to 80% of peak heart rate). Persons with severe lung disease may need to intersperse rest periods with exercise and may also require supplemental oxygen during training. Training may be better tolerated and optimal benefits gained

Cystic Fibrosis: Exercise Programming

Modes	Goals	Intensity/ Frequency/Duration	Time to Goal
Aerobic • Large muscle activities (walking, biking, rowing, swimming, jogging)	• Increase $\dot{V}O_2$peak, peak work rate, and endurance • Decrease $\dot{V}_E$, HR, and RPE, and increase SaO_2 at a given work rate. • Increase respiratory muscle endurance • Facilitate mucus clearance	• 60-85% peak heart rate (Karvonen) • 3-4 days/wk; sicker patients may need 2 daily sessions • Start at 10 min, build in 1-min increments to 20-30 min • Monitor HR, or SaO_2 in hypoxemic persons • RPE/dyspnea scales sometimes useful • Emphasize duration over intensity	• 2-3 mo or more
Functional • Activity-specific	• Increase/maintain function and ADLs	• Optimal programming not known	
Strength • Large muscle activities	• Increase strength and endurance • Decrease steroid myopathy • Decrease air trapping	• Start with 3 sets of 10 reps, light resistance • Optimal programming unknown	• 6-12 wk or more

Medications	Special Considerations
• Bronchodilator premedication may enhance training effect in persons with a response to bronchodilators. • Steroid myopathy may not reverse with training, and may cause diabetes/hypertension complications for exercise. • Supplemental O_2 may enhance training effect due to increased oxygenation causing decreased HR.	• Monitor SaO_2 at the beginning of the program to determine the level of O_2 supplement. • Severe disease can cause hypertrophic pulmonary osteoarthropathy and bone pain during exercise. • Beware of the risk and presence of diabetes. • End-stage lung disease may cause cor pulmonale and severely limit training intensity.

if training is performed after chest physiotherapy and bronchodilator therapy (in persons who have a positive response to bronchodilator therapy). Standard exercise equipment may need to be adapted to fit children and smaller individuals. Clients should be encouraged to adopt lifestyle changes that include aerobic activities such as walking, jogging, biking, and swimming (see the Cystic Fibrosis: Exercise Programming table). Exercise intensity may need to be altered during an exacerbation of pulmonary infection commonly experienced by individuals with CF. At such times, clients are most likely to attain their target heart rates at a less intense work rate.

Special Considerations

Exercise training in a supervised and monitored setting is not necessary for the majority of persons with CF. However, it may be prudent initially to monitor oxyhemoglobin saturation in hypoxemic persons to determine the desired amount of oxygen supplementation. Some persons with CF may also have asthma or exercise-induced asthma and may require inhaled bronchodilator or sodium cromolyn therapy prior to physical activities that might provoke bronchoconstriction. Despite losing excessive salt through sweating, people with CF appear to be able to maintain adequate thermoregulation during shorter periods of exercise in the heat. Longer periods of exercise in the heat may warrant increased fluid and dietary salt intake.

Some persons with more severe lung disease may experience bone or joint pain in the legs, particularly in the knees. The pain may be attributed to hypertrophic pulmonary osteoarthropathy, seen as an elevated periosteum upon X ray examination.

With increasing age, it is estimated that nearly 50% of persons with CF develop impaired glucose tolerance and that 6 to 10% develop overt diabetes. The risk of diabetes increases with each decade of life and may be exacerbated by oral corticosteroid treatment. Exercise testing and training for these individuals should follow the recommendations outlined in chapter 21.

Finally, some persons with severe or end-stage lung disease may have evidence of cor pulmonale (right ventricular hypertrophy) and even right ventricular failure. For these individuals, submaximal exercise testing may be indicated, and exercise training should be of low intensity and aimed at improving functional capacity with respect to activities of daily living.

CASE STUDY Cystic Fibrosis

A 14-year-old female with CF complained of having trouble keeping up with her friends when shopping at the mall. CF was suspected at birth when she was born with meconium ileus, and it was subsequently verified by a sweat test. She was pancreatic insufficient and took pancreatic enzyme supplements with meals and snacks. She had a history of frequent exacerbations of pulmonary infections that have required two-week hospitalizations for each episode. She missed approximately five days of school per month because of fatigue from coughing a lot during the night and had to be excused from class about three times per week because of excessive coughing. The cough was sometimes productive, more so after she did chest physiotherapy (twice a day). Her appetite was diminished, and she thought she had lost some weight recently (5 lb [2.3 kg]).

S: "I get short of breath and cough a lot when I walk between classes at school."

O: Vitals: Height: 5'0" (1.52 m) Weight: 85 lb (38.56 kg) BMI: 16.68 kg/m²
HR: 98 contractions/min BP: 110/80 mmHg Respiration: 20 breaths/min

Thin adolescent female; cannot talk without getting dyspneic

Pectus excavatum, increased thoracic diameter, digital clubbing

Resting oxyhemoglobin saturation: 96% (room air)

FVC: 80% of predicted

FEV_1: 40% of predicted (10% decrease from 1 mo ago)

A: 1. Cystic fibrosis with severe airway obstruction
2. Exacerbation of pulmonary infection
3. Chronic undernutrition with recent weight loss

P: 1. Increase chest physical therapy to qid.
2. Prescribe inhaled aerosolized tobramycin 80 mg bid.
3. Prescribe a high-calorie liquid nutrient at snack time bid.
4. Evaluate exercise tolerance via progressive graded exercise test (consider 6-min walk if oxyhemoglobin desaturates during graded exercise test).
5. Follow up in 3 wk.
6. Repeat exercise testing when clinically stable to provide basis for developing an exercise prescription promoting cardiorespiratory endurance.
7. No exercise program is recommended until exacerbation of CF is resolved.

Suggested Readings

Cerny, F.J., T.P. Pullano, and G.J. Cropp. 1982. Cardiorespiratory adaptations to exercise in cystic fibrosis. *American Review of Respiratory Diseases* 126 (2): 217-20.

Godfrey, S. 1974. *Exercise testing in children.* Philadelphia: W.B. Saunders.

Nixon, P.A. 1996. Role of exercise in the diagnosis and management of pulmonary disease in children and youth. *Medicine and Science in Sports and Exercise* 28 (4): 414-20.

Nixon, P.A., M.L. Joswiak, and F.J. Fricker. 1996. A six-minute walk test for assessing exercise tolerance in severely ill children. *Journal of Pediatrics* 129: 362-66.

Nixon, P.A., D.M. Orenstein, S.E. Curtis, and E.A. Ross. 1990. Oxygen supplementation during exercise in cystic fibrosis. *American Review of Respiratory Disease* 142 (4): 807-11.

Nixon, P.A., D.M. Orenstein, S.F. Kelsey, and C.F. Doershuk. 1992. The prognostic value of exercise testing in patients with cystic fibrosis. *New England Journal of Medicine* 327: 1785-88.

Orenstein, D.M., K.G. Henke, D.L. Costill, C.F. Doershuk, P.J. Lemon, and R.C. Stern. 1983. Exercise and heat stress in cystic fibrosis patients. *Pediatric Research* 17: 267-69.

Orenstein, D.M., and P.A. Nixon. 1989. Patients with cystic fibrosis. In *Exercise in modern medicine*, edited by B.A. Franklin, S. Gordon, and C.G. Timmis, 204-14. Baltimore: Williams & Wilkins.

Orenstein, D.M., and B.E. Noyes. 1993. Cystic fibrosis. In *Principles and practice of pulmonary rehabilitation*, edited by R. Casaburi and T.L. Petty, 439-58. Philadelphia: W.B. Saunders.

Schneiderman-Walker, J., S.L. Pollock, M. Corey, D.D. Wilkes, G.J. Canny, L. Pedder, and J.J. Reisman. 2000. A randomized controlled trial of a 3-year home exercise program in cystic fibrosis. *Journal of Pediatrics* 136: 304-10.

Wood, R.E., T.F. Boat, and C.F. Doershuk. 1976. State of the art: Cystic fibrosis. *American Review of Respiratory Disease* 113: 833-78.

CHAPTER 19

Lung and Heart-Lung Transplantation

David J. Ross, MD
UCLA School of Medicine

Overview of the Pathophysiology

Since the first human lung transplant was attempted in June 1963 by Hardy and colleagues, over 8,000 lung and heart-lung transplant procedures have been performed. One-year actuarial survival now approaches 75 to 80% after lung transplantation, which compares favorably with the sobering 18 days as witnessed for the initially reported case. Since the introduction during the early 1980s of cyclosporine, a calcineurin inhibitor-type of immunosuppressive medication, lung and heart-lung transplantation have became clinically successful endeavors for myriad end-stage cardiopulmonary diseases.

The physiologic responses observed posttransplant, however, reflect not the attributes of the allograft lung but rather an admixture of responses as determined by the nature of each patient's native lung disease, state of conditioning, and type of transplant procedure (e.g., single or bilateral lung, heart-lung transplant). Furthermore, potential adverse effects of immunosuppressive drugs may affect the physiologic responses to exercise after transplantation. A thorough discussion regarding the clinical management of these complicated patients is beyond the scope of this text; however, familiarity with their complex exercise physiology should aid exercise prescription and successful rehabilitation.

The type of surgical procedure is determined in light of several key factors: the native cardiopulmonary disease, recipient age, and scarcity of donor organs. In the United States, approximately 74,000 patients currently await solid organ transplantation, while nearly 4,000 specifically require either lung or heart-lung organ donation. Therefore, single lung transplant (SLT) procedures are frequently pursued for older recipients who suffer from either the spectrum of diseases associated with interstitial pulmonary fibrosis or emphysema. Condi-

tions associated with significant pulmonary vascular disease (e.g., primary pulmonary hypertension, Eisenmenger's complex, sarcoidosis) may be approached with either single or bilateral lung transplantation but generally do not require an en bloc heart-lung transplant except in situations involving complex congenital heart disease. Pulmonary diseases characterized by chronic airway suppuration (e.g., cystic fibrosis, bronchiectasis) require bilateral lung transplantation to thereby eliminate both native lungs that pose a serious risk for posttransplant infection during immunosuppression.

The conventional surgical approach to either single or bilateral lung transplantation entails anastomosis of proximal mainstem bronchus (or bronchi, for bilateral), pulmonary artery, and reestablishing pulmonary venous effluent by means of anastomosis of a left atrial "cuff." SLT is accomplished via a traditional posterolateral thoracotomy incision, while an extensive transverse bilateral anterior thoracosternotomy (clam shell incision) is utilized for bilateral grafts. Heart-lung transplantation involves the en bloc implantation of bilateral lungs and heart via a median sternotomy incision. During these surgical procedures, most centers do not perform revascularization of the bronchial arterial circulation while patients are similarly rendered "extrinsically denervated" from autonomic influences and are devoid of normal pulmonary lymphatic drainage. The physiologic responses observed after transplant, therefore, may be significantly affected by these fundamental physiologic differences.

Effects on the Exercise Response

Clinical investigations have suggested the following alterations in function that may impact the exercise response observed posttransplantation:

- Bronchial hyperresponsiveness to either inhaled methacholine, hypertonic saline aerosol, or exercise has been demonstrated in a significant number of lung transplant recipients. Hyperresponsiveness may relate to either extrinsic cholinergic pulmonary denervation or airway inflammation such as during allograft rejection or infection.

• Abnormal mucociliary clearance may relate to a physical impediment imposed by the bronchial anastomosis. Additionally, studies have suggested bronchial mucosal abnormalities characterized by altered epithelium, decreased ciliary beat frequency, and alteration in mucous rheology.

• Cardiac sympathetic denervation after combined heart-lung transplantation, similar to isolated orthotopic heart transplantation, can reduce the achieved maximum exercise heart rate, peak oxygen consumption ($\dot{V}O_2$peak), peak oxygen pulse, and lactate threshold. Cardiac reinnervation later occurs in a proportion of such patients and is associated with improved chronotropic and inotropic cardiac responses and enhanced oxygen delivery to exercising skeletal muscles.

• Altered pulmonary vascular permeability may occur soon after lung transplantation and relate to "ischemia reperfusion" graft injury or, later in their clinical course, during episodes of rejection and associated perivascular inflammation. Physiologic consequences of an increased pulmonary vascular permeability and interstitial edema may include a decline in spirometric indices, increased wasted ventilation, and increased ventilation-perfusion inequality and gas exchange.

• Altered respiratory pattern (i.e., disproportionate increase in tidal volume at a reduced respiratory rate), consistent with the absence of vagal-mediated inflation inhibition (Hering-Breuer Reflex), has been detected after combined heart-lung and bilateral lung transplantation. Stable heart-lung recipients with normal graft function, however, manifest an appropriate response of ventilation to exercise or progressive hypercapnia. Furthermore, pulmonary denervation does not impede the normal tachypneic response to either an increased elastic impedance or intrinsic pulmonary restriction. By contrast, the hypercapnic ventilation response may appear blunted relatively soon after lung transplantation when specifically performed for end-stage hypercapnic chronic obstructive pulmonary disease, but subsequently returns toward normal. Further, the detection of inspiratory resistive loads appears normal after combined heart-lung transplantation, despite the absence of pulmonary afferent innervation.

• Abnormal pulmonary function tests are frequently observed after both heart-lung and isolated pulmonary transplantation. Heart-lung transplant recipients often have a mild restrictive ventilatory defect that may relate to volumetric constraints of the recipient chest cavity and thoracic musculature. The elastic behavior or pressure-volume relationships after uncomplicated lung transplantation appear relatively normal. Values for vital capacity and maximum expiratory flow rates are expectedly less after single (approximately 60% of predicted normal value) versus bilateral or heart-lung transplantation.

Effects of Exercise Training

Despite attaining higher spirometric values after single or bilateral lung or combined heart-lung transplantation, cardiopulmonary exercise studies have demonstrated the following:

• Values for $\dot{V}O_2$peak (approximately 45-55% of predicted) and maximum work rate in these recipients are reduced.

• An abnormally reduced "threshold" for lactate, ventilation, and standard bicarbonate are observed in association with reduction in maximal tolerable exercise capacity, although this cannot be ascribed to factors such as cardiac dysfunction, anemia, or limitations imposed by pulmonary vasculature or lung mechanics.

• Quadriceps muscle biopsies and 31P-magnetic resonance spectroscopy after clinical lung transplantation have suggested a decrease in proportion of type I fibers and reduced skeletal muscle oxidative capacity and reduced intracellular pH. No difference has been detected in the activities of glycolytic enzymes, while transplant recipients demonstrate a higher reliance on glycolytic non-oxidative metabolism. Therefore, alteration in fiber proportion and reduced mitochondrial activity may indeed contribute to the exercise limitation witnessed after lung transplantation.

• Immunosuppressant medications may potentially contribute to an alteration in exercise physiology. Systemic glucocorticoids have well-described adverse effects on peripheral skeletal muscle and are commonly administered to patients suffering from a spectrum of pulmonary diseases prior to transplant, as well as in combination therapies posttransplantation.

Glucocorticoids can induce a selective atrophy of type II fibers; however, because these are the major source for lactate production in exercising skeletal muscle, one would not expect corticosteroids to cause inordinate intracellular acidosis. Calcineurin inhibitor-type immunosuppressive medications (e.g., cyclosporine or tacrolimus) have been shown to inhibit skeletal muscle mitochondrial respiration in vitro and diminish endurance exercise time in rats. The mechanism involved is not entirely clear but may relate to diminished mitochondrial calcium efflux with subsequent mitochondrial dysfunction. No impact on fiber size has yet been attributed to cyclosporine, although reduction in capillarity of limb musculature may further contribute to the reduction in aerobic capacity.

Lung and Heart-Lung Transplantation: Exercise Testing

Methods	Measures	Endpoints	Comments
Aerobic Cycle (ramp protocol 10-15 watts/ min; staged protocol 25 watts/3-min stage) Treadmill (1 MET/3-min stage)	• 12-lead ECG, HR • BP • Respired gas analysis • Blood lactate • RPE, dyspnea scales (0-10) • Pulse oximetry or arterial PO_2	• Serious dysrhythmias • >2 mm ST-segment depression • T-wave inversion with significant ST change • SBP > 250 mmHg or DBP > 115 mmHg • Maximum ventilation • $\dot{V}O_2$peak • Lactate/ventilatory threshold	• Atrial arrhythmias common early posttransplant. • Heart-lung transplant may be associated with cardiac denervation. • Lung transplant may be associated with absent Hering-Breuer reflex. • Very reduced transitional thresholds for lactate and HCO_3.
Endurance 6-min walk	• Distance	• Note vitals, dyspnea index, SaO_2 at rest stops	• Useful measure in assessing pretransplant severity of illness and posttransplant progress.
Strength Isokinetic/Isotonic	• Peak torque • Maximum number of reps		• Decreased muscle mass/force related to corticosteroids.
Flexibility Sit and stretch	• Hip, hamstring, lower back flexibility		• Post-thoracotomy pain may restrict flexibility.
Neuromuscular Gait analysis Balance			• Tremors and possible myopa- thy with calcineurin inhibitors. • Decreased visual acuity due to cataracts or diabetes.
Functional Sit to stand Stair climbing Lifting	• Perform tests if clinically indicated		

Medications

Many of the following medications are used for either immunosuppression or as prophylaxis to thereby prevent potential posttransplant complications:

• Calcineurin-inhibitor immunosuppressive medications (e.g., cyclosporine, tacrolimus), TOR inhibitors (e.g., rapamycin), antimetabolites (e.g., azathioprine, methotrexate, mycophenolate mofetil)
• Loop and thiazide diuretics: May contribute to electrolyte abnormalities and muscle weakness.
• Antihypertensive medications (e.g., beta blockers, ACE inhibitors, calcium-channel blockers)
• Antibiotics (e.g., quinolone-type [e.g., ciprofloxacin], trimethoprim sulfamethoxazole, antiviral [e.g., ganciclovir sodium, acyclovir])

(continued)

Medications *(continued)*

- HMG CoA reductase inhibitor medications (e.g., "statins") for hyperlipidemia posttransplant: May cause muscle pain or severe muscle injury with potential kidney failure.
- Calcineurin inhibitors: May cause tremor, neuropathy or myopathy, electrolyte abnormalities (decreased magnesium and increased potassium), renal tubular metabolic acidosis, or kidney failure.
- TOR inhibitors: May cause bleeding tendency (decreased platelets) and hyperlipidemia.
- Beta blockers: May reduce heart rate response to exercise.
- Calcium-channel blockers: May cause leg swelling or hypotension.
- Quinolone antibiotics: May cause tendinitis and tendon rupture.
- Antiviral medications: May have associated neurotoxicity.
- Many medications may cause anemia or leukopenia. The spectrum of adverse medication effects may impact exercise capacity or muscle function.

• The physiologic differences in exercise physiology and aerobic capacity notwithstanding, one preliminary study after lung transplantation has demonstrated significant benefits from formal exercise conditioning. After a six-week program whereupon training intensity ranged from 30 to 60% of maximum heart rate reserve, improvements were observed in minute ventilation, cardiac reserve, and $\dot{V}O_2$peak. Congruent with these findings, recent studies of similarly immunosuppressed heart transplant recipients have also highlighted the benefits of structured exercise training. Therefore, to mitigate the potential adverse effects of immunosuppressive medications and the frequent preexistent state of deconditioning, structured exercise rehabilitation programs may offer significant clinical advantages.

Management and Medications

Pulmonary transplantation offers a renewed sense of hope and quality of life for enumerable patients with end-stage cardiopulmonary diseases. Nevertheless, the required chronic immunosuppressive medications represent a double-edged sword after transplant. Although decreasing the incidence of acute graft rejection, such medications may heighten the risk of developing opportunistic infection, malignancy, osteoporosis, hypertension, diabetes mellitus, and associated toxicity. The exercise physiologist should be cognizant of these potential complications and maintain vigilance accordingly. Notable complications for the posttransplant patient may include the following:

• Acute allograft rejection and dysfunction are often heralded by increased subjective sensation of dyspnea, reduction in spirometric function, and gas exchange. Expeditious evaluation of the patient for possible transbronchoscopic biopsy and therapy is imperative.

• Pneumonia, although often related to typical community-acquired viral or bacterial infections, may be attributed to opportunistic or atypical pathogens caused by chronic immunosuppressive medications. Routine patient vaccination with polyvalent pneumococcal and annual influenza vaccines are recommended.

• Systemic hypertension is often related to adverse effects of glucocorticoids and calcineurin inhibitor-type medications. Patients often will require antihypertensive medications with frequent dosage adjustments. However, significant elevation in blood pressure may indicate a toxic blood level range for either cyclosporine or tacrolimus versus potential worsening renal function related to these medications.

• Osteoporosis, related to both systemic glucocorticoids and calcineurin inhibitor-type immunosuppressants, poses a significant risk for vertebral and hip fracture after transplantation. Newer prophylactic strategies for osteoporosis include calcium supplementation, hormonal replacement therapy, bisphosphonates, as well as exercise, strength, and balance training.

• Chronic anemia is usually related to suppression of the bone marrow by immunosuppressive medications. However, various viral infections (e.g., Parvovirus B19, herpesvirus) may sometimes be responsible. Severe reductions in hemoglobin concentration may affect the patient's peak exercise tolerance and ventilatory threshold.

• Bronchiolitis obliterans syndrome (BOS) or chronic graft rejection represents the Achilles' heel of lung transplantation and may affect two-thirds of recipients by five years. Progressive small airway fibrosis and obliteration result in an inexorable decay in lung function over time that frequently is refractory to augmented immunosuppressive therapies. Recurrent respiratory tract infections and abnormalities of larger airways (i.e., bronchiectasis) frequently ensue.

• Abnormalities of glucose tolerance and metabolism, related to immunosuppressive medications, may complicate the clinical course of these patients. Excessive weight gain and potential diabetic complications may be favorably impacted by regular exercise and nutritional counseling.

Lung and Heart-Lung Transplantation: Exercise Programming

Modes	Goals	Intensity/ Frequency/Duration	Time to Goal
Aerobic • Large muscle activities (walking, cycling, swimming)	• Increase $\dot{V}O_2$peak and endurance • Increase lactate and ventilatory thresholds • Decrease sensitivity to dyspnea • Develop more efficient breathing patterns • Restore ADLs	• THR 60-80% of peak HR • RPE 11-13/20 (comfortable pace) • Monitor dyspnea • 1-2 sessions/day • 3-7 days/wk • 20-30 min/session (shorter intermittent exercise sessions may be necessary initially) • Emphasize duration over intensity	• Variable, 3-12 mo (depending on posttransplant medical/ surgical complications)
Strength • Free weights • Isokinetic/Isotonic machines	• Increase maximal number of reps • Increase isokinetic torque/ work • Increase lean body mass	• Low resistance, high reps • 2-3 days/wk	• Variable, 3-12 mo
Flexibility • Stretching • Tai chi	• Increase ROM	• Daily	
Neuromuscular • Walking and balance exercises • Breathing exercises	• Improve gait and balance • Decrease muscle weakness and myopathy	• Daily	
Functional • Activity-specific exercises	• Restore ADLs • Return to work • Improve quality of life • Restore sexuality	• Daily	

Medications	Special Considerations
• See exercise testing table.	• RPE and dyspnea are the preferred methods of monitoring intensity. Many clients are unable to achieve a training HR yet demonstrate physiologic improvement. • Musculoskeletal complaints, postsurgical chest wall pain, and osteoporosis are common posttransplant complications. • Myopathy involving respiratory and peripheral muscles may be related to calcineurin inhibitors and corticosteroid medications. Severe muscle pain may indicate a serious complication of "statin"-type lipid-lowering medications. • "Bronchial hyperresponsiveness" posttransplant may contribute to exercise-related bronchospasms and dyspnea. • Clients usually respond to exercise optimally in mid to late morning, due to adverse effects (e.g., nausea, fatigue) of morning medication schedules. • Avoid extremes in ambient temperature and humidity caused by frequent use of antihypertensive and diuretic medications. • Supplemental O_2 may be required either early posttransplant or subsequent to graft complications. *(continued)*

Medications (continued)	Special Considerations (continued)
	• New or worsening SaO_2 responses to exercise may indicate organ rejection or infection and should be communicated to the transplant team. • Anxiety, depression, and/or fear are common effects of dyspnea or medications such as corticosteroids.

• Bronchial anastomosis complications may significantly affect clinical outcomes after lung transplantation. Fortunately, neither dehiscence nor bronchovascular fistula complications are presently common. However, development of bronchial anastomotic stricture or stenosis usually caused by exuberant scar tissue formation may both impair spirometric function and the normal "mucociliary escalator." Posttransplant inflammation involving airway cartilage rings may contribute to bronchomalacia, whereupon dynamic airway collapse may limit expiratory flow rates. Potential remedies may include endobronchial laser photoresection of granulation tissue and/or deployment of a bronchial stent to thereby maintain the bronchial lumen. Furthermore, localized infections of the anastomosis (e.g., fungal) may require therapy with systemic or inhaled aerosol antibiotics. Bronchoscopic assessment is generally required to establish a definitive diagnosis and, thus, direct the appropriate therapies.

Recommendations for Exercise Testing

The primary objectives for exercise testing are two-fold: (1) to assess the severity of exercise impairment prior to organ transplant or determine progression of disease and urgency for transplantation and (2) to characterize exercise limitations posttransplantation. Pretransplant assessment of $\dot{V}O_2$max or 6-min walk distance correlate with severity of illness for cystic fibrosis, for example, and the associated risk of death while awaiting transplantation. Posttransplant testing may be valuable in determining whether exercise limitation is related to graft dysfunction, occult cardiac disease, peripheral muscle weakness, or a persistent state of deconditioning.

During either era, pre- or posttransplantation, the principal objectives for exercise testing are similar (also see the Lung and Heart-Lung Transplantation: Exercise Testing table on page 119):

• assess severity of disease or progression;

• assess maximal physical work capacity and state of aerobic fitness;

• observe cardiorespiratory and metabolic responses to exercise;

• observe oxyhemoglobin saturation during exercise;

• provide a basis for prescribing exercise within safe limits; and

• assess changes in fitness and cardiorespiratory responses to exercise that occur with disease progression or medical/surgical interventions.

Recommendations for Exercise Programming

The principal goals of exercise training, both pre- and posttransplantation, are to improve aerobic fitness and alleviate the sense of dyspnea. Exercise prescriptions should be tailored to the type of native lung disease, level of patient fitness, and posttransplant allograft spirometric function (see the Lung and Heart-Lung Transplantation: Exercise Programming table on page 121). Pretransplant patients with pulmonary arterial hypertension, for example, may be predisposed to development of right ventricular ischemia, arterial oxygen desaturation, and syncope during exertion. Exercise of moderate intensity (60-80% of peak heart rate) should be targeted for approximately 20 to 30 min. Beta blockers received posttransplant may limit exercise heart rate response; therefore, assessment of perceived exertion may be preferable. Patients should be encouraged to adopt healthy lifestyle modifications that incorporate aerobic activities, balanced diet, and maintenance of appropriate body weight.

Special Considerations

All patients after organ transplantation and certain patients prior to transplant require chronic immunosuppression, which poses an increased risk for serious infection. Isolation of such patients from the general population in rehabilitation programs is generally not warranted, although one should be cognizant of the potential risks for transmission of respiratory pathogens from other clients. Maintaining cleanliness of all exercise equipment and patient avoidance of potential ill contacts during these sessions should be emphasized. Potential for impaired glucose tolerance or systemic hypertension as an adverse effect of immunosuppressive medications should be monitored during exercise and related to the referring physician. Significant deterioration in exercise tolerance or arterial oxygen saturation from prior baseline values may represent a harbinger of allograft rejection, cytomegalovirus, or other posttransplant opportunistic infections. Such data may be of crucial importance to the organ transplant team in determining the need for expeditious clinical evaluation and bronchoscopic lung biopsy. The clinical value in maintaining excellent lines of communication with the transplant team is of paramount importance.

CASE STUDY Lung Transplantation

A 45-year-old woman underwent bilateral sequential lung transplantation three years ago for interstitial pulmonary fibrosis complicated by severe secondary pulmonary hypertension with right-sided heart failure. She initially improved quite dramatically with respect to both spirometric lung function and exercise tolerance, and went home (to Kuwait) approximately three months posttransplant on standard triple-drug immunosuppression (i.e., cyclosporine, mycophenolate mofetil, and prednisone). She returned for reevaluation complaining of progressive shortness of breath and recurrent respiratory tract infections with methicillin-resistant Staphylococcus aureus and Pseudomonas aeruginosa. She also complained of severe low back pain after sustaining a "slip and fall" injury.

S: "I can't breathe again, and my back hurts."

O: Middle-aged woman, on oxygen, breathless and extremely fatigable with minimal exertion

Breath sounds: Bilateral basilar crackles and musical inspiratory and expiratory rhonchi
Thoracolumbar spine: Mildly tender to palpation, with decreased ROM for flexion and extension
Neurologic examination: Normal
Pulse oximetry: 95% arterial oxygen saturation on 3 l/min O_2 via nasal prongs
Chest X rays: Bibasilar scarring and probable dilated and thickened larger airways or bronchiectasis
Spirometry: Significant decreases in FVC and FEV_1; severe obstructive ventilatory defect
Spine X rays: Multiple compression fractures of T7, T9, and L1
Spine MRI scan: No evidence of malignancy

A: 1. BOS, or chronic graft rejection
2. Recurrent respiratory tract infection caused by bronchiectasis and recent exacerbation
3. Osteoporosis with multiple vertebral compression fractures
4. Severe exercise intolerance

P: 1. Intravenous antibiotic treatment of current respiratory infection is needed.
2. Prescribe aerosolized antibiotic prophylaxis for chronic bronchiectasis.
3. Treat osteoporosis pharmacologically.
4. Additional immunosuppression to prevent further loss of lung function from chronic rejection (e.g., tacrolimus and methotrexate) is necessary.
5. Prescribe outpatient pulmonary rehabilitation.

Exercise Program
Goals:
1. Improve functional capacity to increase and maintain ADLs
2. Alleviate dyspnea; improve strength and balance/coordination
3. Pulse oximetry during exercise to determine supplemental oxygen requirements

(continued)

CASE STUDY   Lung Transplantation (continued)

Mode	Frequency	Duration	Intensity	Progression
Aerobic	3 days/wk	20-30 min/ session	THR (110 contractions/ min) RPE 12/20	Progress as tolerated over 6-wk program
Strength (all major muscle groups)	2 days/wk	2 sets of ≤ 12 reps	To fatigue	Add resistance until 12 reps achieves fatigue
Flexibility	Daily	20-60 s/stretch	Hold below discomfort threshold	Maintain
Neuromuscular (walk drills, breathing exercises)	Daily	Individualized as needed	As tolerated	Maintain
Functional (activity-specific exercises)	Daily	Individualized as needed	As tolerated	Gradual over 3-12 mo
Warm-up/Cool-down	Before and after each session	10 min	RPE <10/20	

Suggested Readings

Biring, M.S., M. Fournier, D.J. Ross, and M.I. Lewis. 1998. Cellular adaptations of skeletal muscles to cyclosporin. *Journal of Applied Physiology* 84: 1967-75.

Garone, S., and D.J. Ross. 1999. Bronchiolitis obliterans syndrome: Review of our knowledge and treatment strategies. *Current Opinion in Organ Transplantation* 4: 254-63.

Grossman, R.F., and J.R. Maurer. 1990. Pulmonary considerations in transplantation. *Clinics in Chest Medicine* 11: 2.

Hokanson, J.F., J.G. Mercier, and G.A. Brooks. 1995. Cyclosporine A decreases rat skeletal muscle mitochondrial respiration in vitro. *American Journal of Respiratory and Critical Care Medicine* 151: 1848-51.

Iber, C., P. Simon, J.B. Skatrud et al. 1995. The Breuer-Hering reflex in humans: Effects of pulmonary denervation and hypocapnia. *American Journal of Respiratory and Critical Care Medicine* 152: 217-24.

Joint Statement of the American Society for Transplant Physicians (ASTP)/American Thoracic Society (ATS)/European Respiratory Society (ERS)/International Society for Heart and Lung Transplantation (ISHLT). 1998. International guidelines for the selection of lung transplant candidates. *American Journal of Respiratory and Critical Care Medicine* 158: 335-39.

Miyoshi, S., E.P. Trulock, H.-J. Schaefers et al. 1990. Cardiopulmonary exercise testing after single and double lung transplantation. *Chest* 97: 1130-36.

Ross, D.J., P.F. Waters, A. Mohsenifar et al. 1993. Hemodynamic responses to exercise after lung transplantation. *Chest* 103: 46-53.

Schwaiblmair, M., W. von Scheidt, P. Uberfuhr et al. 1999. Functional significance of cardiac reinnervation in heart transplant recipients. *Journal of Heart and Lung Transplantation* 18 (9): 838-45.

Stiebellehner, L., M. Quittan, A. End et al. 1998. Aerobic endurance training program improves exercise performance in lung transplant recipients. *Chest* 113 (4): 906-12.

SECTION IV

Metabolic Diseases

Patricia L. Painter, PhD,
FACSM

J. Larry Durstine, PhD,
FACSM

CHAPTER 20

End-Stage Metabolic Disease: Renal Failure and Liver Failure

Patricia L. Painter, PhD, FACSM
University of California, San Francisco

Joanne B. Krasnoff, MS
University of California, San Francisco

Overview of the Pathophysiology

End-stage renal disease (ESRD) is the loss of kidney function to the point of severe reduction of clearance of necessary waste products from the blood. ESRD results in severe metabolic abnormalities that affect nearly all physiologic systems. The following are common consequences of renal failure:

- metabolic acidosis;
- hypertension;
- left ventricular hypertrophy;
- anemia;
- secondary hyperparathyroidism;
- peripheral neuropathy;
- muscle weakness;
- autonomic dysfunction; and
- elevated triglycerides and reduced high-density lipoprotein cholesterol.

Thirty percent of dialysis clients are diabetic. Most dialysis clients are inactive and possess low functional capacities.

End-stage liver disease (ESLD) is characterized by cirrhosis, which is irreversible, and widespread damage to the hepatocytes resulting from an underlying disease. The most common etiologies of cirrhosis include viral disease (hepatitis), alcoholic liver disease, metabolic diseases, disease of the biliary tract, venous outflow obstruction, toxins, and immunologic disease. The damaged and dead hepatocytes are replaced by fibrous tissue, which leads to fibrosis (scarring). Hepatocytes then regenerate in an abnormal pattern surrounded by fibrous tissue. This abnormal liver structure eventually leads to decreased blood flow to and through the liver.

There are many clinical manifestations of cirrhosis, including jaundice, portal hypertension and varices, ascites, hepatic encephalopathy, and ultimately hepatic failure. Individuals with ESLD experience fatigue, muscle wasting, anorexia, and anemia in addition to other symptoms specific to the etiology. Biochemical markers that (1) assess liver function (serum albumin, prothrombin time), (2) excretory function (bilirubin, alkaline phosphatase), and (3) hepatic inflammation (serum aminotransferases: AST, ALT) are monitored. A liver biopsy is used for determining the etiology of the liver disease, as well as for tracking treatment results and disease progression.

Effects on the Exercise Response

Exercise intolerance is well documented in individuals with ESRD treated with dialysis, with the average peak oxygen consumption ($\dot{V}O_2$peak) being about 20 ml $\cdot$ kg^{-1} $\cdot$ min^{-1}. Exercise responses are characterized by a blunted heart rate response and excessive blood pressure increases. The primary reason for termination of exercise is leg fatigue. The limitations to exercise in these individuals could be any one of a number of factors, including the following:

- reduced peak cardiac output caused by a blunted heart rate response;

- reduced oxygen-carrying capacity from anemia; and
- subnormal capacity to extract oxygen related to weakness and structural and functional changes in muscle.

Clients with ESLD also have reduced $\dot{V}O_2$peak, reported to be about 55% age predicted. This may be caused by anemia, bed rest or inactivity, protein-caloric undernourishment, metabolic abnormalities related to lipid and/or carbohydrate metabolism, decrease in muscle mass, and alcoholic myopathy. They exhibit a lower maximal heart rate and reduced muscle strength. Electrolyte abnormalities can cause electrocardiographic changes.

Effects of Exercise Training

The level of exercise tolerance that can be achieved in these individuals is unclear, and it is probable that some individuals on dialysis will not improve their $\dot{V}O_2$peak levels with training. Aerobic exercise training usually improves $\dot{V}O_2$peak by about 20 to 25%. This increase in $\dot{V}O_2$peak is the result of increased oxygen extraction in the muscle because stroke volume or cardiac output does not change after training. Low oxygen delivery to the skeletal muscle is improved by erythropoietin (EPO) therapy that increases hemoglobin as well as $\dot{V}O_2$peak and quality of life. Because $\dot{V}O_2$peak in these persons correlates with muscle strength more closely than with hemoglobin, it is thought that skeletal muscle dysfunction is a major limiting factor for exercise capacity.

It has been reported that exercise training improves blood pressure control, lipid profiles, and psychological profiles in some clients. The peak exercise capacity of many people on dialysis is such that the energy requirements of common activities of daily living are challenging to them. Thus, increasing functional capacity should be a major objective of exercise therapy for people with renal failure. Since limitations may be related to muscle weakness, it is reasonable to try both resistance and aerobic training programs to improve functional capacity.

Exercise counseling for independent home exercise and/or cycling during dialysis has been shown to improve physical performance tests (e.g., sit to stand, gait speed) and self-reported physical functioning as measured with the SF-36 questionnaire.

There is very little exercise training experience in clients with ESLD. One 12-week study (3-4 30-min sessions/week) in persons with chronic hepatitis resulted in a 30% increase in $\dot{V}O_2$peak with no change in liver function tests, indicating no negative training effect on liver function.

Management and Medications

In persons with ESRD, some form of renal replacement therapy is required for maintenance of life. The main form of maintenance therapy is hemodialysis. Other treatment options include peritoneal dialysis and renal transplantation. Medical management issues include assuring adequate dialysis therapy, which is monitored through urea kinetics and other blood testing; adequate blood pressure control, which often requires a variety of antihypertensive agents; control of the anemia using recombinant human EPO; control of secondary hyperparathyroidism through use of phosphate-binding agents; and adequate access for dialysis—that is, either blood access (for hemodialysis via arteriovenous fistula) or peritoneal catheter (for peritoneal dialysis).

Clients may develop any of the following problems:

- congestive heart failure before the initiation of dialysis (due to fluid overload) or in the case of inadequate dialysis or fluid intake indiscretion;
- accelerated atherosclerosis;
- pericardial effusion resulting from inadequate dialysis and uremia;
- abnormal electrocardiogram caused by electrolyte abnormalities or structural changes;
- dysrhythmias from abnormal electrolytes (rare);
- cardiomegaly resulting from fluid and/or pressure overload, coronary artery disease, pericardial disease, uremic toxins, or other conditions;
- renal osteodystrophy resulting from secondary hyperparathyroidism;
- persistent anemia caused by iron deficiency, nonresponse to EPO, or both; and
- peritonitis resulting from catheter infection (in clients treated with peritoneal dialysis).

Many clients are hypertensive and, thus, are treated with antihypertensive agents. During hemodialysis, a complex interaction of antihypertensive medications and dialysis can lead to either inadequate drug levels or severe hypotension. For this reason, antihypertensive medications are often not taken on dialysis days. Nearly all dialysis clients take recombinant EPO for anemia, although hematocrits are only partially corrected (usually up to 35%). Phosphate binders are prescribed for virtually all dialysis clients to prevent hyperparathyroidism and renal osteodystrophy. Insulin is administered to diabetic clients requiring it, with those on peritoneal dialysis receiving medication in their dialysis fluid. Other medications may be required for coexisting medical concerns.

ESRD and ESLD: Exercise Testing

Methods	Measures	Endpoints*	Comments
Aerobic Cycle (ramp protocol 5-25 watts/ min; staged protocol 25-50 watts/3-min stage) Treadmill (1-2 METs/stage)	• 12-lead ECG, HR • BP • RPE (6-20)	• Serious dysrhythmias • >2 mm ST-segment depression or elevation • Ischemic threshold • T-wave inversion with significant ST change • SBP > 250 mmHg or DBP > 115 mmHg • Onset of muscle fatigue	• Most clients terminate exercise test because of skeletal muscle fatigue.
Strength Isokinetic/Isotonic	• 10-12 RM, peak torque		• 1 RM not recommended.
Flexibility Sit and reach	• Distance		• Useful in debilitated individuals.
Neuromuscular Gait analysis Balance			• Indicated for peripheral neuropathy, prosthetic devices, and/or severe muscle wasting.
Functional Timed sit to stand Gait speed Functional lifting tests	• 10 reps • m/s • RPE (6-20)		• Used for assessment of capacity for ADLs. • Useful for ADL assessment.

*Measurements of particular significance; do not always indicate test termination.

Medications	Special Considerations
• Antihypertensive agents: Administer as needed. Depends on dialysis schedule and compliance to fluid restrictions. • Erythropoietin: Used for anemia. Hematocrit should be maintained between 30 and 35%. • ESLD medications: Interferon, ribavirin (hepatitis antivirals), prednisone, and azathioprine (Imuran) beta blocker for autoimmune disease; diuretics for edema; Fosamax for low bone mineral density.	• Hemodialysis patients should be tested on a non-dialysis day. • Clients treated with continuous ambulatory peritoneal dialysis should be tested without fluid in the abdomen. • Do not measure BP in the arm with the arteriovenous fistula (ESRD). • Spontaneous avulsion fractures may be possible in patients with long-standing renal bone disease (usually have been on dialysis > 5 yr). • 30% of dialysis patients are diabetic (see testing table in chapter 21). • Cites may affect ventilation (ESLD). • Esophageal/gastric varices: Avoid Valsalva (ESLD). • Bleeding and bruising are possible due to coagulation disorders (ESLD). • Fatigue is a common concern (ESRD and ESLD).

The management of ESLD focuses on prevention of long-term complications, reduction in mortality, and symptom improvement. Treatment of the underlying liver disease may slow or stop the progression, depending on the etiology. For example, discontinuation of alcohol intake will stop progression of alcoholic cirrhosis. Treatment of metabolic diseases, such as iron overload in hemochromatosis or copper overload in Wilson disease, is also effective in stopping progression. Pharmacological therapy is sometimes effective in chronic viral hepa-

ESRD and ESLD: Exercise Programming

Modes	Goals	Intensity/Frequency/Duration	Time to Goal
Aerobic • Large muscle activities	• Increase aerobic capacity • Increase time to exhaustion • Increase work capacity • Improve BP	• 50-90% peak HR • 50-85% $\dot{V}O_2$peak • Monitor RPE • 4-7 days/wk • 20-60 min/session	• 4-6 mo
Strength • Free weights • Weight machines • Isokinetic machines	• Increase maximal number of reps	• Avoid high weights • Concentrate on low-weight/high-rep program	• 4-6 mo
Flexibility • Stretching/yoga	• Maintain/increase ROM • Improve gait, balance, and coordination		
Functional • Activity-specific exercise	• Increase ADLs • Increase vocational potential • Increase physical self-confidence		

Medications	Special Considerations
• Antihypertensives: Administer as needed (depends on dialysis schedule and compliance to fluid restrictions). • Erythropoietin: Use for anemia; hematocrit should be maintained between 30 and 35%.	• Individuals receiving hemodialysis may not tolerate exercise after dialysis treatment. • Patient treated with continuous ambulatory peritoneal dialysis may be more comfortable exercising without fluid in the abdomen. • Be aware of the arteriovenous fistula and IV access lines. • Spontaneous avulsion fractures may occur in patients with long-standing renal bone disease (usually have been on dialysis > 5 yr). • 30% of dialysis patients are diabetic; see chapter 21 exercise programming table. • Fatigue is a common concern. • Gradual progression is essential. • Patients frequently experience medical setbacks; program may have to be adjusted accordingly. • Exercise during hemodialysis treatment is recommended and should be encouraged when possible (in conjunction with the dialysis unit staff).

titis (B, C), autoimmune hepatitis, primary biliary cirrhosis, and sclerosing cholangitis. Complications of cirrhosis are treated using various techniques, including endoscopic sclerotherapy or rubber band ligation for bleeding esophageal varices and low-sodium diet or diuretic therapy for ascites. Coagulation disorders are often responsive to vitamin K. When clients are unresponsive to all treatments and pharmacological therapies, liver transplantation becomes the final treatment option of ESLD. There is no information on how any of these therapies interact with or are impacted by exercise training.

Recommendations for Exercise Testing

The utility of exercise testing for diagnostic purposes is questioned in these client groups since they are limited primarily by muscle fatigue. Thus, maximal diagnostic exercise testing may not be beneficial for screening before an exercise training program. In most cases, requiring such testing may present an unnecessary barrier to beginning a program of exercise training. Since these individuals experience continuing and intensive medical care, such testing probably does not provide any additional information. If some evaluation is needed, physical performance testing may be most appropriate (see the ESRD and ESLD: Exercise Testing table on page 128).

Recommendations for Exercise Programming

There is no guarantee that all individuals on dialysis or those with ESLD will respond to exercise training with an increase in $\dot{V}O_2$peak or functional capacity. The optimal program of exercise training has not been identified

for either of these client groups. Additionally, the interactions between morbidity, the adequacy of dialysis (or treatments for liver disease) and other unknown factors, and the response to exercise training have not been completely defined. The chronicity of the disease and the multiple medical problems presented in these individuals often become the focus of the health care professionals who are caring for them. Information or referral for exercise training in the past has typically not been part of the traditional care routine. Although it is difficult to integrate an exercise program into an already complex and intensive medical schedule, exercise training does provide the only possible chance to increase or at least maintain functional capacity in these individuals. Increased awareness of the potential exercise benefits for individuals with ESRD or ESLD on the part of the medical community is needed (see the ESRD and ESLD: Exercise Programming table on page 129).

CASE STUDY End-Stage Renal Disease

A 64-year-old African-American female with ESRD secondary to hypertension had been treated with hemodialysis for 18 months and referred for exercise training evaluation. She retired from an office job upon starting dialysis treatments, which were 3 hours, 3 times a week (540 min/wk). She tolerated dialysis well and had a synthetic graft in her upper arm as an access for dialysis treatments. The graft had been declotted twice in the past two years and was working well. She had a history of coronary artery disease, which was effectively treated with PTCA 3 years ago.

Presently, the client is doing well and has been evaluated for living-related transplant from her daughter. She currently does no regular physical activity and has no exercise history. The daughter is athletic and very interested in getting her mother started on an exercise program.

S: "I have been gradually getting weaker since starting dialysis. My leg muscles are weak and there are times when I am afraid of falling. I have difficulty climbing stairs and tire easily when shopping. I would like to get stronger before my transplant. I have also heard that exercise may help my blood pressure and I would like to take fewer drugs for my blood pressure."

O: Vitals: Height: 4'11" (1.5 m)   Weight: 165 lb (75 kg)   BMI: 33.4 kg/m²
HR: 82 contractions/min   BP: 156/92 mmHg

Elderly, overweight woman, appearing to lack energy

Ambulates slowly, but does not appear short of breath

Medications: EPO, Diltiazem, Multivitamins, Phosphate binders

Labs:
  Albumin: 3.3 mg/dl
  Hematocrit: 32%
  Total cholesterol: 148 mg/dl
  kT/v (indicator of adequacy of dialysis): 1.6 (average in her dialysis unit is 1.38)

Graded exercise test:
  6-min walk: 919.5 ft (280 m); 3 rest stops during the test
  Sit to stand (10 cycles): 37.58 s (51% age-predicted norm)
  Gait speed (20 m): 66.9cm/s (52.3% of normal for age)

Self-reported physical function (SF-36 scores):
  Physical functioning: 36/100
  Physical composite scale: 35.5 (normal: 50.0)

A: 1. ESRD secondary to hypertension, treated with hemodialysis
2. CAD s/p (PTCA 3 years ago)
3. Exercise intolerance (decreased strength and endurance)
4. Hypertension
5. Secondary hyperparathyroidism
6. Renal osteodystrophy

P: 1. Initiate muscular strengthening.
2. Prescribe a cardiovascular exercise program.

Exercise Program

Goals:

1. Improved muscular strength, endurance, and balance

2. Short-term goals (1 mo):
Walk around block at home 3 times continuously without stopping
Climb 1 flight of stairs without stopping
Reevaluate

3. Long-term goals (6 mo):
Walk 2 mi (3.2K) continuously
Climb 1 flight of stairs 3 times continuously

Mode	Frequency	Duration	Intensity	Progression
Aerobic (walk short distances, bike)	5-7 days/wk	As tolerated	As tolerated	Walk 1 block in 1st wk; then increase by 1/2 block/wk, as tolerated
Strength (all major muscle groups)	3 days/wk	1 set of 10-12 reps	Therabands™	Increase to 3 sets of 10-12 reps over 4 wk; increase to stronger color bands as tolerated
Flexibility (all major muscle groups)	3 days/wk	20 s/stretch	Maintain each stretch below discomfort threshold	
Warm-up/Cool-down	Before and after each session	5-10 min	RPE 7-9/20	

Suggested Readings

Beyer, N., M. Asdahl, B. Strange, P. Kirkegaard, B.A. Hansen, T. Mohr, and M. Kjaer. 1999. Improved physical performance after orthotopic liver transplantation. *Liver Transplantation and Surgery* 5 (4): 301-9.

Diesel, W., T.D. Noakes, C. Swanepoel, and M. Lambert. 1990. Isokinetic muscle strength predicts maximum exercise tolerance in renal patients on chronic hemodialysis. *American Journal of Kidney Diseases* 16: 109-14.

Goldberg, A.P., E.M. Geltman, J.M. Hagberg, J.R. Gavin, J.A. Delmez, R.M. Carney, A. Naumowicz, M. Holdfield, and H.R. Harter. 1983. Therapeutic benefits of exercise training for hemodialysis patients. *Kidney International* 516: S303-9.

Johansen, K. 1999. Physical functioning and exercise capacity in patients on dialysis. *Advances in Renal Replacement Therapy* 6 (2): 141-48.

Krasnoff, J., and P.L. Painter. 1999. The physiologic consequences of inactivity and bed rest. *Advances in Renal Replacement Therapy* 6 (2): 124-32.

Krasnoff, J.B. 2001. Liver disease, transplant, and exercise. *Clinical Exercise Physiology* 3 (1): 27-34.

Moore, G.E., K.R. Brinker, and J. Stray-Gundersen. 1993. Determinants of $\dot{V}O_2$ peak in patients with end-stage renal disease: On and off dialysis. *Medicine and Science in Sports and Exercise* 25: 18-23.

Painter, P.L. 1999. Exercise after renal transplantation. *Advances in Renal Replacement Therapy* 6 (2): 159-64.

Painter, P.L. 1988. Exercise in end-stage renal disease. *Exercise and Sport Sciences Review* 16: 305-39.

Painter, P.L., L. Carlson, S. Carey, S.M. Paul, and J. Myll. 2000. Physical functioning and health-related quality-of-life changes with exercise training in hemodialysis patients. *American Journal of Kidney Diseases* 35 (3): 1-12.

Painter, P.L., and K. Johansen. 1999. Introduction: A call to activity. *Advances in Renal Replacement Therapy* 6 (2): 107-9.

Painter, P.L., and G.E. Moore. 1994. The impact of rHu erythropoetin on exercise capacity in hemodialysis patients. *Advances in Renal Replacement Therapy* 1 (1): 55-65.

Painter, P.L., A.L. Stewart, and S. Carey. 1999. Physical functioning: Definitions, measurement and expectations. *Advances in Renal Replacement Therapy* 6 (2): 110-23.

Ritland, S., N. Foss, and S. Skrede. 1982. The effect of standardized work load on "liver tests" in patients with chronic active hepatitis. *Journal of Gastroenterology* 17: 1013-16.

Robertson, H.T., N.R. Haley, M. Guthrie, D. Cardenas, J.W. Eschbach, and J.W. Adamson. 1990. Recombinant erythropoietin improves exercise capacity in anemic hemodialysis patients. *American Journal of Kidney Diseases* 15: 325-32.

CHAPTER 21

Diabetes

W. Guyton Hornsby, Jr., PhD, CDE, FACSM
West Virginia University

Ann L. Albright, PhD, CDE
University of California, San Francisco

Overview of the Pathophysiology

Diabetes is a chronic metabolic disease characterized by an absolute or relative deficiency of insulin that results in hyperglycemia. Current thinking is that anyone who has a blood glucose level higher than 120 mg/dl has diabetes. The recent history of someone's average blood glucose can be estimated by measuring the glycosylated hemoglobin (HbA_1c). Individuals with diabetes are at risk for developing microvascular complications, including retinopathy and nephropathy; macrovascular disease; and various neuropathies (both autonomic and peripheral). Silent ischemia is common in persons with diabetes, particularly if the disease is longstanding (see chapter 6 for management of this problem). Several distinct forms of diabetes are known to exist, and for classification purposes they have been divided into the following major categories.

Type 1 Diabetes Mellitus

In type 1 diabetes mellitus, there is an absolute deficiency of insulin caused by a marked reduction in insulin-secreting beta cells of the pancreas. Consequently, insulin must be supplied by injection or an insulin pump. Those with type 1 diabetes are prone to developing ketoacidosis when marked hyperglycemia occurs from inadequate insulin. The cause of type 1 diabetes is thought to involve an autoimmune response directed at the beta cells that ultimately leads to their destruction in genetically susceptible individuals. The factors that trigger the autoimmune response have not been specifically identified but may include viruses or toxins. The precise nature of the genetic influence in the pathogenesis of type 1 diabetes is also unclear, but the histocompatibility (human lymphocyte antigen) types DR3 and DR4 are associated with increased risk for type 1 diabetes. This form of diabetes usually occurs before the age of 30 but can occur at any age. Of the estimated 16 million people with diabetes mellitus in this country, approximately 5 to 10% have type 1 diabetes.

Type 2 Diabetes Mellitus

Individuals with type 2 diabetes are considered to have a relative insulin deficiency because they may have elevated, reduced, or normal insulin levels but still present with hyperglycemia. The pathophysiology of type 2 diabetes remains unclear and is probably multifactorial. In this form of diabetes, peripheral tissue insulin resistance and defective insulin secretion are common features. With insulin resistance, glucose does not readily enter the insulin-sensitive tissues (primarily muscle and adipose tissue), and blood glucose rises. The increase in blood glucose causes the beta cells of the pancreas to secrete more insulin in an attempt to maintain a normal blood glucose concentration. Unfortunately, this additional endogenous insulin is usually ineffective in lowering blood glucose and may further contribute to insulin resistance. In some people, the beta cells may become exhausted over time and insulin secretion decreases.

The mechanisms underlying insulin resistance remain unclear but probably involve defects in the binding of insulin to its receptor and in post-receptor events such as glucose transport. Obesity significantly contributes to insulin resistance, and the majority (80%) of people with type 2 diabetes are obese at onset. Several varieties of abnormalities in insulin secretion have been identified, but virtually all people with type 2 diabetes have lost the acute (first) phase insulin release. Insulin therapy may or may not be required, depending on the degree of functional insulin and/or insulin sensitivity/responsiveness remaining. Those with type 2 diabetes do not develop ketoacidosis except under conditions of unusual stress (e.g., trauma). Type 2 diabetes is clearly genetically influenced, because it occurs in identical twins with almost total concordance. The onset is insidious, with few or no classic symptoms, and many people go undiagnosed until organ damage has occurred. This form of diabetes usually occurs after the age of 40, although a small number of people under the age of 30 have a form of type 2 diabetes called maturity-onset diabetes of youth. Type 2 diabetes affects approximately

85 to 90% of the 16 million people with diabetes mellitus.

Gestational Diabetes

Gestational diabetes occurs during pregnancy because of the contra-insulin effects of pregnancy. Gestational diabetes is usually diagnosed by an oral glucose tolerance test (OGTT) performed between 24 and 28 weeks of gestation. Risk factors for the development of gestational diabetes include family history of gestational diabetes, previous delivery of a large birth weight baby, and obesity. The term *gestational diabetes* does not apply to those who have diabetes prior to pregnancy or to those with type 2 diabetes who may have been undiagnosed until pregnancy. The classic characteristic of gestational diabetes is that it resolves postpartum. This characteristic separates it from previously undiagnosed type 2 diabetes that remains following pregnancy. Approximately 50% of the women who develop gestational diabetes develop type 2 diabetes later in life.

Other Specific Types of Diabetes

Certain endocrinopathies, genetic syndromes, infections leading to β-cell destruction, reactions to drugs or toxic chemicals, uncommon forms of immune-mediated diabetes, diseases of the exocrine pancreas, and genetic defects in β-cell function and in insulin action can result in rather rare forms of diabetes. Many of these conditions have been identified and are classified as other specific types of diabetes. These types may or may not require insulin treatment, depending on the pathophysiology of the condition and the level of normal insulin secretion and insulin action. These conditions include the following:

- endocrinopathies such as acromegaly, Cushing's syndrome, glucagonoma, and pheochromocytoma;
- genetic syndromes such as Down syndrome, Klinefelter's syndrome, and Turner's syndrome;
- cell destruction by viruses such as coxsackievirus B, cytomegalovirus, adenovirus, mumps, and congenital rubella;
- reactions to drugs or chemicals such as nicotinic acid, glucocorticoids, thiazides, adrenergic agonists, thyroid hormone, Dilantin, β-interferon, and Vacor (rat poison);
- uncommon forms of immune-mediated diabetes such as "stiff man" syndrome and conditions with anti-insulin receptor antibodies;
- diseases of the exocrine pancreas such as pancreatitis, neoplasia, and cystic fibrosis;
- defects in β-cell function such as maturity-onset diabetes of the young (MODY); and

- genetic defects in insulin action such as type A insulin resistance, leprechaunism, and Rabson-Mendenhall syndrome.

Impaired Glucose Tolerance and Impaired Fasting Glucose

Impaired glucose tolerance (IGT) and impaired fasting glucose (IFG) are intermediate metabolic conditions between normoglycemia and frank diabetes. The upper limit of normal fasting glucose has been set at 109 mg/dl and the value used for the provisional diagnosis of diabetes is greater than 125 mg/dl. A confirmed fasting glucose between 110 and 125 mg/dl is recognized as IFG and a 2-hour value on an OGTT falling between 140 and 200 mg/dl may be recognized as IGT. Those with IGT and IFG are at increased risk for developing type 2 diabetes, but progression to diabetes is not a certainty.

Effects on the Exercise Response

Under normal conditions in people without diabetes, there is a precise coordination of hormonal and metabolic events that results in maintenance of glucose homeostasis. Insulin and counter-regulatory hormone concentrations in people with diabetes do not respond to exercise in the normal manner, and the balance between peripheral glucose utilization and hepatic glucose production may be disturbed. The effect of diabetes on a single exercise session is dependent on several factors, including:

- use and type of medication to lower blood glucose (insulin or oral hypoglycemic agents);
- timing of medication administration;
- blood glucose level prior to exercise;
- timing, amount, and type of previous food intake;
- presence and severity of diabetic complications;
- use of other medication secondary to diabetic complications; and
- intensity, duration, and type of exercise.

Effects of Exercise Training

Exercise is considered by many to be one of the cornerstones of diabetes care. An exercise training program has the potential to provide several benefits for the diabetic. These benefits may include the following:

- Possible improvement in blood glucose control. Exercise should be a part of diabetes therapy (in addition to diet and medication) to improve blood glucose control for those with type 2 diabetes, but is not considered a component of treatment in type 1 diabetes to lower blood glucose. Those with type 1 diabetes are encouraged to exercise to gain other benefits, but blood glucose must be in reasonable control (< 250 mg/dl, no ketones) if the individual is to exercise safely.

• Improved insulin sensitivity/lower medication requirement. Exercise training results in improved insulin sensitivity, and for many with diabetes this translates into a reduction in dose of insulin or oral agents.

• Reduction in body fat. Weight loss increases insulin sensitivity and may allow those with diabetes to reduce the amount of insulin or oral hypoglycemic agents needed. Exercise coupled with moderate caloric intake is considered the most effective way to lose weight.

• Cardiovascular benefits. Regular exercise decreases the risk of cardiovascular disease. It is likely that this is true to some extent for persons with diabetes.

• Stress reduction. Stress can disrupt diabetes control by increasing counter-regulatory hormones, ketones, free fatty acids, and urine output, making stress reduction an important part of diabetes care.

• Prevention of type 2 diabetes. Epidemiological studies have indicated that exercise may play a role in preventing type 2 diabetes. Those with IGT, gestational diabetes, or a family history of type 2 diabetes may especially benefit from a regular aerobic exercise program.

Nearly everyone with diabetes can derive some benefit from an exercise program, although not all benefits will necessarily be realized by each person with diabetes. Careful monitoring of blood glucose and attention to balancing food intake and medication are necessary for the person to participate safely in an exercise program.

Management and Medications

The management of diabetes depends on the form of diabetes, blood glucose goals, and the presence and severity of diabetic complications. One goal of diabetes management is to normalize blood glucose to the extent that it is safe to do so. This is accomplished by insulin, oral agents for type 2, or both, if necessary; by an individual nutrition care plan; and by participation in a regular exercise program as appropriate.

As the vast majority of morbidity and mortality in diabetes is related to macrovascular disease, medical management must also focus on reducing risk of cardiovascular disease. Medications used in diabetes manage-

ment not only include glucose-lowering agents but also often include aspirin, ACE inhibitors, other antihypertensives, lipid-lowering agents, and pain medications. (See chapter 12 on hypertension and chapter 22 on hyperlipidemia for information on these medications.) Insulin and oral hypoglycemic agents are the primary means for proper medical management of diabetes.

• Insulin allows glucose to enter the cells of insulin-sensitive tissue. There are several different types of insulin available pharmaceutically that vary in onset, peak, duration, and source (see table 21.1 on page 136).

• Oral agents for type 2 diabetes are medications that help the pancreas secrete more insulin, alter carbohydrate absorption, reduce liver glycogenolysis, and/or increase insulin sensitivity (see table 21.2 on page 136).

The most significant effect of both insulin and oral hypoglycemic agents on exercise testing and exercise training is their ability to cause hypoglycemia. Attention to timing of medication, food intake, and blood glucose level before and after exercise is necessary. If exercise is of long duration (i.e., > 60 min), blood glucose should be tested during exercise.

Recommendations for Exercise Testing

Recommendations for exercise testing depend on age, duration of diabetes, and presence of diabetic complications (see the Diabetes: Exercise Testing table on page 137). Exercise testing using protocols for populations at risk for coronary artery disease (CAD) is recommended in people who:

• have type 1 diabetes and are over the age of 30;
• have had type 1 diabetes longer than 15 years;
• have type 2 diabetes and are over age 35;
• have either type 1 or type 2 diabetes and one or more of the other CAD risk factors;
• have suspected or known CAD; and/or
• have any microvascular or neurological diabetic complications.

People with diabetes who do not meet any of these criteria may be tested with use of protocols for the general healthy population. The primary objectives of exercise testing in those with diabetes are to:

• identify the presence and extent of CAD and
• determine appropriate intensity range for aerobic exercise training.

Recommendations for Exercise Programming

The exercise prescription for people with diabetes must be individualized according to medication schedule, presence and severity of diabetic complications, and goals and expected benefits of the exercise program. Physical activity for those without significant complications or limitations should include appropriate endurance and resistance exercise for developing and maintaining cardiorespiratory fitness, body composition, and muscular strength and endurance (see the Diabetes: Exercise Programming table on page 138). Food intake with exercise must be considered for type 1 individuals. In general, 1 hour of exercise requires an additional 15 g of carbohydrate either before or after exercise. If exercise is vigorous and of longer duration, an additional 15 to 30 g of

Table 21.1   Types of Insulin

Insulin type	Onset (hr)	Peak (hr)	Effective duration (hr)
Rapid acting			
Lispro (Humalog)	< 0.25	0.5-1.0	2-4
Short acting			
Regular	0.5–1.0	2–3	3-6
Intermediate acting			
Lente	3-4	4-12	12-18
NPH	1-4	4-10	10-16
Long acting			
Ultralente*	6-10	Unknown	18-20
Glargine (Lantus)	1-2	Unknown	24

*Ultralente insulin is purportedly long acting, but the pharmacokinetics of human Ultralente are not dramatically different from Lente or NPH in the vast majority of individuals.

Table 21.2   Oral Agents Used for Treatment of Diabetes

Type/Generic name	Trade name	Usual daily dose (mg)	Duration (hr)
Sulfonylureas			
Acetohexamide	Generic name only	250-1500	12-18
Chlorpropamide	Diabinase	100-750	60+
Glimepiride	Amaryl	1-4	12-24
Glipizide	Glucotrol, Glucotrol XL	2.5-40	16-24
Glyburide	DiaBeta, Glynase, PresTab, Micronase	1.25-20	12-24
Tolazimide	Tolinase	100-1000	10-16
Tolbutamide	Orinase	500-3000	6-10
Biguanides			
Metformin	Glucophage	500-2550	12-24
Sulfonylurea/Biguanide			
Glyburide/Metformin	Glucovance	1.25/250-20/2000	12-24
Alpha-Glucosidase Inhibitors			
Acarbose	Precose	25-100 tid	4
Miglitol	Glyset	25-100 tid	2-3
Thiazoladinediones			
Pioglitazone	Actos	15-45	Unknown
Rosiglitazone	Avandia	4-8	Unknown
Meglitinides			
Nateglinide	Starlix	60-120 tid	1-2
Repaglinide	Prandin	0.5-4 tid	1-2

Diabetes: Exercise Testing

Methods*	Measures	Endpoints**	Comments

Aerobic
Cycle
(ramp protocol 17 watts/
min; staged protocol 25–50
watts/3-min stage)
Treadmill
(1-2 METs/stage)
	• 12-lead ECG, HR	• Serious dysrhythmias
		• >2mm ST-segment
		  depression or elevation
		• Ischemic threshold
		• T-wave significant ST
		  change
			• High risk for CAD.

	• BP	• SBP > 250 mmHg or DBP > 115 mmHg	
	• RPE (6-20)	• Onset of peripheral pain	

Strength
Isokinetic/Isotonic
	• Maximum number of
	  reps, peak torque
			• Excessive BP increases may be
			  problematic if mascrovascular
			  complications exist.

Flexibility Goniometry Sit and reach	• Distance	• Full ROM	

Strength
Gait analysis
Balance
			• Indicated for peripheral
			  neuropathy and/or prosthetic
			  devices.

*Methods of exercise testing are conservative because of the high risk of underlying cardiovascular disease and other chronic complications. More aggressive methods may be indicated for athletes or active patients without complications.

**Measurements of particular significance; do not always indicate test termination.

Medications	Special Considerations
• Insulin/hypoglycemic agents: May result in hypoglycemia. • Antihypertensives: See appendixes A, B, and C. • Lipid-lowering agents: See appendixes A, B, and C.	• Test should be postponed if blood glucose concentration is > 250 mg/dl and ketones are present. • If blood glucose is < 100 mg/dl, carbohydrate should be ingested, and consider delaying the test until the blood glucose is > 100 mg/dl. • Autonomic neuropathy is common; may be associated with silent ischemia, postural hypotension, and/or blunted HR response to exercise. • Peripheral neuropathy is common; may cause numbness, tingling in extremities, Charcot's joint, and reduced balance. • Microvascular complications may be affected by excessively high BP. • Peripheral vascular disease may result in intermittent claudication and/or infections or ulcers in the lower extremities with poor wound healing. • Insulin and meal schedule should be considered when testing. • Hypoglycemia can still occur several hours after exercise. • If angina and/or silent ischemia are present, see chapter 6.

carbohydrate every hour may be required. Exercise is contraindicated if:

- there is active retinal hemorrhage or there has been recent therapy for retinopathy (e.g., laser treatment);
- illness or infection is present;
- blood glucose is above 250 mg/dl and ketones are present (blood glucose should be lowered before initiation of exercise); or
- blood glucose is 80 to 100 mg/dl because the risk of hypoglycemia is great (in this situation, carbohydrate should be eaten and blood glucose allowed to increase before initiation of exercise).

Exercise precautions include the following:

- keeping a source of rapidly acting carbohydrate available during exercise;
- consuming adequate fluids before, during, and after exercise;
- practicing good foot care by wearing proper shoes and cotton socks, and inspecting feet after exercise; and
- carrying medical identification.

Diabetes: Exercise Programming

Modes	Goals	Intensity/ Frequency/Duration	Time to Goal
Aerobic • Large muscle activities	• Increase aerobic capacity • Increase time to exhaustion • Increase work capacity • Improve BP response to exercise • Reduce cardiovascular risk factors	• 50-90% peak HR* • 50-85% $\dot{V}O_2$peak* • Monitor RPE** • 4-7 days/wk • 20-60 min/session	• 4-6 mo
Strength • Free weights • Weight machines • Isokinetic machines	• Increase maximal number of reps • Improve performance for patients interested in competition	• Low-resistance, high repetitions for most clients • High resistance OK for athletes with well-controlled diabetes	• 4-6 mo
Anaerobic • High-intensity intervals	• Only for athletes in good diabetic control	• Same as healthy athletes	
Flexibility • Stretching/yoga	• Maintain/increase ROM • Improve gait	• Limited data available; 2-3 sessions/wk may suffice	• 4-6 mo
Neuromuscular • Yoga	• Improve balance • Improve coordination	• Limited data available; 2-3 sessions/wk may suffice	
Functional • Activity-specific exercise	• Increase ADLs • Increase vocational potential • Increase physical self-confidence	• Individualized to each client	

*Lower-intensity activity may be advisable if complications are present and/or diabetes is of long duration. The majority of persons with type 2 diabetes will benefit from low- to moderate-intensity physical activity of 40-70% $\dot{V}O_2$max.

**Using RPE is especially useful in persons whose HR has been altered by autonomic neuropathy or medications.

Medications	Special Considerations
•See exercise testing table.	•A snack and/or insulin dosage change may be needed 30-60 min before exercise. •Monitor blood glucose before and after exercise. •Exercising late in the evening increases risk of nocturnal hypoglycemia. •If angina and/or silent ischemia are present, see chapter 6. •Observe for exaggerated BP response.

CASE STUDY Diabetes Mellitus

A 70-year-old man with type 2 diabetes mellitus suffered a stroke 10 months ago during a six-vessel coronary artery bypass graft surgery. He suffered a right-sided paralysis and alexia without agraphia. He had completed 4 months of stroke rehabilitation and was ambulatory with assistance because of a noticeable right-side weakness. He was referred by his endocrinologist for continued improvement in strength and functional ability. The client complained of weakness and inability to perform activities of daily living.

S: "I hate not being able to do the things I want to do."

O: Vitals: Height: 5'10" (1.78 m)   Weight: 180 lb (81.6 kg)   BMI: 25.75 kg/m²
          HR: 55 contractions/min   BP: 140/82 mmHg

Elderly male, hemiplegic on the right

Weak right upper and lower extremity in all muscles

Decreased passive ROM in right shoulder

Labs:
  Fasting glucose: 148 mg/dl
  HbA$_1$c 8.1% (normal range: 3.8-6.3%)
  Triglycerides: 222 mg/dl
  Total cholesterol: 175 mg/dl
  HDL: 27 mg/dl
  LDL: 104 mg/dl

Graded exercise test (recumbent cycle ergometer, 25 watts/2-min stage):
  Peak work rate: 75 watts
  Total time: 6 min
  Peak RPE: 14/20
  Peak HR: 82 contractions/min
  Peak BP: 184/74 mmHg
  VO$_2$max (estimated): 20.7 ml · kg^{-1} · min^{-1}
  ECG: Sinus rhythm at rest and throughout exercise and recovery
  No dysrhythmias and no report of chest discomfort

Body composition:
  Fat: 28.2% (BodPod)

Medications: Verapamil, Aspirin, Insulin

A: 1. Type 2 diabetes mellitus
    2. Cerebrovascular accident with right hemiparesis
    3. CAD
    4. Decreased ROM of the right shoulder

(continued)

CASE STUDY Diabetes Mellitus (continued)

P:
1. Initiate post-stroke rehabilitation.
2. Prescribe a comprehensive diabetes program including diabetes management and cardio-vascular risk reduction.

Exercise Program
Goals:

1. Improved ambulation with progressive strengthening of lower extremities
2. Increased strength and ROM in right shoulder
3. Improved aerobic conditioning
4. Education (client and spouse) on glucose management during exercise
5. Short-term goals (1 mo):
   Safely perform the timed "get up and go" test < 20 s
   Be able to do ≥ 20 min aerobic exercise
6. Long-term goals (6 mo):
   Safely perform the timed "get up and go" test < 10 s
   Be able to do ≥ 45 min aerobic exercise
   Walk unassisted on treadmill
   Be able to do resistance exercises unassisted

Mode	Frequency	Duration	Intensity	Progression
Aerobic (recumbent bike, arm ergometer, rower, Schwinn Air-Dyne™ [arms only])	3 days/wk	5 min/apparatus to orient and assess exercise tolerance	Determine tolerable "comfortable" limits to establish baseline	Add 1-2 min/day up to 15 min/apparatus Increase intensity after 15 min achieved
Strength (all major muscle groups, emphasis on right side)	3 days/wk	2-3 sets of 10-15 reps	~40-50% 1RM with right-side assistance	Increase to 18-20 reps, then to ~50-60% 1RM Remove assistance as tolerated
Flexibility (all major muscle groups)	Daily with assistance	Hold each stretch for 6-10 s	Maintain stretch below discomfort point	Increase to 20 s as tolerated Add rotator cuff stretch
Neuromuscular				
Functional (get up and go)	Intermittent			For reassessment tests
Warm-up/Cool-down	Before and after each session	5-10 min	Below talk test level RPE 7-9/20	

Special precautions:
- Conduct glucometer tests before and after exercise.
- Beware of hypoglycemia during and after exercise.
- Protect against falls.
- Be attentive to signs or complaints of shoulder pain with arm exercise.

Follow-Up
The physician adjusted insulin dosing to 16 U NPH + 6 U regular insulin before breakfast on exercise days, and 18 U NPH + 8 U regular insulin on non-exercise days. The pre-evening meal dose was reduced to 8 U NPH insulin on all days. The client was not allowed to exercise on any day when the insulin had not been adjusted for exercise. He also was not allowed to leave the exercise facility with a blood glucose under 80 mg/dl.

After 12 weeks, he could do all resistance and treadmill exercise without assistance. The client made such good progress in the first 2 or 3 weeks that the "get up and go" test was not repeated. After 6 months, the HbA$_1$c was 7.1%; episodes of mild hypoglycemia were occurring only on rare occasions. He was regularly exercising for 15 min at the following levels:

Schwinn Air-Dyne™: 25 watts

Treadmill: 1.7 mph, 0% grade

Rower: 10 watts

Recumbent cycle ergometer: 35 watts

Suggested Readings

American College of Sports Medicine. 2000. Position stand: Exercise and type 2 diabetes. *Medicine and Science in Sports and Exercise* 32: 1345-60.

American Diabetes Association. 2001. Position statement: Nutrition recommendations and principles for people with diabetes mellitus. *Diabetes Care* 24 (supplement 1): S44-47.

American Diabetes Association. 2001. Position statement: Diabetes mellitus and exercise. *Diabetes Care* 24 (supplement 1): S51-55.

American Diabetes Association. 1994. *The fitness book for people with diabetes*, edited by W.G. Hornsby. Richmond, VA: American Diabetes Association.

Buse, J.B. 2000. Progressive use of medical therapies in type 2 diabetes. *Diabetes Spectrum* 13: 211-20.

Graham, C., and P. Lasko-McCarthey. 1988. Exercise options for persons with diabetic complications. *Diabetes Educator* 16: 212-20.

Ruderman, N., and J.T. Devlin. (in press). *The health professional's guide to diabetes and exercise*, 2nd ed. Richmond, VA: American Diabetes Association.

Ruderman, N.B., and S.H. Schneider. 1992. Diabetes, exercise and atherosclerosis. *Diabetes Care* 15: 1787-93.

Sherman, W.M., and A.L. Albright. 1992. Exercise and type II diabetes. *Exercise and Sports Science Exchange* 4 (37): 1-5.

The Expert Committee on the Diagnosis and Classification of Diabetes Mellitus. 2001. Report of the expert committee on the diagnosis and classification of diabetes mellitus. *Diabetes Care* 24 (supplement 1): S5-20.

CHAPTER 22

Hyperlipidemia

J. Larry Durstine, PhD, FACSM
University of South Carolina

Geoffrey E. Moore, MD, FACSM
McGill University

Paul D. Thompson, MD, FACSM
Hartford Hospital

Overview of the Pathophysiology

Lipids are not soluble in an aqueous solution such as plasma and must combine with various proteins (apolipoproteins) to form the micelle particles. Lipoproteins are spherical in shape with apolipoproteins surrounding a lipid core that contains triglyceride, phospholipid, and free and esterified cholesterol. Lipoproteins are separated by ultracentrifugation into different gravitational density ranges. There are four principal lipoprotein classes:

- Chylomicrons are derived from intestinal absorption of exogenous (dietary) triglyceride.

- Very low density lipoprotein (VLDL or pre-β-lipoprotein) is synthesized in the liver and is the primary transport mechanism for endogenous triglyceride.

- Low-density lipoprotein (LDL or β-lipoprotein) represents the final stage in the catabolism of VLDL and is the principal carrier of cholesterol. Intermediate-density lipoprotein (IDL) and lipoprotein(a) are subfractions of LDL.

- High-density lipoprotein (HDL or α-lipoprotein) is involved in the reverse transport of cholesterol and is typically studied as two separate subfractions: HDL_2 and the more dense HDL_3.

Triglyceride and cholesterol move between the intestine, liver, and extrahepatic tissue by a complex transport system with plasma lipoproteins as the prominent element. This system is facilitated by several im-portant enzymes: lipoprotein lipase (LPL), hepatic lipase, lecithin-cholesterol acyltransferase (LCAT), and cholesterol ester transfer protein (CETP). These enzymes and lipoproteins interact to create several metabolic pathways. Chylomicrons, VLDL, IDL, and LDL are involved in the pathways that move lipids from the intestine or liver to peripheral tissues. HDL, however, is involved in the reverse cholesterol transport (i.e., from the peripheral tissues back to the liver). Variations in these pathways, from genetic and lifestyle factors, can change blood lipoprotein concentration and influence coronary artery disease (CAD) risk.

A variety of environmental, genetic, and pathologic factors can alter cholesterol and triglyceride transport. Some factors are gender, age, body fat distribution, dietary composition, cigarette smoking, some medications, genetic inheritance, and routine participation in physical activity. When these factors combine to yield elevated blood lipid and lipoprotein concentrations, the condition is referred to as dyslipidemia and has several forms:

- Hyperlipidemia indicates elevated blood triglyceride and cholesterol.

- Hypertriglyceridemia denotes only elevated triglyceride concentration.

- Hypercholesterolemia implies only elevated blood cholesterol concentration.

- Hyperlipoproteinemia or dyslipoproteinemia denotes elevated lipoprotein concentrations. Hyperlipoproteinemia is associated with genetic abnormalities or may be secondarily related to an underlying disease such as diabetes mellitus, renal insufficiency, hypothyroidism, biliary obstruction, dysproteinemia, or nephrotic kidney disease.

When one considers risk of CAD and peripheral arterial disease, the principal concerns are hypertriglyceridemia (elevated VLDL triglyceride), hypercholesterolemia (increased LDL cholesterol [LDL-C]), and mixed hyperlipidemia (increased LDL-C and VLDL triglyceride).

Effects on the Exercise Response

Generally, dyslipidemia does not alter the exercise response to a single session of exercise unless the dyslipidemia is longstanding and has led to CAD or secondary illness. When this occurs, the secondary disease process alters the exercise response in accordance with that problem (e.g., angina and claudication). In such cases, attention must be given to the exercise response in view of these other conditions. Possible exceptions to this rule include individuals with genetic disorders. Individuals who have extraordinarily high lipid concentrations may have inadequate oxygen supply to vital tissues such as heart or brain and be at great risk for stroke, myocardial infarctions, or both. Medical management to gain control of the dyslipidemia before the client begins an exercise program would be prudent, and in these cases exercise should be supervised. In addition, because dyslipidemic clients may have prescribed medications for other conditions, the type and dose of these medications should be noted before the person undergoes exercise testing or training.

Effects of Exercise Training

Regular participation in physical activity can bring about beneficial changes in persons with normal lipid and lipoprotein concentrations as well as most persons with dyslipidemia. These changes include the following:

- Triglyceride concentrations are generally lower.
- HDL cholesterol (HDL-C) concentrations are typically higher (but not always).
- Enzyme activity (LPL, LCAT, and CETP) in the metabolism of lipoproteins is increased.

These exercise training changes will enhance reverse cholesterol transport and can be augmented further by a low-fat diet, weight loss, and reduction in adiposity. Thus, exercise training can directly (e.g., by increased LPL activity) or indirectly (e.g., by reductions in body weight and body fat) improve blood lipid and lipoprotein profiles.

Congenital deficiencies in lipid transport can cause abnormal blood lipid and lipoprotein profiles, and these clients may have a substantially different response to routine physical activity from that seen in healthy individuals. For example, exercise training does not amplify LPL activity in clients with LPL deficiency; nor does HDL concentration increase in individuals with low HDL (hypoalphalipoprotein syndrome). The mechanisms responsible for changes in dyslipidemic conditions as a consequence of exercise training are unclear and in many cases are likely to be different from those reported for healthy subjects.

Management and Medications

Current treatment guidelines for the management of plasma lipids and lipoproteins have been provided by the National Cholesterol Education Program Adult Treatment Panel III (NCEP). Though dietary modification, weight loss, and exercise are recommended as initial therapy for at least six weeks, the primary therapy for reducing lipid and lipoprotein levels is pharmacological. Pharmacological therapy is highly effective and generally well tolerated. In contrast, hygienic therapy, including diet, exercise, and weight loss, is greatly limited by patient adherence and effectiveness. The occasional patient can achieve desired lipid levels by hygienic therapy alone, but in clinical practice, this is unfortunately the exception and not the rule. Nevertheless, because exercise can profoundly decrease plasma triglycerides and improve glucose intolerance, which contributes to dyslipidemia, we recommend daily exercise programs for all patients under treatment for lipid disorders. We consider hygienic therapy with diet, weight loss, and exercise to be adjunctive to pharmacological therapy but extremely important for the following reasons.

- Low-fat and high-carbohydrate diets lower HDL-C and increase triglyceride concentrations.
- Exercise diminishes these effects of diet on HDL-C and triglyceride concentrations.
- Low-calorie diets that cause weight loss decrease total cholesterol and LDL-C, and increase HDL-C.
- The effects of low-calorie diets are complex (e.g., low-calorie diets decrease HDL-C in obese women but increase HDL-C in distance runners).

Lipid-lowering medications act by a variety of mechanisms but generally have few hemodynamic or electrocardiographic effects. A combination of lipid-lowering drugs is frequently used. This practice can cause substantial reductions in dyslipidemia with reductions in cost and side effects while compliance is enhanced. A major risk of combination therapy is muscle toxicity and damage (rhabdomyolysis) with use of fibric acid derivatives or niacin and hepatic hydroxymethylglutaryl coenzyme A (HMG CoA) reductase inhibitors. Recent data suggest that exercise potentiates the propensity to develop drug-induced muscle damage.

HMG CoA reductase inhibitors inhibit the enzyme hydroxymethylglutaryl (HMG). CoA reductase, or *statins*, should be selected as the initial medical therapy for most lipid and lipoprotein disorders. They are extremely effective, have been demonstrated to reduce primary and secondary CAD events in multiple trials, and are well tolerated. Five statins are presently available in the United States: fluvastatin, lovastatin, pravastatin, atorvastatin, and simvastatin. More powerful statins are in development. Currently, available agents at their maximal doses can reduce LDL-C by 20 to 60%. They also reduce triglycerides by as much as 40% and increase HDL-C by 6 to 10%. The primary mechanism of action is to reduce cholesterol synthesis that results in a compensatory increase in LDL receptors. The combined effect is to decrease LDL-C. Many patients and physicians are concerned about inducing hepatic injury with these drugs, but this has rarely been an important issue.

The most important clinical side effect of these medications is muscle discomfort. In addition to symptomatic muscle complaints, these agents can produce asymptomatic elevations of creatine phosphokinase (CPK). Such elevations of CPK are exacerbated by eccentric exercise, making such elevations possibly more frequent in cardiac rehabilitation participants. No other lipid-lowering medications have side effects with such direct implications for CAD patients participating in exercise programs. The exercise-induced CPK elevations can reach high levels (as high as 21,000 U/l) without significant sequelae. Rare patients have experienced frank rhabdomyolysis with vigorous exercise. Rhabdomyolysis with statins usually occurs when statins have been combined with other agents such as fibric acid derivatives, niacin, cyclosporine, macrolide antibiotics such as erythromycin, and azole derivatives.

Bile acid sequestrants medications are administered as a powdered resin dissolved in liquid or as tablets. The tablets often do not contain sufficient resin to be effective except with multiple tablets. Resins inhibit the intestinal reabsorption of bile and its transport in the portal circulation to the liver. This loss of bile stimulates the upregulation of hepatic LDL receptor activity that reduces plasma LDL-C levels. These drugs are most effective when given with the fattiest meal because at this point, they are most likely to encounter bile in the gut. The major side effects of bile acid sequestrants are constipation, bloating, and flatulence. These medications also interfere with the absorption of fat-soluble vitamins and other medications. A newer tablet form of these drugs, colesevelam, is designed not to interfere with the absorption of other medications.

Hyperlipidemia: Exercise Testing

Methods	Measures	Endpoints*	Comments
Aerobic Cycle (ramp protocol 17 watts/min; staged protocol 25-50 watts/3 min stage) Treadmill (1-2 METs/3-min stage)	• 12-lead ECG, HR	• $\dot{V}O_2$peak/work rate • Serious dysrhythmias • >2 mm ST-segment depression or elevation • Ischemic threshold • T-wave inversion with significant ST change	• See testing tables in chapters 12 and 21.
	• BP, rate pressure product	• SBP > 250 mmHg or DBP > 115 mmHg • Exaggerated or hypotensive response	
	• RPE (6-20)	• Volitional fatigue	
Endurance 6-min walk	• Distance	• Note time, distance, symptoms at rest stops	• Useful for deconditioned persons.

*Measurements of particular significance; do not always indicate test termination.

Medications	Special Considerations
• HMG CoA reductase inhibitors and fibric acid used together may cause muscle damage.	• High risk of cardiac and arterial insufficiency. • Xanthomas may cause biomechanical problems. • Very high triglyceride/cholesterol may cause intravascular sludging and ischemia.

Fibric acid derivatives are useful as single agents for reducing elevated triglyceride levels. Gemfibrozil and fenofibrate are currently available in United States. These drugs are well tolerated with few side effects. They tend to increase LDL-C slightly in patients with hypertriglyceridemia because they increase LPL activity and facilitate the catabolism of VLDL to LDL. Fibric acid derivatives should be used with extreme caution in patients using statins concurrently because this combination can produce rhabdomyolysis. Most physicians should avoid this combination altogether and refer such patients to specialty lipid clinics.

Niacin or nicotinic acid is extremely useful in patients with low HDL-C levels with or without elevated triglycerides. Niacin has multiple potential areas of action but has a main effect in inhibiting lipolysis. Lipolysis inhibition reduces the quantity of plasma free fatty acids and their available transport to the liver, and reduces their subsequent synthesis into triglyceride. Niacin has the largest effect of any of the lipid agents in increasing HDL-C and can also reduce LDL-C concentrations. Because niacin inhibits lipolysis and because lipolysis is greatest during periods of fasting such as overnight, the most important niacin dose is the bedtime dose. Sustained-release formulations of niacin designed solely for nocturnal administration are available.

Niacin may be poorly tolerated because it often produces cutaneous flushing and lowers blood pressure, but this can be reduced by use of slow-release formulations. Also, since the flushing is prostaglandin mediated, the effect can be minimized by the simultaneous administration of aspirin or other prostaglandin inhibitors. All patients being treated for lipid disorders should receive aspirin as well so that the combination of aspirin and sustained-release niacin is an effective approach to the problem of flushing. In addition to cutaneous flushing, niacin can produce a reversible hepatitis, activate gout and peptic ulcers, and it can lead to glucose intolerance.

All individuals treated with niacin should have liver function tests performed at least every four months. Hepatitis can occur with both regular-release and sustained-release niacin but is 10 times more frequent with the sustained-release form. Patients should stop taking the medication and contact their physician if they develop frequent nausea, vomiting, unexpected weight loss, or other potential signs of hepatitis.

Stanol esters are food additives approved by the Food and Drug Administration as substitutes for butter and margarine. Stanol esters interfere with the absorption of dietary and biliary cholesterol from the intestine, and their effect on biliary cholesterol makes them effective even among persons on low-cholesterol diets. Their effect on plasma cholesterol is maximal at three servings daily and is not augmented by additional doses. They are also stable up to 400° F so that they can be substituted for butter and margarine in cooking.

Some medications used to treat other medical problems also affect plasma lipid and lipoprotein. These include beta antagonists (beta blockers), thiazide diuretics, oral hypoglycemic agents, insulin, estrogen, and progesterone.

- Beta blockers may increase triglyceride concentrations and reduce HDL-C concentrations, with the exception of those with intrinsic sympathomimetic activity.

Hyperlipidemia: Exercise Programming

Modes	Goals	Intensity/Frequency/Duration	Time to Goal
Aerobic •Large muscle activities	•Increase work capacity •Increase endurance •Decrease cholesterol and triglyceride concentrations •Increase daily caloric expenditure •Decrease adiposity	•40-70% of peak work rate or RPE 11-16/20 •Monitor HR or RPE •40-60 min/session (or 2 sessions/day of 20-30 min) •Emphasize duration rather than intensity	•4 mo (fitness) •9-12 mo (lipids) •Increase duration over intensity

Medications	Special Considerations
•See appendixes A, B, and C. •See exercise testing table.	•Obesity may limit training choices. •See exercise testing table and exercise programming table for people with obesity (chapter 23).

- Thiazide diuretics may increase total plasma cholesterol, VLDL cholesterol, LDL-C, and triglyceride without an effect on HDL-C concentration.

- Oral hypoglycemic agents or insulin therapy may reduce triglyceride and increase HDL-C in diabetic individuals in whom blood glucose is not well controlled. These benefits are secondary to the improvement in blood glucose.

- Levothyroxine increases hepatic LDL receptor activity and thereby lowers LDL-C in clients who are hypothyroid. This medication may produce elevations of heart rate and blood pressure as well as cardiac dysrhythmias, and can lead to angina in patients with CAD.

- Sex steroids in combination (as in oral contraceptives) tend to increase cholesterol depending on the estrogen-progesterone ratio.

- Estrogens tend to raise HDL-C and VLDL triglyceride concentrations, especially in postmenopausal women.

- Progesterone decreases triglyceride as well as HDL-C concentrations.

To date, few studies have examined the interaction of these medications with exercise training. Some preliminary results suggest that exercise training may attenuate the increased triglyceride concentration and reduced HDL-C concentrations associated with the use of beta blockers. Thus, it is possible that exercise may counteract the adverse effect of some medications.

Recommendations for Exercise Testing

If the dyslipidemia condition is congenital, but the client does not have any signs or symptoms of some other primary condition (e.g., CAD or renal insufficiency), exercise testing can follow normal protocols used for populations at risk for CAD. However, if signs or symptoms of other primary diseases are present, exercise testing should follow recommendations for that particular disorder (see the Hyperlipidemia: Exercise Testing table on page 144).

The primary objectives of exercise testing are to:

- uncover hidden CAD;

- determine functional capacity; and

- determine appropriate intensity range for aerobic exercise training.

Recommendations for Exercise Programming

The exercise prescription for the client with dyslipidemia should be adjuvant to therapy that restricts energy intake and dietary fat consumption as well as the appropriate therapy of lipid-lowering medications. Presently available information suggests that there may be different energy expenditure thresholds for different lipids and lipoproteins. For example, triglyceride concentrations are lower in hypertriglyceridemic men after 2 weeks of aerobic exercise (45 min/day) on consecutive days, whereas total plasma cholesterol concentration usually remains unchanged even after 1 year of exercise training. On the other hand, HDL-C concentrations are frequently increased by exercise regimens requiring 1000 to 1200 kcal of energy expenditure/wk (minimal training period of 12 wk). Inactive subjects may also have a lower threshold than physically active persons for change in HDL-C concentration. In any case, inactive persons may expect a favorable change in blood lipids within several months (see the Hyperlipidemia: Exercise Programming table on page 145).

The primary goal for exercise training is to expend calories by exercise training with exercise that is

- performed at moderate intensities (40-70% of maximal functional capacity),

- performed often (preferably 5 days/wk), and

- performed once a day, although exercising twice a day may be necessary to increase total energy expenditure and may be useful in persons with time constraints or severe exercise intolerance from chronic disease or morbid obesity.

CASE STUDY **Dyslipoproteinemia**

A 58-year-old woman with type III hyperlipidemia was having trouble controlling her cholesterol. She had attempted many dietary changes but had not been taking medications to lower her cholesterol. She was short of breath after walking 500 ft (152.4 m) down a hallway and complained of fatigue that prevented her from doing many things her friends could do.

S: "I've made a lot of dietary changes, but I can't improve my cholesterol."

O: Vitals: Height: 5'5" (1.65 m)   Weight: 180 lb (81.6 kg)   BMI: 30 kg/m²
   HR: 85 contractions/min   BP: 126/88 mmHg

Tired appearance (bags under eyes)

Palmar xanthomas

Labs:
   Hemoglobin: 14.2 g/dl
   Hematocrit: 38.0%
   Fasting glucose: 110 mg/dl
   Total cholesterol: 630 mg/dl
   Triglycerides: 796 mg/dl

Graded exercise test (Bruce protocol):
   Peak work rate: 3.40 mph @ 14% grade
   Total treadmill time: 6:40
   Test termination from leg fatigue
   Peak HR: 160 contractions/min
   Peak BP: 190/95 mmHg
   Peak RPE: 19
   $\dot{V}O_2$max: 23.4 ml · kg⁻¹ · min⁻¹
   Peak Respiratory Exchange Ratio: 1.10
   ECG: Sinus rhythm at rest and throughout exercise and recovery, 1 mm of upsloping ST change that resolved after 1 min of recovery
   No dysrhythmias
   No report of chest discomfort

Body composition:
   Fat: 28.5% (skin folds)

Medications: None

A: 1. Type III hyperlipidemia

   2. Deconditioning with easy fatigability

P: 1. Begin hyperlipidemia management with diet and exercise for 6 wk.

   2. After 6 wk, reevaluate for medical management.

Exercise Program
Goals:

   1. Short-term (1 mo):
   Be able to walk 1mi (1.6K) < 20 min
   Climb 1 flight of stairs 3 consecutive times

   2. Long-term (6 mo):
   Return to work part time
   Be able to walk 3 mi (4.8K)

Mode	Frequency	Duration	Intensity	Progression
Aerobic (walking or biking)	4-5 days/wk	20 min/session to start	THR 134-141 contractions/min (65-75% HRR) RPE 13-15/20	Add 5 min of activity every wk to 45 min Increase intensity every 2 wk to 75-85%
Strength (all major muscle groups)	3 days/wk		1 set of 10-12 reps	Add weight as needed to maintain comfortable resistance for 10-12 reps

(continued)

CASE STUDY Dyslipoproteinemia (continued)

Mode	Frequency	Duration	Intensity	Progression
Flexibility (all major muscle groups)	3 days/wk		Maintain each stretch for 20 s or below discomfort point	
Warm-up/Cool-down	Before and after each sesson	5-10 min	RPE 7-9/20	

Special precautions:
- Avoid Valsalva maneuver.
- Stay hydrated.

Follow-Up

After 6 weeks, her total cholesterol was 678 mg/dl, triglycerides were 397 mg/dl, HDL-C was 43 mg/dl, and LDL-C was 556 mg/dl. She had been trying to follow an American Heart Association low-fat diet. Gemfibrozil (600 mg bid) was prescribed. After 5 weeks on gemfibrozil, her total cholesterol was 218 mg/dl, triglycerides were 135 mg/dl, HDL-C was 68 mg/dl, and LDL-C was 135 mg/dl. The patient attended 80% of the supervised exercise sessions and reported that in the last 4 weeks had begun to exercise in addition to the supervised sessions. She was not short of breath after a 500-ft (152.4-m) walk and had no complaints of fatigue. After 12 weeks of exercise programming, her graded exercise test (Bruce protocol) time was 7:35. Estimated $\dot{V}O_2$max was 26.5 ml · kg^{-1} · min^{-1}.

Suggested Readings

Bruce, C., R.A. Chouinard Jr., and A.R. Tall. 1998. Plasma lipid transfer proteins, high-density lipoproteins, and reverse cholesterol transport. *Annual Review of Nutrition* 18: 297-330.

Chong, P.H., and B.S. Bachenheimer. 2000. Current, new and future treatments in dyslipidaemia and atherosclerosis. *Drugs* 60 (1): 55-93.

Durstine, J.L., P.W. Grandjean, P.G. Davis, M.A. Ferguson, N.L. Alderson, and K.D. DuBose. 2001. The effects of exercise training on serum lipids and lipoproteins: A quantitative analysis. *Sports Medicine* 31 (15): 1033-62.

Durstine, J.L., and P.D. Thompson. 2001. Exercise in the treatment of lipid disorders. *Cardiology Clinics* 19 (3): 471-88.

Executive Summary of the Third Report of the National Cholesterol Education Program (NCEP). 2001. Expert panel on detection, evaluation, and treatment of high blood cholesterol in adults (Adult Treatment Panel III). *Journal of the American Medical Association* 285 (19): 2486-97. [Online]. Available: **www.nhlbi.nih.gov/chd**.

Kwiterovich P.O., Jr. 2000. The metabolic pathways of high-density lipoprotein, low-density lipoprotein, and triglycerides: A current review. *American Journal of Cardiology* 86 (12A): 5L-10L.

Oliver, M.F., K. Pyorala, and J. Shepherd. 1997. Management of hyperlipidaemia. Why, when and how to treat. *European Heart Journal* 18 (3): 371-75.

Shepherd, J. 2001. Economics of lipid-lowering in primary prevention: Lessons from the West of Scotland Coronary Prevention Study. *American Journal of Cardiology* 87 (5A): 19B-22B.

Superko, H.R. 2001. Lipoprotein subclasses and atherosclerosis. *Frontiers in Bioscience* 1 (6): D355-65.

Superko, H.R. 2000. Hypercholesterolemia and dyslipidemia. *Current Treatment Options in Cardiovascular Medicine* 2 (2): 173-87.

Tall, A.R. 1998. An overview of reverse cholesterol transport. *European Heart Journal* 19 (supplement A): A31-35.

CHAPTER 23

Obesity

Janet P. Wallace, PhD, FACSM

Indiana University

Overview of the Pathophysiology

Obesity is excess body fat frequently resulting in a significant impairment of health. The prevalence of obese and overweight adults varies depending on the measurement technique. According to the Centers for Disease Control (CDC) Behavioral Risk Factor Surveillance System, 35.3% of all men and 33.2% of all women in the United States were found to be overweight in 1999. This represents a 14% increase in the prevalence of overweight for men and a 19% increase for women since 1995. The prevalence of obesity has increased from 11.6% of the nation's population in 1990 to 19.7% in 1999. More evident is the prevalence of overweight children and adolescents, which has increased 27% in the last decade to reach 13 to 14% in 1999. This increase in the prevalence of obesity has not only led to the American Heart Association to affirm obesity as a primary risk factor for heart disease but is also the basis for which the CDC declared diabetes an epidemic. In addition, many obese persons are at risk for diabetes.

Although the causes of obesity include hypothalamic, endocrine, and genetic disorders, diet and physical inactivity are the primary causes of the more common form of obesity found in the United States. The accumulation of excess fat is not just a simple balance of caloric intake and caloric expenditure. Caloric intake and expenditure may be likened to opposing forces balanced on a fulcrum of physiological and metabolic functions that control fat storage and fat release. The balance can be altered by the lifestyle factors of diet and physical inactivity, but once the fulcrum of the balance is displaced, the caloric balance between intake and expenditure may no longer be even. Excess dietary fat, sugar, and physical inactivity, in combination, are the lifestyle factors that contribute to the instability of caloric balance. This altered physiological fulcrum in obesity includes

- increased fasting insulin,
- increased insulin response to glucose,
- decreased insulin sensitivity,
- decreased growth hormone,
- decreased growth hormone response to insulin stimulation,
- increased adrenocortical hormones,
- increased cholesterol synthesis and excretion, and
- decreased hormone-sensitive lipase.

Altered insulin function may be a primary mechanism in the etiology and maintenance of obesity.

Obesity has been defined with many systems, most commonly height/weight tables, body mass index (BMI), and body fat percentage. More recently, an estimate of the distribution of body fat has been utilized.

- Height/weight tables: People are considered obese when they weigh more than 20% above their desirable weight as listed in the tables.

- BMI: Although different BMI standards have been published for increased risk of disease for men (>27.8 kg/m^2) and women (27.3 kg/m^2), a combined categorization has been derived from the epidemiological literature, measured in body weight (kg)/height (m^2):

  Acceptable range (low risk): 20.0-25.0 kg/m^2

  Mildly overweight (increased risk): 25.1-27.0 kg/m^2

  Moderately overweight/obese: 27.1-30.0 kg/m^2

  Markedly overweight/obese: 30.1-40.0 kg/m^2

  Morbidly obese: > 40.0 kg/m^2

Epidemiological evidence has been developed and provides the basis for classification of disease risk based on BMI and waist circumference. This classification is presented in table 23.1 (page 149).

- The following percentages of body fat are for men and women.

	Men	Women
Minimal fat	5%	8%
Below average	5-15-%	14-23%
Above average	16-25%	24-32%
At risk	> 25%	> 32%

Table 23.1 Classification of Disease Risk Based on Body Mass Index (BMI) and Waist Circumference

| | BMI (kg/m²) | Disease risk[1] relative to normal weight and waist circumference[2] | |
		Men ≤ 102 cm Women ≤ 88 cm	Men > 102 cm Women > 88 cm
Underweight	< 18.5	. . .	. . .
Normal[3]	18.5-24.9	. . .	. . .
Overweight	25.0-29.9	Increased	High
Obesity class			
I	30.0-34.9	High	Very high
II	35.0-39.9	Very high	Very high
III	> 40.0	Extremely high	Extremely high

Adapted from Expert Panel. 1998. Executive summary of the clinical guidelines on the identification, evaluation, and treatment of overweight and obesity in adults. *Archives of Internal Medicine* 158: 1855-67.

1. Disease risk for type 2 diabetes, hypertension, and cardiovascular disease. Ellipses indicate that no additional risk at these levels of BMI was assigned.
2. A gender-neutral value for waist circumference (> 100 cm) has also been suggested as an index of obesity.
3. Increased waist circumference can also be a marker for increased risk even in persons of normal weight.

- Obesity classification systems have also been based on phenotype, fat cell morphology, and health status:
  - Phenotype:
    Type I: Excess body mass or percentage fat
    Type II: Excess subcutaneous truncal-abdominal fat (android)
    Type III: Excess abdominal visceral fat
    Type IV: Excess gluteal-femoral fat (gynoid)
  - Cell morphology:
    Hyperplastic obesity
    Hypertrophic obesity
  - Health status:
    Mild obesity
    Morbid obesity

Obesity increases not only the risk of disease but also the severity of disease. The distribution of body fat may contribute more to disease than total body fat. Upper body fat distribution has been associated with increased risk of coronary artery disease (CAD), hypertension, hyperlipidemia, and diabetes, as well as hormone and menstrual dysfunction. Truncal adipocytes have a higher metabolic activity than other sites. This increased activity has been associated with glucose intolerance, hypertension via increased sodium retention, sympathetic nervous system activation, increased intracellular calcium, and hypertrophy of smooth muscle vessels. Abdominal adipocytes are associated with increased very low density lipoprotein, triglyceride, and adipose lipoprotein lipase activity. Thus, excess fat in specific deposits may contribute more to the diseases associated with obesity. Body fat distribution can be estimated by the measurement of waist-to-hip

ratio, although this ratio is not well standardized. The most common and most often recommended technique may be the ratio of the minimal waist to the largest gluteus. Standards for this method of calculating waist-to-hip ratio are as follows:

- Lower body fat distribution for men: < 0.776
- Lower body fat distribution for women: < 0.776
- Upper body fat distribution for men: > 0.913
- Upper body fat distribution for women: > 0.861

Effects on the Exercise Response

The effects of obesity on exercise testing are not always straightforward. The obvious effect of obesity on exercise testing is low physical work capacity because of excess body weight. Because obesity is associated with other diseases, however, any of the confounding influences of these diseases may be involved in exercise testing. For example, obese adults have a higher risk of CAD and may exhibit myocardial ischemia during exercise testing. A hypertensive response to exercise testing may be exhibited despite the absence of hypertension at rest. Consideration of glucose intolerance is essential for the obese diabetic client.

Effects of Exercise Training

Exercise training is effective in reducing body weight in moderate obesity, but may not be as effective in morbid obesity. When body weight is reduced through regular dynamic exercise, body fat is reduced, while lean body weight is either maintained or increased. Populations with low lean body weight are the most likely to gain lean body weight with exercise training. This excludes the obese because in these people, lean weight is increased only to support the excess fat. On the other hand, resistance training can increase the lean body weight of almost any population.

Physical activity affects body fat distribution by promoting regional fat loss in the abdominal sites. Fat loss through exercise is more efficient for individuals with upper body fat distribution. The resultant reduction of regional fat in the abdominal sites significantly decreases the risk of the diseases associated with upper body fat distribution.

Physical activity may be one of the most important factors in the maintenance of weight loss. This maintenance may occur directly through increases in energy expenditure, or the positive behavior change of exercise could act indirectly by influencing the participant to decrease caloric intake. The influence of physical activity on food intake is unclear in human studies. Non-obese people may increase food intake with exercise, whereas obese people may not.

The effects of exercise training on metabolism are not well established. Metabolic rate, including the caloric cost of physical activity, does decline with weight reduction via caloric restriction. In the starvation state, however, the maintenance of metabolic rate through exercise may not always counteract the reduction mediated by food restriction. In any case, exercise training has profound effects on glucose metabolism in both the moderately and the morbidly obese. These include

- decreased fasting glucose;
- decreased fasting insulin;
- increased glucose tolerance; and
- decreased insulin resistance.

These changes have been found, in some instances, without changes in body weight or body fat. Other reports show that the more dramatic changes in glucose

Obesity: Exercise Testing

Methods	Measures	Endpoints*	Comments
Aerobic Cycle (ramp protocol 17 watts/min; staged protocol 25-50 watts/3-min stage) Treadmill (1-2 METs/3-min stage)	• 12-lead ECG, HR • BP, rate pressure product • RPE (6-20)	• Serious dysrhythmias • >2 mm ST-segment depression or elevation • Ischemic threshold • T-wave inversion with significant ST change • SBP > 250 mmHg or DBP > 115 mmHg • Volitional fatigue	• Clients are at higher than normal risk for CAD/hypertension.
Flexibility Goniometry	• ROM		• Used to determine joints that need stretching.
Neuromuscular Gait analysis Balance			• Useful in identifying individuals with poor balance who may require more supervision during exercise, and to assess improvement in balance after training and/or weight reduction.

*Measurements of particular significance; do not always indicate test termination.

Medications	Special Considerations
• For clients with hypertension, refer to chapter 12. • For clients with diabetes, refer to chapter 21. • For clients with hyperlipidemia, refer to chapter 22.	• Increased risk of orthopedic injury. • Increased risk of cardiovascular disease. • Increased risk of heat intolerance.

metabolism occurred in those who exhibited the greatest reduction in deep abdominal fat.

Management and Medications

Reduction of fat weight with the preservation of lean body weight is the primary objective of obesity management. The individual who is most likely to be successful in weight loss:

- is slightly or moderately obese;
- has upper body fat distribution;
- has no history of weight cycling;
- has a sincere desire to lose weight; and
- became overweight as an adult.

Behavioral change focuses on dietary and activity habits toward weight reduction, whereas more invasive interventions have been used in morbid or extreme obesity (BMI > 40).

Dietary objectives are:

- reduction in total calories; and
- reduction in fat intake.

Physical activity objectives are:

- increase in daily activity; and
- physical conditioning.

Other medical techniques include the following:

- starvation diets;
- gastroplasties;
- jejunoileal bypass;

Obesity: Exercise Programming

Modes	Goals	Intensity/ Frequency/Duration	Time to Goal
Aerobic •Large muscle activities (walking, rowing, cycling, water aerobics)	•Reduce weight •Increase functional performance •Reduce risk of CAD	•50-70% $\dot{V}O_2$peak •Monitor RPE and HR •5 days/wk •40-60 min/session (or 2 sessions/ day of 20-30 min) •Emphasize duration rather than intensity	•9-12 mo •Increase duration over intensity
Flexibility •Stretching	•Increase ROM	•Daily or at least 5 sessions/wk	
Functional •Activity-specific exercise	•Increase ease of performing ADLs •Increase vocational potential •Increase physical self-confidence		

Medications	Special Considerations
•For clients with hypertension, refer to chapter 12. •For clients with diabetes, refer to chapter 21. •For clients with hyperlipidemia, refer to chapter 22.	•Use low-impact modes of activity. •There is increased risk of hyperthermia. •Equipment modification may be necessary (e.g., wide seats on cycle ergometers and rowers). •Strength training may serve as a valuable adjunct to aerobic training when trying to maintain lean body weight. Begin with guidelines listed in chapter 4 programming table. For further strength gain, heavier resistance with fewer reps may be employed as the client adapts to the program. •See text for multiple environmental precautions to prevent injury. •Goal setting and decisional balance are important behavioral interventions.

- jaw wiring;
- intragastric balloons;
- fat excision; and
- anti-obesity medications.

There are prescription and over-the-counter medications for weight control that act by suppressing appetite. Medications approved by the Food and Drug Administration (FDA) include sympathomimetic drugs (medications that stimulate the sympathetic nervous system) such as amphetamines, other synthetic amines, isoindoles, and caffeine. Serotonin uptake inhibitors have been tried as appetite suppressants but do not have FDA approval for that purpose. The contribution these pharmacologic appetite suppressants make to weight loss in obese persons is not well understood, but it is thought that these agents have little clinical value. Thyroid hormone has been used in the past, but because drug-induced hypothyroidism can cause dangerous cardiovascular side effects as well as osteoporosis, thyroid hormone should not be used to control weight. Antidepression medications have also been used in weight reduction.

Recommendations for Exercise Testing

Evaluation of the client who is obese includes more than just exercise testing. Additional assessments include medical and weight histories, motivation and readiness for change, nutrition and eating habits, and body composition. Body composition assessment includes a measure of the extent of obesity, distribution of body fat, and a reasonable target weight. An additional assessment for potential for injury would also be prudent.

Although obesity is now considered one of the major risk factors for safety in exercise testing, exercise testing is not always necessary for obese adults who want to start an exercise program. Nevertheless, exercise testing plays an important role in the optimal management of exercise treatment for persons who are obese. The primary objective of exercise testing with individuals who are obese is exercise prescription. Disease diagnosis is a secondary, yet essential, objective. A determination of physical work capacity is important for selecting the intensity of exercise (see the Obesity: Exercise Testing table on page 151).

Recommendations for Exercise Programming

Although the primary objective of exercise in the treatment of obesity is to expend more calories, the optimal

approach to increase energy expenditure is debatable. The exercise prescription must optimize energy expenditure yet minimize potential for injury. On the other hand, exercise should be enjoyable and practical and should fit into the lifestyle of the individual.

The energy expenditure of the actual exercise as well as that of the recovery period, excess postexercise oxygen consumption (EPOC), should be considered in the total energy expenditure for a single exercise session. The debate is whether 2 or more short sessions a day will produce a higher total energy expenditure (exercise + EPOC) than 1 longer session of the same intensity. The use of two or more shorter sessions has been recommended because the elevated energy expenditure of recovery may be sustained for a longer period of time than after a single session, even though longer. On the other hand, the single longer exercise session may have an advantage for substrate utilization and for ease of incorporation into some individuals' lifestyles.

Substrate utilization may not be important for weight reduction. The literature supports total calories expended, rather than calories from fat or carbohydrate stores, to be fundamental to body fat reduction. For this reason, recommendations for both types of prescriptions are listed (see the Obesity: Exercise Programming table):

- Mode:
  Non-weight-bearing exercise
  Walking
  Increase in daily living activities
  Resistance training
- Frequency: Daily or at least 5 sessions/week
- Duration: 40 to 60 min/day or 20 to 30 min twice daily
- Intensity:
  50 to 70% of peak oxygen consumption ($\dot{V}O_2$peak)
  Exercise intensities of 70 to 85% of $\dot{V}O_2$peak can be prescribed providing the risk of injury is minimal

Exercise programs that include high-resistance activities (i.e., free weights, resistance machines) can lead to preferential retention of lean body weight. However, aerobic activity has more potential to decrease fat weight than does resistance training because the former can be sustained for a longer time, allowing more energy to be expended.

Special Considerations

Exercise will not be effective if the client is not motivated or ready to make the necessary changes. Motivational strategies are often required to help clients move into readiness for change. These strategies can include

- goal setting and
- decision/balance sheets.

Injury prevention is the most important consideration in exercise for adults who are obese. In fact, physical injury may be one of the primary reasons for discontinuation of exercise. Excess body weight may exacerbate existing joint conditions. Another concern is thermoregulation. The following considerations and guidelines are relevant for exercise programming in obese populations:

- Prevention of overuse injury
- Injury history

- Adequate flexibility, warm-up, and cool-down sessions
- Gradual progression of intensity and duration
- Use of low-impact or non-weight-bearing exercises
- Thermoregulation
- Neutral temperature and humidity
- Times of day (e.g., should be cool)
- Adequate hydration
- Clothing (e.g., should be loose fitting)

Other considerations may be dependent on associated diseases that coexist with obesity.

CASE STUDY Obesity

A 54-year-old woman entered a weight-loss program wanting to lose weight, feel better, be able to cross her legs, not always be out of breath, enjoy her grandson, wear "normal" clothes, and stop falling down. She had been overweight for 37 years and wanted to lose 143 to 154 lb (65-70 kg). She had a history of weight cycling (44-77 lb [20-35 kg]) during the past 15 years. She could not remember the number of times she had dieted, although she had tried most popular techniques, including fad diets. She was hospitalized 4 years ago for severe depression. On more than one occasion, her mother and father had made discouraging remarks about her weight.

She wrote the following notes on her intake form: "I am morbidly obese and it's frightening and adds to my severe depression and low self-esteem. Sometimes I think my life insurance money would help my daughter and grandson more than me. I have been suicidal several times due to stress and depression. A lot is weight related. These feelings began in college. I hate my body."

S: "This weight loss clinic is my last hope."

O: Vitals: Height: 5'1" (1.55 m) Weight: 267.5 lb (121.37 kg) BMI: 50.5 kg/m²
   HR: 85 contractions/min BP: 140/88 mmHg

Morbidly obese woman in no acute distress

Past history: Irritable bowel syndrome; osteoarthritis of the spine and lower extremities; several falls resulting in 2 left leg fractures; a prior sleep apnea study inconclusive

Family history: Heart disease, hypertension, and diabetes at advanced ages

Social history: Her usual day was stressful in the broadcast industry; she worked so frantically that she reported, "Sometimes my blood pressure rises and I get dizzy or see flashing lights."

Medications: Lotensin, Prozac, Ativan, Pempro, Klonopin, Adipex, Imodium AD, Bentyl

Abdominal girth: 125.1 cm

Waist-to-hip ratio: 81:6

Body composition: % body fat was not determined

Total cholesterol: 234 mg/dl
  HDL: 51 mg/dl
  Triglycerides: 230 mg/dl
  Fasting blood glucose: 103 mg/dl

FVC: 2.29 l

FEV$_1$: 1.76 l (77% of FVC)

Cycle ergometry:
   Peak work rate: 600 kpm
   Peak HR: 160 contractions/min
   Peak BP: 276/90 mmHg
   ECG response: Normal without ectopy; no symptoms of cardiac ischemia
24-hour diet recall and 2-day diet diary:
   Total caloric intake: 1240 kcal/day
   Protein intake: 60 g/day (19% of total calories)
   Carbohydrate intake: 106 g (34% of total calories)
   Fat intake: 63 g (46% of total calories)
   Vitamin and mineral intake: 6-115% of dietary goals
Psychometric evaluations:
   Internal locus of control
   Self-efficacy good for walking 1 mi (1.6K)
Diet readiness assessment:
   Path clear with respect to goals and attitudes
   Moderate tendency to eat because food is available
   Alternates between out-of-control eating and strict dieting
   Bingeing habits require attention
   Sometimes eats in response to emotional highs and lows
   External motivation beneficial

A: 1. Morbid obesity with poor eating and physical activity habits

2. History of major depression with probable anxiety disorder

3. Low aerobic capacity

4. Exaggerated BP response to exercise

P: 1. Prescribe a diet program for weight loss.

2. Institute an exercise program to increase caloric expenditure.

3. Identify multiple psychological support systems.

Exercise Program

Goals:

1. Increase physical activity without injury

2. Improve eating habits:
   Total calories: 1900 cal/day, with lower fat and higher carbohydrate intakes
   Exercise: Substitute walking for snacks

3. Improve self-esteem

4. Weekly counseling sessions; monthly meetings with dietitian and/or support group

5. Continue psychotherapy

(continued)

CASE STUDY Obesity *(continued)*

Mode	Frequency	Duration	Intensity	Progression
Aerobic (stationary cycling, water aerobics)	2 days/wk (in center) 5 days/wk (at home)	To start: 15-20 min/session or 2 sessions/day of 10-15 min	Talk test limit (must be able to carry on a conversation)	Increase as tolerated to 30-40 min/session Gradually increase ADLs to 30 min/day May consider 2 sessons/day
Strength				
Flexibility				
Neuromuscular				
Functional				
Warm-up/Cool-down				

Suggested Readings

Atkinson, R.L., and J. Walberg-Rankin. 1994. Physical activity, fitness, and severe obesity. In *Physical activity, fitness, and health*, edited by C. Bouchard, R.J. Shephard, and T. Stephens, 696-711. Champaign, IL: Human Kinetics.

Buskirk, E.R. 1993. Obesity. In *Exercise testing and exercise prescription for special cases: Theoretical basis and clinical application*, edited by J.S. Skinner, 185-210. Philadelphia: Lea & Febiger.

Hill, J.O., H.J. Drougas, and J.C. Peters. 1994. Physical activity, fitness, and moderate obesity. In *Physical activity, fitness, and health*, edited by C. Bouchard, R.J. Shephard, and T. Stephens, 684-95. Champaign, IL: Human Kinetics.

National Insititutes of Health (NIH) and National Heart, Lung, and Blood Institute (NHLBI). 1998. Clinical Guidelines on the identification, evaluation, and treatment of overweight and obesity in adults: Evidence report. Bethesda, MD: NIH NHLBI. [Online]. Available: **www.nhlbi.nih.gov**.

Verrill, D., E. Shoup, L. Boyce, B. Fox, A. Moore, and T. Forkner. 1994. Recommended guidelines for body composition assessment in cardiac rehabilitation: A position paper by the North Carolina Cardiopulmonary Rehabilitation Association. *Journal of Cardiopulmonary Rehabilitation* 14: 104-21.

Wallace, J.P., P.G. Bogle, K.T. Murray, and W.C. Miller. 1994. Variation in the anthropometric dimensions for estimating upper and lower body obesity. *American Journal of Human Biology* 6: 699-709.

CHAPTER 24

Frailty

Connie Bayles, PhD, FACSM
University of Pittsburgh

Overview of the Pathophysiology

Physical decline associated with aging can be attributed to a number of complex interactions, including normal aging, disease, and disuse. Frail health can be found across the entire age spectrum, but adults who are elderly are especially prone to becoming frail (weak, vulnerable, slight). The frail older adult is generally identified as having one or more of the following: extreme old age, some type of disability, and the presence of multiple chronic diseases or geriatric syndromes. Adults who are older and frail are more dependent, recover slowly from illness, undergo more falls and injuries, have more acute illnesses, and are more often institutionalized or hospitalized. All these factors can result in increased mortality. The most rapidly growing elderly population group is the oldest of the old. According to the U.S. Census Bureau, this group numbered 3 million in 1994 and is expected to climb to 19 million in 2050.

Many older adults who are considered frail tend to have the most serious health problems and disabilities and/or are functionally impaired. Functional impairment for the elderly means a restriction in or lack of ability to perform the activities of daily life required for independent living.

The elderly are often confronted with disease that results in disuse and may accelerate the development of frailty. The body is in constant change throughout life, with changes occurring in the cardiovascular, respiratory, nervous, musculoskeletal, renal, and metabolic systems as part of the normal aging process (see table 24.1). Along

Table 24.1 Physiological Changes Associated With Aging

System	Function	Change
Cardiovascular	Resting HR	No change
	Maximal HR	Decrease
	Resting cardiac output	Decrease
	Maximal cardiac output	Decrease
	Resting SV	Decrease
	Maximal SV	Decrease
	Resting BP	Increase
	Exercise BP	Increase
	$\dot{V}O_2$peak	Decrease
Respiratory	Residual volume	Increase
	Vital capacity	Decrease
	Total lung capacity	No change
	Respiratory frequency	Increase
Nervous	Reaction time	Decrease
	Nerve conduction time	Increase
	Sensory deficits	Increase
Musculoskeletal	Muscular strength	Decrease
	Muscle mass	Decrease
	Flexibility	Decrease
	Balance	Decrease
	Bone density	Decrease

(continued)

157

Table 24.1 (continued)

System	Function	Change
Renal	Kidney function Acid-base control Glucose tolerance Drug clearance Cellular water	Decrease Decrease Decrease Decrease Decrease
Metabolic	Basal metabolic rate Lean body mass Body fat	Decrease Decrease Increase

Table 24.2 Common Medical Disorders That Contribute to Frailty in Elderly Individuals

System	Medical disorder
Cardiovascular	Hypertension, hypotension, coronary artery disease, valvular heart disease, failure, dysrhythmia, peripheral arterial disease
Pulmonary	Asthma, chronic pulmonary disease, pneumonia
Musculoskeletal	Arthritis, degenerative disk disease, polymyalgia rheumatica, osteoporosis, degenerative joint disease
Metabolic/endocrine	Diabetes, hypercholesterolemia
Gastrointestinal	Dental disorder, malnutrition, incontinence, diarrhea
Genitourinary	Urinary tract infection, cancer
Hematologic/immunologic	Anemia, leukemia, cancer
Neurological	Dementia, Alzheimer's disease, cerebrovascular disease, Parkinson's disease, disorders
Eye and ear	Cataracts, glaucoma, hearing disorders
Psychiatric	Anxiety disorders, hypochondria, depression, alcoholism

with normal aging, the presence of multiple chronic medical disorders also contribute to increased physical decline (see table 24.2). The presence of these diseases does not, in itself, define frailty but may place an individual at greater risk of becoming frail.

Effects on the Exercise Response

Persons who are elderly and frail are faced with a variety of medical problems that can put them at risk for a medical emergency during exercise testing. As a result, the following should be kept in mind with respect to exercise testing in persons who are frail.

• Preliminary tests such as Independent Activities of Daily Living (IADL), Activities of Daily Living (ADL), Mini Mental State, the Geriatric Depression Scale, and the Nutritional Risk Index may be helpful to review before testing.

• Medical history and present medications should be reviewed before the person undergoes testing.

• Exercise tests should be individualized, starting at low work rates, and in many cases should incorporate longer warm-up periods. Various modes of testing should be considered to meet the needs of the client.

• Since older frail persons will usually take a longer time to reach a steady state, the exercise test should focus on longer work stages with increases in grade rather than speed.

• Caution should be taken that the exercise stages are not too long because older frail persons fatigue more quickly. Nevertheless, if the test is needed for diagnostic purposes, a more aggressive protocol may be used.

• Older frail persons are susceptible to dehydration and insulin insensitivity, and care should be taken to identify physiological features associated with these conditions.

Effects of Exercise Training

Physical activity appears to be of critical importance for delaying the metabolic disorders associated with aging. In older populations, physical activity can produce increased muscle strength and endurance as well as maximal aerobic power. Flexibility, coordination, and balance are also improved, resulting in a decreased risk for falling while enhancing mobility. Also, exercise has been shown to increase socialization and self-esteem. These benefits have important implications for the frail elderly in maintaining or promoting independence in daily living activities.

Management and Medications

The elderly and frail person is usually taking more medications than are people in any other segment of the population. Since renal excretion of chemicals is reduced in the elderly, drugs will remain in the body for longer periods of time. This increases the importance of recognizing conditions such as polypharmacy and self-medication. Exercise professionals working with this group must be able to identify individuals who do not follow medication instructions. Before developing an exercise program for an elderly person, a comprehensive list of the client's medications is necessary.

Many medications have side effects. Side effects and the type of medicines associated with these side effects include the following:

- dizziness (sedatives, hypnotics, anticonvulsants, tricyclic antidepressants, anti-psychotics);
- confusion and/or depression (sedatives, hypnotics, anticonvulsants, anti-psychotics, antidepressants, diuretics, antihypertensives);
- fatigue and weakness (beta blockers, diuretics, tricyclic antidepressants, anti-psychotics, barbiturates, benzodiazepines, antihistamines, antihypertensives);
- postural hypotension (tricyclic antidepressants, anti-psychotics, antihypertensives, diuretics, nitrates, narcotic analgesics, vasodilators, levodopa);
- involuntary muscle movements (anti-psychotics, levodopa, tricyclic antidepressants, adrenergics);
- urinary incontinence (benzodiazepines, barbiturates, phenothiazines, chlorpromazines, anticholinergics, diuretics); and
- increases in heart rate (anti-glaucoma agents/miotics, bronchodilators/anti-asthmatic agents).

Recommendations for Exercise Testing

Cardiorespiratory, strength, neuromuscular, flexibility, and functional performance tests enable the exercise professional to assess the current functional levels of participants and are important for developing an appropriate exercise program. The client who has cardiac problems and exhibits coronary heart disease risk factors should be assessed by a graded exercise test. Various testing modalities, including treadmill and cycle tests, can be used depending upon the client's medical status. For clients who are free from any coronary heart disease and who have physician clearance, a simple 6- or 12-min test or 20-ft (6.1-m) walk test is recommended (see the Frailty: Exercise Testing table on page 160). Heart rate, blood pressure, ratings of perceived exertion, and distance walked are monitored and recorded to ensure a proper exercise prescription.

Maintaining or improving muscle strength can improve functional ability in persons who are elderly. A handheld dynamometer is often used to assess muscle strength because it is easy to use and is a reliable means of obtaining an objective measurement of strength. Baseline measures of strength enable the exercise professional to chart progress and provide feedback to participants as they progress in an exercise program.

In the development of a physical activity program for individuals who are frail and elderly, neuromuscular and functional performance tests are sometimes important for use in evaluating progress. Information obtained from gait, balance, and coordination tests enables the exercise professional to plan appropriate intervention programs as well as to target those individuals who are at risk for falling. Flexibility training can increase joint flexibility and mobility. The goniometer is an important tool for measuring flexibility, and information gained from such tests can be employed as feedback that participants can use to note improvements.

Recommendations for Exercise Programming

The exercise prescription for persons who are elderly and frail should reflect medical and social needs. Past exercise experience and the setting of goals are major contributors to the success of a program. Because in many instances persons who are elderly have lost the freedom to make choices, the choice of activity by the participant is very important. Compliance to exercise programming is enhanced when the exercise professional and the client work together.

Frailty: Exercise Testing

Methods	Measures	Endpoints*	Comments
Aerobic Cycle (ramp protocol 17 watts/min; staged protocol 25-50 watts/3-min stage) Treadmill (low-level protocol such as Naughton, Balke, Ware)	• 12-lead ECG, HR • BP, rate pressure product • RPE (6-20) • METs	• Serious dysrhythmias • >2 mm ST-segment depression or elevation • Ischemic threshold • T-wave inversion with significant ST change • SBP > 250 mmHg or DBP > 115 mmHg	
Endurance 6- or 12-min walk	• Distance • Speed	• Volitional fatigue • Unsteadiness	• 6- or 12-min walk good for measuring progress in exercise programs.
Strength Handheld dynamometer	• 3 RM		• Used to determine intensity of strength training and progress in stength training programs. • Sometimes contraindicated in people with osteoporosis.
Neuromuscular 20-ft (6.1-m) walk Chair stand 1-legged stance 8-step tandem gait 360° turn	• Number of steps • Mobility/balance	• Volitional fatigue • Unsteadiness	• Walk tests are good for measuring gait and balance disorders and progress in exercise programs.
Flexibility Sit and reach Goniometer	• Distance		

*Measurements of particular significance; do not always indicate test termination.

Medications	Special Considerations
May be taking one or more of the following (see appendixes A, B, and C for effects): • Diuretics • Antihypertensives • Anti-anginal agents • Antiarrhythmic agents • Psychotropic medications • Insulin • Anticoagulants	• Observe client for balance difficulties to prevent falls. • Clients may be prone to fractures caused by osteoporosis. • Increased risk of cardiovascular and cerebrovascular diseases. • Low tolerance for hot and cold environments: reduced effectiveness of sweating; susceptible to heat cramps, exhaustion, stroke, and dehydration. • Make sure that regular medication schedule is followed. • Assess client for any cognitive deficits. • Adapt the test if client is using an assistive device.

Frailty: Exercise Programming

Modes	Goals	Intensity/ Frequency/Duration	Time to goal
Aerobic •Large muscle activities (walking, cycling, rowing, swimming; chair exercise may be indicated for some clients)	•Increase functional capacity and independence	•Monitor RPE (intensity should not be main focus) •3-5 days/wk •5-60 min/session	•~3 mo
Strength •Low-level, progressive resistance exercise (free weights, weight machines, isokinetic machines) •Ball machines	•Increase overall muscular strength •Decrease risk of falling •Increase hand strength	•Start program without weight; add weight slowly •3 days/wk •~20 min/session	•~3 mo
Flexibility •Stretching/yoga	•Increase ROM	•20 s/stretch	
Neuromuscular •1-foot stand •Stair climbing •Practice falling techniques •Balloon activity •Tandem gait •Chair stand exercise	•Increase neuromuscular coordination, gait, balance, flexibility, and lower body strength •Prevent falls •Increase hand-eye coordination and reaction time		

Medications	Special Considerations
•See exercise testing table.	•Target HR should not be main focus. •Avoid ballistic exercises. •Avoid neck circumduction. •Avoid isometric and static resistance exercises. •See exercise testing table.

Prescribing the mode of exercise for persons who are elderly must be done with care. The primary goal for this population is to increase functional capacity and independence. Medical history and past exercise experience are important indicators of the type of exercise to be recommended. Although walking is the easiest and least expensive form of exercise, this activity may not be best for everyone (see the Frailty: Exercise Programming table). Cycling, swimming, and chair activities are most appropriate for people with degenerative joint disease, hip replacements, and knee replacements. Low-level strength training programs in the frail elderly can incorporate ankle and wrist weights as an essential component. Flexibility, eye-hand coordination, reflex training, and fall prevention activities are also important.

CASE STUDY Frailty

An 81-year-old female presented complaining of increasing shortness of breath during exertion. She lived in an assisted-living facility and had a past medical history of chronic obstructive pulmonary disease, diabetes, osteoarthritis, and cataracts. She smoked 2 to 3 packs of cigarettes/day but denied any alcohol abuse. She had been a homemaker and had held a variety of jobs as well. She had never participated in any formal exercise program but sought advice because of problems with shortness of breath.

(continued)

CASE STUDY   Frailty (continued)

S: "I need help because I can't breathe when I walk."

O: Vitals: Height: 4'10" (1.47 m)   Weight: 140 lb (63.5 kg)   BMI: 29.38 kg/m²

Woman of an elderly appearance

Kyphotic; barrel chest; digit clubbing

Echocardiogram: Mild left ventricular hypokinesis and mild right ventricular hypertrophy

Graded exercise test:
  Test terminated after 7 min because of fatigue and shortness of breath
  ECG: Frequent PACs, couplets, and a 4 contraction run of SVT, but no ischemia
  Peak HR: 120 contractions/min
  Peak BP: 140/80 mmHg
  Peak exercise capacity: 4 METs
  VO_2peak: 14 ml $\cdot$ kg^{-1} $\cdot$ min^{-1}

Assessments:
  IADL score: 8 (normal: > 10)
  ADL score: 85 (normal: > 85)
  Mini Mental State score: 30 (good: > 24)
  Yesavage depression scale: 3 (< 4 is normal)
  Nutritional Risk Index: 8 (normal: < 4)

Medications: Proventil inhaler, Atrovent inhaler, Proventil tabs, Theo-Dur, Lasix, Vitamin K, Amoxicillin for a respiratory tract infection

A: 1. Exercise intolerance caused by multiple chronic diseases (COPD, diabetes, osteoarthritis, and mild obesity) and deconditioning

P: 1. Exercise program with supplemental oxygen is necessary.
  2. Refer client to nutritionist for weight-loss diet.
  3. Diabetes education is recommended.
  4. Recommend a smoking-cessation program.

Exercise Program

Goals:

  1. Adjust to using oxygen with ADLs and exercise
  2. Daily physical activity
  3. Reevaluation after 1 mo

Mode	Frequency	Duration	Intensity	Progression
Aerobic	5-6 days/wk	As tolerated to start	As tolerated	Increase over 1 mo to 40 min/session
Strength (all major muscle groups)	3 days/wk	1 set of ≤ 10 reps	Therabands™	Achieve 1 set of 10 reps for all muscle groups
Flexibility (all major muscle groups)	3 days/wk	20-60 s/stretch	Maintain stretch below discomfort point	
Neuromuscular				
Functional				
Warm-up/Cool-down	Before and after each sesson	10-15 min		

Suggested Readings

Abrass, I.B. 1990. The biology and physiology of aging. *Western Journal of Medicine* 153: 641-45.

American College of Sports Medicine. 2001. *ACSM's resource manual for guidelines for exercise testing and prescription.* Edited by J. Roitman, M. Herridge, M. Kelsey, T. LaFontaine, L. Miller, M. Wegner, M. Williams, and T. York. 4th ed. Philadelphia: Lippincott Williams & Wilkins.

American College of Sports Medicine. 2000. *ACSM's guidelines for exercise testing and prescription.* Edited by B. Franklin, M. Whaley, and E. Howley. 6th ed. Philadelphia: Lippincott Williams & Wilkins.

Chapron, D.J., and R.W. Besdine. 1987. Drugs as an obstacle to rehabilitation of the elderly: A primer for therapists. *Topics in Geriatric Rehabilitation* 2 (3): 63-81.

Duke University Center for the Study of Aging and Human Development. 1978. *Multidimensional functional assessment: The OAR's methodology.* Durham, NC: Duke University.

Folstein, M.F., S. Forstein, and P.R. McHugh. 1975. Mini Mental State: A practical method for grading the cognitive state of patients for the clinician. *Journal of Psychiatric Research* 12: 189-98.

Fried, L.P. 1994. Frailty. In *Principles of geriatric medicine and gerontology,* edited by W.R. Hazzard, E.L. Bierman, J.P. Blass, W.H. Ettinger, and J.B. Halter, 1149-55. New York: McGraw-Hill.

Lord, S., R. Clark, and I. Webster. 1991. Physiological factors associated with falls in an elderly population. *Journal of the American Geriatric Society* 39 (12): 1194-1200.

Mahoney, F.I., and D.W. Barthel. 1965. Functional evaluation: The Barthel Index. *Maryland State Medical Journal* 14: 61-65.

Schwartz, R.S., and D.M. Buchner. 1994. Exercise in the elderly: Physiologic and functional effects. In *Principles of geriatric medicine and gerontology,* edited by W.R. Hazzard, E.L. Bierman, J.P. Blass, W.H. Ettinger, and J.B. Halter, 95-105. New York: McGraw-Hill.

Silverstone, B. 1994. Public policies on aging: Reconsidering old-age eligibility. *Gerontologist* 34 (6): 724-25.

Tinetti, M.E. 1986. Performance-oriented assessment of mobility problems in elderly patients. *Journal of the American Geriatric Society* 34: 119-26.

Tinetti, M.E., and S.F. Ginter. 1988. Identifying mobility dysfunctions in elderly patients: Standard neuromuscular examination or direct assessment? *Journal of the American Medical Association* 259: 1190-93.

U.S. Census Bureau, Economics and Statistical Administration. 1995. *U.S. Department of Commerce May 1995 report.* Washington, DC: U.S. Government Printing Office.

Vitti, K.A., C.M. Bayles, W.J. Carender, J.M. Prendergast, and F.J. D'Amico. 1993. A low-level strength training exercise program for frail elderly adults living in an extended attention facility. *Aging, Clinical and Experimental Research* 5 (5): 363-69.

Wolinshy, F.D., J.M. Prendergast, D.K. Miller, R.M. Coe, and M.N. Chavez. 1985. Preliminary validation of a nutritional risk measure among the elderly. *American Journal of Preventive Medicine* (March): 53-59.

Yesavage, J.A. 1992. Depression in the elderly: How to recognize masked symptoms and choose appropriate therapy. *Postgraduate Medicine* 91 (1): 255-61.

SECTION V

Immunological/ Hematological Disorders

Geoffrey E. Moore, MD, FACSM
J. Larry Durstine, PhD, FACSM

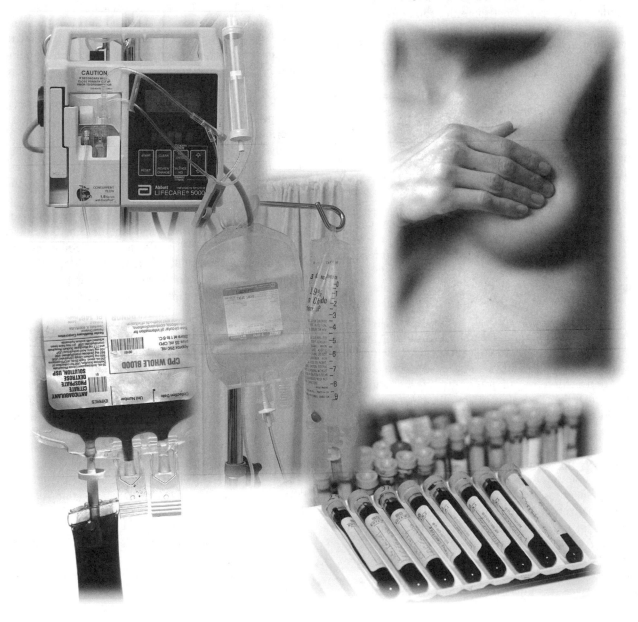

CHAPTER 25

Cancer

Anna L. Schwartz, PhD, ARNP
University of Washington

Overview of the Pathophysiology

Cancer is not a single disease; it is a collection of hundreds of diseases that share the common feature of excessive, uncontrolled cellular proliferation and the potential for these cells to spread to distant anatomical sites (e.g., metastasis). The initial symptoms of cancer can be either local, such as the cough of the person with lung cancer, or systemic, as in the drenching night sweats of Hodgkin's lymphoma. After treatment, the symptoms of cancer can result from the progression of the illness or the side effects of treatment. Treatment of cancer can include surgery, radiation, chemotherapy, and immunotherapy, either singly or in combination, and can be designed to attempt a cure or remission, or for control of disease and relief of symptoms. Cancer is cured when a remission is thought to be permanent, but many cancers are considered cured if the client does not have a recurrence within five years after treatment. Recurrence of cancer occurs when a few cancer cells escape being eradicated and subsequently grow back over time.

Virtually all individuals with cancer can benefit from rehabilitation and exercise. As the prior paragraph suggests, the goals of exercise therapy may differ depending on whether a client is receiving initial treatment for a new diagnosis, is in remission, or is receiving treatment for a recurrence. Moreover, the response to exercise and adaptability to training is influenced by whether the individual has local or metastatic disease, and on the side effects of the particular form of treatment. The specific roles and applications of exercise programming are therefore exquisitely complex in persons with cancer, the full scope of which cannot be covered in this brief discussion. Exercise management for persons with cancer requires extensive individualization by the exercise specialist. There is great reason for everyone with cancer to have hope, since Lance Armstrong's three consecutive victories in the Tour de France proves that it is indeed possible to have advanced cancer, undergo extensive treatment, and go on to achieve extraordinary levels of human performance.

Effects on the Exercise Response

Persons with cancer, as well as those who have survived it, may have disease- or treatment-specific physical limitations that pose challenges to exercise. Tumors can involve any part of the body, and their effect on the exercise response is directly related to the tissues affected. Pain is common when a tumor involves the musculoskeletal system; shortness of breath is common with lung involvement; neural deficits and seizures are common when the central nervous system and brain are involved; and anemia is common when bone marrow is affected. Easy fatigability is common in advanced cancer. The specific effects of cancer on the exercise response are determined by the tissue(s) affected and by the extent of involvement. The result is often exercise intolerance, but the limiting factors can be varied.

The side effects of anticancer therapy also affect the exercise response. These can be acute onset with treatment, but are often delayed onset and permanent (see table 25.1). Amputations cause permanent disability; radiation and chemotherapy can cause permanent scar formation in joints and lung and heart tissues; and drug-induced cardiomyopathies and anemia can cause a permanent limitation in cardiovascular function.

Effects of Exercise Training

Exercise training is safe and beneficial for cancer patients when the exercise is individualized to suit the individual's characteristics. For those undergoing therapy for cancer, exercise training should have the objectives of maintaining strength, endurance, and level of function. For cancer survivors (in remission or after cure), exercise training should have the objective of returning them to their former level of physical and psychological function. Studies have shown that regular, moderate-intensity aerobic exercise during cancer therapy results in reduced levels of fatigue, greater body satisfaction, maintenance of body weight, improved mood, less side effect severity, and a higher quality of life.

Aerobic and resistance exercise programs have the potential to improve bone remodeling and reduce muscle

Table 25.1 Acute and Chronic Treatment Effects

Treatment	Acute effects	Chronic effects
Surgery	Pain Fatigue Limited ROM	Pain Loss of flexibility Nerve damage
Radiation	Pain Fatigue Skin irritation Pulmonary Inflammation	Loss of flexibility Cardiac and/or lung scarring Fractures
Chemotherapy	Fatigue Nausea Anemia Nerve damage Muscle pain Weight gain	Cardiomyopathy Lung scarring Nerve damage Fatigue Bone loss Leukemia
Immunotherapy	Weight gain or loss Fatigue Flu-like syndrome Nerve damage	Nerve damage Myopathy

weakness and the muscle-wasting effects of glucocorticoids that are often part of the treatment regimen.

Significant improvements in functional ability, as measured by a 12-min walk, have been observed in clients who participated in an aerobic exercise program. In contrast, clients who followed the common dictum to "get more rest" showed a greater than 25% decline in functional ability in eight weeks. Persons undergoing intensive cancer therapy benefit from low- to moderate-intensity exercise, physical therapy, and occupational therapy. Despite the significant fatigue cancer patients experience, exercise appears to reduce fatigue and improve functional ability, mood, and quality of life.

The effects of exercise in persons with cancer have been best studied in women with breast cancer. Exercise training by breast cancer patients receiving treatment results in the following:

- improved shoulder range of motion;
- reduced fatigue, nausea, and other treatment-related side effects;
- improved functional ability;
- improved ability to maintain body weight;
- enhanced body-image and sense of control; and
- improved mood and quality of life.

The effects of exercise on children receiving cancer treatment have not been studied. However, survivors of childhood leukemia have been observed to have mild, persistent cardiovascular compromise as a result of therapy. This does not usually impair function at moderate exercise levels but may hinder elite-level athletic performance. Nonetheless, aerobic capacity and submaximal performance of both children and adults should significantly improve after routine exercise training programs. A concern with adult cancer survivors is that they are more likely to have co-morbid conditions such as coronary artery disease, high blood pressure, diabetes, or high blood lipids. Some cancer treatments also increase risks for cardiovascular disease and death from myocardial infarction. These conditions may actually influence exercise management more than the history of cancer does.

Management and Medications

Cancer treatment usually includes some combination of surgery, chemotherapy, radiation therapy, and/or immunotherapy. The most common problems encountered with each treatment category are:

- surgery can cause pain, loss of flexibility, amputation, and motor and sensory nerve damage; and
- radiation can cause loss of flexibility in irradiated joints and cardiac or lung scarring, or both.

Chemotherapy involves several drugs, each of which have characteristic side effects:

- vinca alkaloids (vincristine, Velban): peripheral nerve damage;
- daunorubicin (Cerubidine): cardiomyopathy;

Cancer: Exercise Testing

Methods	Measures	Endpoints*	Comments
Aerobic Cycle (ramp protocol 17 watts/ min; staged protocol 25-50 watts/3-min stage) Treadmill (1-2 METs/3-min stage)	• 12-lead ECG, HR • BP, rate pressure product • RPE (6-20)	• $\dot{V}O_2$peak/work rate • Serious dysrhythmias • >2 mm ST-segment depression or elevation • Ischemic threshold • T-wave inversion with significant ST change • SBP >250 mmHg or DBP >115 mmHg • Exaggerated or hypotensive response	• See exercise testing tables in chapters 12 and 21.
Endurance 6- to 12-min walk	• Distance	• Volitional fatigue	
Strength Isokinetic/Isotonic	• 1RM • 3RM	• Maximum voluntary contraction • Maximum number of reps • Peak torque	
Flexibility Goniometry Sit and reach		• Angle of flexion/extension • Distance	
Functional ADLs Sit to stand Stair climbing			• Use to determine level of assistance needed.
Neuromuscular Gait analysis Balance	• Gait and balance measures as appropriate for client		• Use to determine level of assistance needed.

*Measurements of particular significance; do not always indicate test termination.

Medications	Special Considerations
• Glucocorticoids: May cause muscle weakness and wasting. • Growth factors: May cause bone pain. • Chemotherapy and immunotherapy: May cause anemia, fatigue, and nausea. Some drugs cause myopathies, neuropathies. • Radiation therapy: Can cause skin breakdown that may be irritated with perspiration, muscle and joint constriction, and cardiopulmonary myopathies.	• Clients are often in debilitated state. • Clients on treatment may be limited by muscle weakness and/or pain from tumor, surgery, or therapy. • The disease itself may limit a client's ability to walk or perform other tests and may necessitate alternative modes of testing. • May need to adapt exercise to client. • Be aware of Hickman catheters, Port-a-caths, and other access lines. • Assess client before each exercise session; an acute change in general health status is a contraindication to exercise. • If platelet count is < 50,000/mm^3, consider risk of bleeding (see chapter 31). • Consider risk of cardiovascular co-morbidity, especially when anemic (see chapter 30).

Cancer: Exercise Programming

Modes	Goals	Intensity/ Frequency/Duration	Time to Goal
Aerobic • Large muscle activities (walking, rowing, cycling, water aerobics)	• Improve/maintain work capacity • Control body weight • Improve mood • Reduce fatigue • Improve quality of life	• Symptoms limited; moderate intensity • Exercise at least every other day • 15-40 min/session	
Strength • Free weights • Weight machines • Isokinetic machines • Therabands™ • Circuit training	• Maintain or improve strength in arms, legs, and trunk • Increase maximal voluntary contraction, peak torque, and power	• Symptom-limited intensity • 50% of 1RM • 2-3 days/wk for 20-30 min • 2-3 sets of 3-5 reps, building to 10-12 reps	
Flexibility • Stretching	• Increase/maintain ROM • Decrease stiffness from disuse	• 5-7 days/wk	• 6-12 wk
Functional • ADLs • Gait and balance exercise	• Maintain as much independence as possible • Return to work • Improve gait • Improve balance	• Daily	

Medications	Special Considerations
• Glucocorticoids: Cause muscle weakness and wasting. • Growth factors: Often cause bone pain. • Chemotherapy and immunotherapy: Cause anemia, fatigue, and nausea. Some drugs cause myopathies and neuropathies. • Radiation therapy: Can cause skin breakdown that may be irritated with perspiration, muscle and joint constriction, and cardiopulmonary myopathies.	• See exercise testing table. • Intensity, frequency, and duration recommendations are difficult to make. Very little research is available. The guidelines presented in chapters 4, 5, and 6 can be used with caution and may need adjustment according to treatment and state of disease. • Clients are often in a debilitated state and need progressive exercise programs. • Clients on treatment are often limited by muscle weakness and/or pain from tumor, surgery, or therapy. • The disease itself may limit a client's ability to walk or perform other tests and may necessitate alternative modes of testing and training. • May need to adapt exercise to client. • Be aware of Hickman catheters, Port-a-caths, and other access lines. • Gradual progression is essential for all cancer clients and survivors. • Exercise programs may need to be adjusted for changes in medical condition.

- doxorubicin (Adriamycin): cardiomyopathy;
- mitoxantrone (Novantrone): cardiomyopathy;
- bleomycin (Blenoxane): pulmonary fibrosis;
- corticosteroids (Decadron, prednisone): myopathy; and
- many others: anemia.

Recommendations for Exercise Testing

Exercise testing is appropriate for persons actively receiving therapy and persons whose cancer is in remission. Individuals actively receiving treatment are generally capable of completing exercise testing, and then following an exercise prescription based on functional ability and limitations that may be disease or treatment related. For clients who have completed therapy, regular exercise is important to maintain or improve function and prevent the development of diseases associated with disuse.

Formal exercise testing should be individualized to the client with attention to the disease, type of treatment, and physical limitations (see Management and Medications section). For example, persons actively receiving treatment who are anemic will have reduced aerobic performance because of reduced oxygen-carrying capacity. Exercise testing can be useful to quantitatively monitor progress during training and rehabilitation.

Depending on the functional ability of a client, exercise testing can usually be performed using standard protocols. Persons receiving treatment or who have completed treatment may be extremely deconditioned or may have experienced significant changes in body weight (either increases or decreases), and may require low-level exercise protocols. Submaximal and subjective symptom-limited treadmill tests are well tolerated, even by debilitated clients, and provide information on aerobic capacity. If 12-lead ECG monitoring is used during exercise testing, the data may be helpful not only to assess aerobic capacity, submaximal endurance, strength, and functional performance, but may also determine whether there are other co-morbid conditions such as coronary artery disease (see the Cancer: Exercise Testing table on page 168).

Recommendations for Exercise Programming

Recommendations for exercise programming are dependent on whether the person is actively receiving cancer treatment, is a survivor cured or in remission, or is being treated for recurrent or metastatic disease (see the Cancer: Exercise Programming table on page 169). For individuals receiving treatment or with recurrent, localized disease, the goal is to preserve and possibly even improve function. For survivors, the goal is to return to a healthy, active lifestyle and make exercise an integral part of everyday life. For individuals with recurrent or metastatic disease, the goals need to be tailored to the person's current level of function. In the setting of metastatic cancer, the goal may be to maintain mobility and independence in the home. Many persons will have disease- or treatment-specific limitations to exercise that necessitate accommodating the mode of exercise to the client's limitation (e.g., needs of amputees, requirement for portable oxygen).

The optimal frequency, duration, and time course of adaptation are not known. There appears to be a dose-response relationship of exercise to fatigue, with less fatigue being experienced in persons who exercise for a duration of more than 10 min, and for clients who exercise at least every other day. The dose-response of exercise in cancer clients needs more study to further determine important prescribing guidelines. Longitudinal exercise studies of women with breast cancer, clients receiving peripheral stem cell transplant, and clients with malignant melanoma all demonstrate that persons adapt to exercise, become more physically fit, and experience less mood disturbance and an improved quality of life.

As noted, the side effects of anticancer treatment can be acute or delayed in onset. Therefore, distinct issues must be addressed in exercise programming for persons who are actively receiving treatment versus survivors. During radiation therapy, for example, a client may experience radiation dermatitis, a reddening of the skin that is painful and often limits motion. Radiation therapy can also cause an acute inflammatory response in lung tissue that can impair oxygen transfer. The effects of radiation can also have a delayed onset, occurring months to years after therapy. For example, radiation can cause lung scarring many months after therapy (which also impairs lung function). Chemotherapy and immunotherapy also have acute and long-term side effects that need to be considered when planning exercise prescriptions. Virtually all anticancer drugs cause fatigue and declines in blood cell counts. Exercise prescriptions should consider where a client is in treatment and accommodate for periods of increased fatigue, and for cycles of treatment. Since most individuals are treated with combinations of surgery, radiation, chemotherapy, and immunotherapy, the exercise specialist is likely to encounter a combination of treatment-related problems.

Special Considerations

It is important, especially for clients actively receiving chemotherapy, that the client's general health status is assessed before each exercise session. Persons with uncontrolled vomiting or diarrhea should postpone the exercise session. Individuals with neutropenic fever should postpone the exercise session until the source of infection is determined and appropriate therapy has been started. Exercise prescription for clients with thrombocytopenia (platelet count < 50,000/mm³) must consider the risk of bleeding (see chapter 31). Steps should be taken to prevent falls and increases in blood and intracranial

pressure. Exercise should probably be limited to low-intensity walking, stationary cycling, and flexibility exercises. Although no studies have examined the effects of exercise in cancer clients with coronary artery disease, logic would suggest that these persons should decrease their exercise intensity during periods of anemia, possibly when hemoglobin levels reach 10 g/dl. Exercise programs may need to be adjusted for changes in the individual's condition and treatment plan.

CASE STUDY Cancer

A 47-year-old female had a stage III infiltrating ductal carcinoma of the left breast. She underwent a modified radical mastectomy, chemotherapy with Adriamycin and Taxotere (ending 3 months prior to the initial consultation), as well as radiation therapy (ending 2 wk prior to the consultation). She was well enough to work 3 to 4 hours in the morning but had fatigue of 6/10 (0 = no fatigue; 10 = extreme fatigue), noting that she tired quickly with activities such as house cleaning and daily chores. She was unable to do much after 4 p.m., making it difficult to prepare evening meals. She was doing self-massage to the surgical site and stretching at least twice a day. She reported being too busy to attend a regular exercise program. She denied cough, swelling, pain, tingling, or myalgia. She had to rest after climbing a flight of stairs.

S: "I feel OK, but I'm always tired."

O: Vitals: HR: 81 contractions/min   BP: 148/81 mmHg   Weight: 179.9 lb (77.5 kg)

Lungs clear, mastectomy incision site

Radiation dermatitis resolving

No lymphedema, extremities neurologically intact

12-min walk: 1215 ft (370.3 m)

Overhead press 1RM: 7 kg

Leg press 1RM: 40 kg

A: 1. Breast cancer, post-mastectomy/radiation/chemotherapy

2. Moderate exercise intolerance (low endurance and weakness)

P: Prescribe an aerobic exercise program.

Exercise Program
Goal:

Regain functional capacity

Mode	Frequency	Duration	Intensity	Progression
Aerobic	3-4 days/wk	12 min/session	RPE 11-13/20 (avoid exhaustion)	Increase to 30 min in 8 wk
Strength (all major muscle groups)	3 days/wk	1 set of 6-12 reps	To fatigue, but avoid exhaustion	Increase as tolerated
Flexibility (all major muscle groups)	3 days/wk	20-60 s/stretch	Maintain stretch below discomfort point	
Neuromuscular				
Functional				
Warm-up/Cool-down	Before and after each sesson	10-15 min	RPE 10/20	

Suggested Readings

Demark-Wahnefried, W., V. Hars, M.R. Conaway, K. Havlin, B.K. Rimer, G. McElveen, and E.P. Winer. 1997. Reduced rates of metabolism and decreased physical activity in breast cancer patients receiving adjuvant chemotherapy. *American Journal of Clinical Nutrition* 65: 1495.

Dimeo, F.C., S. Fetscher, W. Lange, R. Mertelsmann, and J. Keul. 1997. Effects of aerobic exercise on the physical performance and incidence of treatment-related complications after high-dose chemotherapy. *Blood* 90: 3390-94.

Dimeo, F.C., M.H.M. Tilmann, H. Bertz, L. Kanz, R. Mertelsmann, and J. Keul. 1997. Aerobic exercise in the rehabilitation of cancer patients after high dose chemotherapy and autologous stem cell transplantation. *Cancer* 79: 1717-22.

MacVicar, M.G., and M.L.Winningham. 1986. Promoting the functional capacity of cancer patients. *Cancer Bulletin* 38: 235-39.

McTiernan, A., C. Ulrich, C. Kumai, R. Schwartz, J. Mahloch, R. Hastings, J. Gralow, and J.D. Potter. 1998. Anthropometric and hormone effects of an eight-week exercise-diet intervention in breast cancer patients: Results of a pilot study. *Cancer Epidemiology, Biomarkers & Prevention* 7: 477-81.

Mock, V., M.B. Burke, P. Sheehan, E.M. Creaton, M.L. Winningham, S. McKenney-Tedder, L.P. Schwager, and M. Leibeman. 1994. A nursing rehabilitation program for women with breast cancer receiving adjuvant chemotherapy. *Oncology Nursing Forum* 21: 899-907.

Mock, V., K.H. Dow, C.J. Meares, P.M. Grimm, J.A. Dienemann, M.E. Haisfield-Wolfe, W. Quitasol, S. Mitchell, A. Chakravarthy, and I. Gage. 1997. An exercise intervention for management of fatigue and emotional distress during radiotherapy treatment for breast cancer. *Oncology Nursing Forum* 24: 991-1000.

Schwartz, A.L. 2000. Weight change in women who do and do not exercise during adjuvant chemotherapy for breast cancer. *Cancer Practice* 8: 229-37.

Schwartz, A.L. 1999. Fatigue mediates the effects of exercise on quality of life in women with breast cancer. *Quality of Life Research* 8: 529-38.

Schwartz, A.L., M. Mori, R. Gao, L.M. Nail, and M.E. King. 2001. Exercise reduces daily fatigue in women with breast cancer receiving chemotherapy. *Medicine and Science in Sport and Exercise* 33 (5): 718-23.

CHAPTER 26

Acquired Immune Deficiency Syndrome (AIDS)

Arlette C. Perry, PhD, FACSM
University of Miami

Arthur LaPerriere, PhD, FACSM
University of Miami

Nancy Klimas, MD
University of Miami VA Medical Center

Overview of the Pathophysiology

Acquired immune deficiency syndrome (AIDS) is a dynamic and progressive disease that will continue to pose serious health problems well into this century. As of the year 2000, the World Health Organization reported that 36 million adults are infected with the human immunodeficiency virus (HIV), the etiologic agent responsible for AIDS. This represents a 300% increase from 1997. In fact, a total of 5.3 million newly reported cases of HIV infection were recorded in the year 2000. Recently, remarkable gains have been made in the prevention, diagnosis, and treatment of HIV. Nevertheless, despite the tremendous strides made in medical treatments for HIV, a vaccine or cure is still unavailable. Therefore, complementary strategies for the management of HIV, including behavioral intervention such as exercise training, constitute important adjunctive therapy. Significant quantities of scientific evidence indicate that exercise training is not only appropriate but also warranted for many people with HIV.

The body's first line of defense against infectious agents include macrophages and neutrophils, which engulf pathogens, secrete large amounts of different chemicals, and control inflammatory responses. Natural killer cells are also produced by the body to destroy cancer cells. Together these three types of cells make up the innate immune system and act as the body's first line of defense against infectious agents. HIV disease occurs from the selective infection (by HIV) of the immune system's CD4 cell. This lymphocyte is also called the T-helper cell and is part of the body's adaptive immune system. When activated, it divides, conquers, and produces specific reactions in response to infectious agents. T-helper cells along with T-cytotoxic suppressor and B-cells are part of the body's second line of defense, protecting against pathogens that have slipped by the body's first line of defense. T-helper cells are crucial for the normal immune defensive mechanisms. CD4 cells, along with the macrophages, release cytokines, such as various interleukins and tumor necrosis factor (alpha) that activate other cells, as well as potentiate activation of each other. Therefore, the absence of these critical elements will decrease all immune function. Depletion of the CD4 cells, then, results in immunosuppression that leads to:

- increased risk of opportunistic infections;
- decreased food consumption and lean body mass;
- further decreased immune system function and advanced body tissue wasting; and
- disease progression and eventual death.

The progressive clinical nature of HIV disease can be usefully viewed in three dissimilar stages. Important distinctions exist between each stage and are useful for exercise testing and training. The three HIV stages are:

- Stage I: Asymptomatic HIV seropositive;
- Stage II: Early symptomatic HIV; and
- Stage III: AIDS.

In stage I, the individual is infected with HIV and is therefore potentially infectious to others by sexual or bloodborne routes. This person remains relatively healthy and completely free of any symptomatology for HIV disease. Stage I may last 10 or more years depending, perhaps, on the health habits maintained by the individual. During stage II, often referred to as AIDS-related complex (ARC), the number of CD4 cells is moderately diminished, resulting in the development of a variety of intermittent or persistent signs and symptoms that include fatigue, diarrhea, weight loss, fever, and lymphadenopathy. With appropriate management of these early symptoms, most individuals are able to retard disease progression for several years. Stage III, characterized immunologically as a severe depletion of CD4 cells in the presence of malignancy or opportunistic infection, is the most advanced and severe stage of HIV disease. Advances made in antiviral agents and other adjuvant therapies for AIDS-related problems have allowed many to live a relatively high quality of life for numerous years after an AIDS diagnosis.

Effects on the Exercise Response

For individuals who are asymptomatic, HIV infection in most cases does not alter the exercise-related physiological responses to a single session of exercise. At a more advanced stage of immunodeficiency, however, a decrease in exercise performance and training response has been observed. Exercise response to a maximum graded exercise test (GXT) measuring aerobic capacity will vary.

Stage I

- No limitations on maximum graded exercise test for most individuals.
- All metabolic parameters within normal limits for most individuals.

Stage II

- Reduced exercise capacity.
- Reduced oxygen consumption ($\dot{V}O_2$max) and $\dot{V}O_2$ at ventilatory threshold and $\dot{V}O_2$pulse.
- Reduced heart rate reserve and breathing reserve.

Stage III

- Dramatically reduced exercise capacity (maximum graded exercise test may not be possible for all individuals).
- More severe $\dot{V}O_2$ limitations than in stage II.
- Altered neuroendocrine responses.

The reasons for a reduced exercise capacity are not fully understood, but such reduction may be the result of symptoms secondary to HIV infection. Many individuals who are HIV positive will terminate a graded exercise test because of physical exhaustion, muscular fatigue, or both.

Effects of Exercise Training

Exercise is safe and beneficial for most individuals infected with HIV, although a full understanding of the risks and benefits of exercise training has not yet been reached. Short-term exercise sessions can result in an increase in the number of CD4 cells, neutrophils, and cells mediating natural immunity in HIV-seropositive patients. In addition, active seronegative individuals show higher rates of natural killer cell activity than sedentary controls. Moderate aerobic exercise enhances immunosurveillance and protection against upper respiratory tract infection, a condition commonly observed in persons with HIV/AIDS. This is probably related to the summation of positive acute effects that occur during each exercise session. Surveys show that athletes report fewer colds and sick days than non-athletes and that in activities such as brisk walking, there are reportedly fewer days lost to upper respiratory tract infections in seronegative individuals.

In HIV-positive individuals, aerobic exercise combined with strength training may result in improvements in lean body mass, oxidation and endurance capacity, cognitive and physical energy needed for daily living, psychological and coping skills, mood, and physical function for a prolonged period of time. For most HIV-positive individuals, this will result in an improvement in quality of life, which may be the most important benefit of regular physical exercise for HIV-infected individuals.

In addition, the following effects of routine moderate exercise regimens are specific to the different stages of HIV disease:

Stage I

- increase in CD4 cells;
- possible delay in onset of symptoms; and
- increase in muscle function and size.

Stage II

- increase in CD4 cells (lesser magnitude of change than in stage I); and
- possible diminished severity and frequency of some symptoms.

Stage III

- unknown effects on CD4 cells; and
- inconclusive effects on symptoms.

AIDS: Exercise Testing

Methods	Measures	Endpoints*	Comments
Aerobic Cycle (ramp protocol 17 watts/min; staged protocol 25-50 watts/3-min stage) Treadmill (1-2 METs/stage)	• 12-lead ECG, HR • BP • RPE (6-20)	• Serious dysrhythmias • >2 mm ST-segment depression or elevation • Ischemic threshold • T-wave inversion with significant ST change • SBP > 250 mmHg or DBP > 115 mmHg • Volitional fatigue	• Indicated for asymptomatic clients or those with early symptoms. Not indicated for those with severe symptoms. • Record time to exhaustion.
Endurance 1-mi walk 6-min walk	• Time elapsed • Distance traveled		
Strength Isokinetic/Isotonic	• 10-12RM • Maximal voluntary contraction		
Flexibility Sit and reach	• Distance		
Neuromuscular Gait analysis Reaction time Balance			• Especially useful for severely symptomatic people.
Functional ADL, performance-based tests	• Individualize to each client		

*Measures of particular significance; do not always indicate test termination.

Medications	Special Considerations
• Antibiotics: No direct effect on exercise, but opportunistic pneumonia risks desaturation. • AZT/DDI: Can cause anemia. • Inhaled bronchodilators: Tachycardia. • Theophylline: Tachycardia. • Thiazide diuretics: Reduced exercise tolerance. • Over-the-counter remedies: Include cardiovascular stimulants (tachycardia/hypertension).	• Fatigue is common and may signify progression of HIV/opportunistic disease or thyroid disease. • Anemia is common. • Muscle wasting/weakness is common. • Scarring from Pneumocystis pneumonia is the most common clinical disorder. Upper respiratory tract infections occur frequently. • Chronic diarrhea can lead to hypovolemia, hyponatremia, and hypoglycemia. • HIV encephalopathy/neuropathy may lead to neuromuscular sequelae. • Strict universal precautions must be followed as outlined by CDC/OSHA. • Body composition analysis may be desirable. • An acute change in general health status since the last visit is a contraindication to exercise.

AIDS: Exercise Programming

Modes	Goals	Intensity/Frequency/Duration	Time to Goal
Aerobic • Large muscle activities	• Increase aerobic capacity • Increase work capacity	• 60-75% HR max • 50-60% VO_2max • RPE 10-14/20 • 3-5 days/wk • 20-60 min/session	• 3-6 mo
Strength • Free weights • Weight machines	• Increase maximal number of reps		• 3-6 mo
Flexibility • Stretching/yoga • Massage therapy	• Increase ROM • Increase neuromuscular excitability • Decrease joint soreness and risk of injury		
Functional • Activity-specific exercise	• Increase ADLs, prevent deterioration • Restore vocational potential • Improve quality of life • Recreation/fun		

Medications	Special Considerations
• See exercise testing table.	• See exercise testing table.

In contrast to moderate-intensity and/or low-volume exercise, intense exercise and/or exercise for prolonged periods of time (e.g., $\geq$ 90 min) can depress immune function acutely. This may occur in the healthy athlete who is not infected with HIV. At the same time, prolonged and/or intense physical activity results in decreased nasal and salivary IgA (an important antibody) concentration, decreased mitrogen-induced lymphocyte proliferation (a measure of T-cell function), decreased natural killer cell cytotoxic activity (the ability to kill infected cells or cancer cells), decreased nasal mucociliary clearance (sweeping movement of cilia), decreased granulocyte oxidative burst activity (killing activity), low lymphocyte blood counts induced by high concentrations of plasma cortisol, and increased plasma concentrations of pro- and anti-inflammatory cytokines (e.g., interleukin-6 and interleukin-1 receptor antagonists).

This acute effect of intense and/or prolonged exercise may represent an "open window" of altered immunity lasting 3 to 72 hours postexercise, which may be a period of vulnerability when viruses and bacteria may render the athlete most susceptible to subclinical or clinical infection. In healthy athletes who are not infected with HIV, intense exercise temporarily depletes T-cell count. Thus, intense exercise and/or prolonged activity over 90 min should be avoided because of its potentially immunosuppressive activity.

Management and Medications

Exercise training is an excellent adjuvant therapy for most persons with HIV, but it should be used in conjunction with nutritional therapy, behavioral interventions, and primary medical treatments. The first FDA-approved drug to combat HIV and AIDS was AZT (zidovudine). This was followed by other nucleoside analogs, which included didanosine (DDI), zalcitabine (DDC), stavudine (D4T), and lamivudine (3TC). These nucleoside analogs work to inhibit replication of the HIV process. In 1997, the FDA approved Combivir, an AZT-3TC combination medicine that enabled people to cut down the number of tablets taken daily.

Protease inhibitors, the second phase of medical treatment, were first approved for HIV use in 1995. These included Invirase followed by Norvir, Crixivan, Viracept, and Agenerase. Protease inhibitors work similarly to nucleoside analogs but inhibit the virus at a later stage in its replication process. Protease inhibitors markedly reduce the viral load and increase the number of the CD4 cells, which markedly reduces HIV infection and AIDS.

The final class of medical treatment, first approved for HIV use in 1996, was reverse transcriptase inhibitors: Viramune followed by Rescriptor and Sustiva. These drugs restrict HIV proliferation in the early stages of replication. Together these drugs have dramatically improved the quality of life and, for many patients, have made the disease more manageable.

The FDA has also approved at least 22 other drugs for HIV and AIDS-related conditions. Among them are Nebupent (aerosolized pentamidine), a fine mist inhaler to prevent Pneumocystis carinii pneumonia, the most common life-threatening infection of people with AIDS. It should be noted that, along with the medical advances from pharmacological treatment, a number of medical complications have been observed. In 1997, for example, the FDA warned that protease inhibitors may contribute to increases in blood sugar and even diabetes, although some individuals taking protease inhibitors have experienced a change in fat distribution with increased fat deposits found in the abdomen, back of the shoulders, breasts, and/or neck, whereas the face and limbs become thinner.

Recommendations for Exercise Testing

All people infected with HIV, regardless of age or stage of disease, and prior to beginning any type of training, should have a complete physical examination and obtain medical clearance to exercise. A comprehensive assessment of aerobic capacity strength, neuromuscular ability, and flexibility is recommended. Measurement of the aerobic component should incorporate symptom-limited tests and can vary depending upon the stage of disease:

Stages I and II
- Maximal aerobic power

Stage III
- Submaximal aerobic power

The primary objectives of the exercise evaluation are to determine:

- functional capacity;
- appropriate intensity range for aerobic exercise training;
- appropriate mode of exercise training;
- potential hazards or contraindications to exercise training;
- perceived exertions and potential psychological stressors; and
- psychomotor skills for appropriate mode of exercise.

The use of a stationary cycle ergometer is strongly encouraged because of neuromuscular complications that develop as the disease progresses, which preclude treadmill testing (see the AIDS: Exercise Testing table on page 175).

Recommendations for Exercise Programming

Exercise training for HIV-infected individuals should be used as an adjuvant therapy as soon as possible after the disease is diagnosed, preferably while still asymptomatic and healthy. The exercise program should be individualized and should integrate the outcomes of the exercise evaluation with the stage of disease, immunological blood work profiles (CD4 count), and medical treatments. Intense exercise and/or prolonged activity over 90 min is not recommended (see the AIDS: Exercise Programming table).

Special Considerations

It should be remembered that HIV is a contagious disease and universal precautions should be followed at all times. Further, because the individual with HIV is at an increased risk for infectious diseases, care should be taken to minimize the risk. Before each exercise session, particularly during the early weeks of training, the individual's general health status should be assessed (e.g., evaluate blood pressure, pulse rate, temperature, body composition, and psychomotor skills, and ask a few simple questions to determine whether exercise is appropriate). For example, an exercise session should be postponed if an individual has diarrhea. Finally, the exercise program should be routinely reassessed and modified as the individual increases in aerobic capacity and/or as the disease progresses. Relapse prevention strategies should be developed so that exercise can be continued on a routine basis.

CASE STUDY   Human Immunodeficiency Virus

A 38-year-old man with HIV had been taking nucleoside analogs, protease inhibitors, and reverse transcriptase inhibitors. He was early symptomatic HIV and had frequent upper respiratory tract infections and a CD4 count of 280, which had been slowly dropping. Before starting triple drug pharmacotherapy, he had frequent diarrhea and muscle wasting but was doing much better. He had even put on weight in his abdomen, neck, and chest. He was sedentary, tired often, and couldn't seem to do the activities he used to do with friends.

S: "I would like to get in better shape and feel more energetic about doing daily activities."

O: Vitals: Height: 5'10" (1.78 m)   Weight: 185 lb (83.91 kg)   BMI: 26.48 kg/m²
             HR: 72 contractions/min   BP: 124/84 mmHg

Tired appearance

Central adiposity; waist circumference: 43 in (109.2 cm)

Labs:
   Hemoglobin: 14.4 g/dl
   Hematocrit: 41%
   Fasting glucose: 100 mg/dl
   Total cholesterol: 260 mg/dl
   Triglyceride: 160 mg/dl

Graded exercise test (modified Bruce protocol):
   Peak work rate: 3.4 mph @ 14% grade
   Total treadmill time: 13 min
   Test termination from leg fatigue
   Peak HR: 192 contractions/min
   Peak BP: 190/95 mmHg
   $\dot{V}O_2$max: 28.5 ml · kg^{-1} · min^{-1}
   ECG: Sinus rhythm at rest and throughout exercise and recovery except for 2 unifocal PVCs during the test
   No other dysrhythmias
   No report of chest discomfort

Body composition: 26% fat (skin folds)

Medications: Combivir, Crixivan, Viramune

A: 1. Deconditioned; fatigues easily

   2. Hyperlipidemic

P: 1. Begin an aerobic training program with proper diet for 6-8 wk to increase energy level.

   2. Add strength training after 4-6 wk to increase lean body mass and reduce % body fat.

   3. Continue to monitor and supervise progress.

Exercise Program

Goals:

   1. Short-term goals (1 mo):
      Walk/jog 1 mi (1.6K) without feeling fatigued and out of breath
      Climb 2 flights of stairs without huffing and puffing at the top

   2. Long-term goals (6 mo):
      Jog 3 mi (4.8K) without feeling fatigued
      Improve body composition
      Reduce central obesity
      Increase muscular strength

Mode	Frequency	Duration	Intensity	Progression
Aerobic (walking/jogging)	3-5 days/wk	10 min to start, increasing to 20 min, then to 30 min, and finally to 45 min	THR 120 contractions/min (60% of peak HR), increasing to 70% peak HR RPE 13-14/20	Add 5 min every 1-2 wk Increase intensity after 2 mo
Strength (all major muscle groups)	3 days/wk		1 set 8-12 reps, increasing to 2 sets	Add weight as needed to maintain RM at 8-12 reps
Flexibility (all major muscle groups)	3 days/wk		Maintain stretch for 10-30 s/stretch or below discomfort point	
Warm-up/Cool-down	Before and after each session	5-10 min	RPE 6-8/20	

Special considerations:
- Stay hydrated.
- Drink sport drinks with carbohydrates before, during, and after exercise.
- Avoid Valsalva maneuver.

Follow-Up

After 8 weeks, his waist circumference dropped, his body fat percentage dropped, and he lost 4 lb (1.8 kg). His CD4 count went up. His cholesterol dropped slightly and TG levels dropped 12 mg/dl. He reported that he was not as fatigued during the day and felt physically stronger. After 12 weeks, he reported fewer upper respiratory tract infections and more energy. He exercised on days other than supervised sessions and continued to lose weight in the abdominal area. After a graded exercise test retest (modified Bruce protocol), he was able to complete stage III and enter into stage IV of the test for 1 min. Peak $\dot{V}O_2$ at 36.1 ml $\cdot$ kg^{-1} $\cdot$ min^{-1}.

Suggested Readings

LaPerriere, A., M.H. Antoni, and N. Schneiderman. 1990. Exercise intervention attenuates emotional distress and natural killer cell decrements following notification of positive serologic status for HIV-1. *Biofeedback and Self-Regulation* 15: 229-42.

LaPerriere, A., M.A. Fletcher, and N. Klimas. 1991. Aerobic exercise training in an AIDS risk group. *International Journal of Sports Medicine* 12: 53-57.

LaPerriere, A., N. Schneiderman, M.H. Antoni, and M.A. Fletcher. 1990. Aerobic exercise training and psychoneuroimmunology in AIDS. In *Psychological perspectives on AIDS*, edited by A. Baum and L. Temoshok. Hillsdale, NJ: Erlbaum.

Nieman, D.C. 1997. Exercise immunology: Practical applications. *International Journal of Sports Medicine* 18 (supplement 1): S91-100.

Nieman, D.C. 1997. Immune response to heavy exertion. *Journal of Applied Physiology* 82: 1385-94.

Nieman, D.C. 1994. Exercise, upper respiratory tract infection and the immune system. *Medicine and Science in Sports and Exercise* 26: 128-39.

Nieman, D.C., B.K. Pederson. 1999. Exercise and immune function: Recent developments. *Sports Medicine* 27: 73-80.

Rigsby, L., R.K. Dishman, A.W. Jackson, G.S. Maclean, and P.B. Raven. 1992. Effects of exercise training on men seropositive for the human immunodeficiency virus-1. *Medicine and Science in Sports and Exercise* 24: 6-12.

Schmitz, H.R., J.E. Layne, and R. Humphrey. 2002. Exercise and HIV infection. In *ACSM's resources for clinical exercise physiology: Musculoskeletal, neuromuscular, neoplastic, immunologic, and hematologic conditions.* Edited by J.N. Myers, W.G. Herbert, and R. Humphrey. 206-18. Philadelphia: Lippincott Williams & Wilkins.

Spence, D.W., M.A. Galantino, K.A. Mossberg, and S.O. Zimmerman. 1990. Progressive resistance exercise: Effect on muscle function and anthropometry of a select AIDS population. *Archives of Physical Medicine and Rehabilitation* 71: 644-48.

Ullum, H., J. Palmø, J. Halkjaer-Kustensen et al. 1994. The effect of acute exercise on lymphocyte subsets, natural killer cells, proliferative response, and cytokines in HIV seropositive persons. *Journal of AIDS* 7: 1122-32.

CHAPTER 27

Abdominal Organ Transplant (Kidney, Liver, Pancreas)

Patricia L. Painter, PhD, FACSM
University of California, San Francisco

Joanne B. Krasnoff, MS
University of California, San Francisco

Overview of the Pathophysiology

The most common organ transplants performed in the United States are kidney, liver, heart (see chapters 11 and 19), and pancreas. Abdominal organ transplant surgery is performed on persons with end-stage liver or kidney failure, whereas pancreas transplant is performed on individuals with type 1 diabetes (usually simultaneously with kidney transplant). The pathophysiology of each of the end-stage diseases requiring transplant differs. Clients in need of a liver transplant have no other therapies for survival, whereas those with end-stage renal disease are typically treated with dialysis until a transplant can be performed. The waiting times for transplant vary from months to several years, and are increasing because of a shortage of organs available from cadaveric sources. (Living donors are possible for those in need of a kidney and in some centers for those needing a liver transplant.) Thus, severe deconditioning can occur during the wait for transplant. The 1- and 5-year survival rates for liver transplantation in the United States are 85 and 75%, 90 and 85% for kidney transplant.

After successful transplantation, most concerns are related to side effects or complications of immunosuppression medications. Except for the case of primary nonfunctioning or rejection of the transplant, the pathology present after transplant is related primarily to side effects of medications with a major concern being infection. Other side effects will include hypertension, hyper-

lipidemia, induced diabetes, corticosteroid-induced muscle weakness, and reduced bone mineral density. Many individuals experience significant and often excessive weight gain that is frequently attributed to increased appetite related to corticosteroid use. However, accumulating evidence suggests that weight gain may be more related to lifestyle factors, specifically increased caloric intake with minimal physical activity, and not necessarily to increased appetite induced by the medication. Posttransplant, most clients experience increased feelings of well-being and have few, if any, dietary restrictions.

Individuals presenting for abdominal organ transplant are typically deconditioned because disease progression prevents significant physical activity. Following transplantation, lifestyle issues are rarely addressed as part of the post-abdominal transplant medical therapy, despite a high prevalence of cardiovascular risk and incidence of cardiovascular complications in the long-term posttransplant course.

Effects on the Exercise Response

Peak oxygen consumption ($\dot{V}O_2$peak) in kidney transplant recipients averages 26 to 30 ml · kg^{-1} · min^{-1} and is close to normal sedentary values. Liver transplant recipients have improved $\dot{V}O_2$peak compared to pretransplant, but remain 10 to 20% lower than age-matched controls. Pancreas-kidney transplant recipients are reported to have $\dot{V}O_2$peak values similar to nondiabetic kidney transplant recipients. With the exception of diabetic kidney transplant recipients, transplant recipients who participate in regular physical activity have higher exercise capacity than those who remain sedentary. Transplant recipients often exhibit exaggerated

Abdominal Organ Transplant: Exercise Testing

Methods	Measures	Endpoints*	Comments
Aerobic Cycle (ramp protocol 5-20 watts/ min; staged protocol 15-25 watts/3-min stage) Treadmill (0.5-2 METs/stage)	• 12-lead ECG, HR • BP, rate pressure product • RPE (6-20) • METs	• Serious dysrhythmias • >2 mm ST-segment depression or elevation • Ischemic threshold • T-wave inversion with significant ST change • SBP > 250 mmHg or DBP > 115 mmHg • Leg fatigue	• Submaximal fitness testing may be appropriate for most clients because cardiac status is, in most cases, known prior to acceptance for transplant. • Leg fatigue is typically the reason for test termination.
Endurance 6-mi walk	• Distance	• Note time and distance at rest stops	• Mainly useful early after transplant.
Strength Isokinetic/Isotonic	• Maximal number of reps • Isokinetic work/peak torque at fast speeds		• Be aware of prior long-standing bone disease in kidney transplant recipients and other persons who have been on long-term glucocorticoid therapy; 1RM test may not be appropriate.
Flexibility Sit and reach			• Pretransplant inactivity may predispose to decreased ROM.

*Measurements of particular significance; do not always indicate test termination.

Medications	Special Considerations
• Prednisone: May cause muscle weakness and wasting, some joint discomfort; associated with excessive weight gain and truncal obesity. • Immunosuppressants (e.g., cyclosporine, azathioprine, FK506): Rare myopathies. • Antihypertensive agents: See exercise testing table in chapter 12 and appendixes A, B, and C. • Lipid-lowering agents: See exercise testing table in chapter 22 and appendixes A, B, and C.	• Persons typically present in a deconditioned state. • Most persons are limited by muscle weakness. • Be aware of steroid-induced diabetes that occurs after transplant (~30% of cases).

blood pressure responses to a single session of exercise. Generally, heart rate responses to exercise are normal, with the exception of the diabetic kidney-only transplant recipients, who exhibit a blunted heart rate response to exercise.

After liver transplant, 6-min walk distances and measures of muscle strength increase but remain low compared to age-expected values. Self-reported physical functioning improves posttransplant and is significantly higher in transplant recipients who are physically active compared to those who remain sedentary.

Effects of Exercise Training

Data suggest that organ transplant recipients are able to achieve normal or above-normal levels of exercise capacity with training. Participants in competitive events at the U.S. and International Transplant Games show impressive performances in a variety of athletic events. Presently, exercise training studies in various transplant populations are limited. Two exercise training studies with kidney transplant recipients indicated significant improvements in exercise capacity (magnitude of change

Abdominal Organ Transplant: Exercise Programming

Modes	Goals	Intensity/Frequency/Duration	Time to Goal
Aerobic •Large muscle activities	•Increase aerobic capacity •Increase time to exhaustion •Increase work capacity •Improve BP •Assist with weight management •Reduce risk of cardiovascular disease	•50-90% peak HR •50-85% $\dot{V}O_2$peak •4-7 days/wk •20-60 min/session •Monitor RPE	•3-6 mo
Strength •Free weights •Isokinetic machines	•Increase maximal number of reps •Reverse steroid-induced muscle wasting and weakness		•4-6 mo
Anaerobic •Interval training	•Improve performance for those interested in competition		
Flexibility •Stretching/yoga	•Maintain/increase ROM	•20 s/stretch	
Functional •Activity-specific exercise	•Increase ADLs •Recreation/fun		

Medications	Special Considerations
•See exercise testing table.	•Most persons present in a deconditioned state limited by muscle weakness. •Progression with resistance training may need to be slower because of prednisone-induced muscle wasting. •Exercise intensity should be reduced to mild levels during rejection episodes. •Vigorous training for competition is possible for those with a good baseline of regular activity. •Steroid-induced diabetes occurs in about 30% of patients. •Low-impact activities may be most appropriate for persons on high doses of prednisone and/or those with joint disease. •Caloric reduction must be a part of weight-management strategy. •Motivation and adherence are major challenges.

was 25-28%). In addition, improved blood pressure control, indications of bone remodeling, and increased muscle strength have been reported. Although muscle weakness may continue to persist, specific resistance training programs increase muscle strength and reduce the fat-to-muscle ratio, presumably counteracting the muscle-wasting effects of glucocorticoid therapy.

Management and Medications

After organ transplant, virtually all persons are treated with immunosuppression therapy to prevent rejection. Medications include glucocorticoids (prednisone), cyclosporine, and azathioprine. Although new immuno-suppressive medications are continually being developed, transplant recipients are always at risk for organ rejection. In addition to the medications, many persons are on prophylactic therapy to reduce infections, antihypertensive therapy, and lipid-lowering medications (see chapters 12 and 22). Liver transplant recipients with recurrent hepatitis C may be treated with antiviral therapies such as interferon or ribavirin, which often result in excessive fatigue.

Recommendations for Exercise Testing

Standard exercise testing protocols are acceptable for transplant recipients. Low-level exercise testing protocols are indicated early posttransplant. The high prevalence of cardiac risk factors and high incidence of cardiovascular disease posttransplantation indicates that a 12-lead ECG should be used during exercise testing (see the Abdominal Organ Transplant: Exercise Testing table on page 181). Since skeletal muscle weakness is prevalent and may result in nonmaximal performances, exercise tests may be of limited diagnostic use. Performance-based testing such as the 6-min walk may be appropriate early posttransplant but later may not accurately reflect exercise capacity or changes with training.

Recommendations for Exercise Programming

Exercise training should begin soon posttransplant and transplant recipients should be encouraged to incorporate physical activity and healthy lifestyle activities into their "new life" routines. Posttransplant, many recipients present in a significantly deconditioned state and may need strength training first to be able to complete aerobic activity (see the Abdominal Organ Transplant: Exercise Programming table). Once aerobic activities are tolerated well, gradual progression should be implemented. Joint discomfort may be experienced by those on high doses of prednisone and during the "taper" phase of the immunosuppressive management. Non-weight-bearing activities may be best tolerated by some, while many recipients are able to progress to jogging and other sporting activities without difficulty.

It is recommended that some low-level activities be continued during rejection episodes to maintain a pattern of activity and counteract muscle-wasting effects of the prednisone doses. Prednisone affects muscle metabolism so that a longer period is necessary for strength gain. Therefore, strength training programs may have to incorporate a slower rate of progression to allow for this longer adaptation time. Liver transplant recipients may experience delayed wound healing and back pain and are at risk for incisional hernias. Liver transplant recipients being treated for recurrent hepatitis C may also experience extreme fatigue. Motivation and adherence to exercise programs remain the major challenges following transplantation.

CASE STUDY Organ Transplantation

A 52-year-old Caucasian man with ulcerative colitis had been sedentary for 2 months after an orthotopic liver transplantation for sclerosing cholangitis. He also had a history of diabetes mellitus. His convalescence was complicated by hepatic artery thrombosis that necessitated a subsequent re-transplant 6 days after the first transplant, and by polymicrobial sepsis/intra-abdominal abscess 3 weeks after the second transplant. After that, he was generally well but had a low energy level, muscle weakness, slept quite a bit at home, and had "enormous" cravings for sweets. He had a 16-year-old son and 19-year-old daughter, so he was anxious to get back to work as a financial planner.

S: "My muscles have turned to fat. I am afraid of falling down the stairs as my balance is not great and my legs are weak. I purchased a commode for the downstairs bathroom because getting on and off the toilet was too much work for my little legs."

O: Vitals: Height: 5'10" (1.78 m) Weight: 140.6 lb (63.8 kg) BMI: 20.12 kg/m²
HR: 92 contractions/min BP: 106/62 mmHg

Tired appearance (bags under eyes), cachectic

Gait slow and unstable

Notably short of breath after walking 500 ft (152.4 m) down the hallway for examination

(continued)

CASE STUDY Organ Transplantation (continued)

Labs:
  Hemoglobin: 10.2 g/dl
  Hematocrit: 30.0%
  Fasting glucose: 125 mg/dl
  Total cholesterol: 181 mg/dl
  HDL: 29 mg/dl
  LDL: 92 mg/dl
  Triglycerides: 302 mg/dl

Graded exercise test (ramp protocol):
  Peak work rate: 3.0 mph @ 10% grade
  Test termination from leg fatigue
  Peak HR: 149 contractions/min
  Peak BP: 166/70 mmHg
  Peak RPE: 19/20
  $\dot{V}O_2$max: 21.3 ml · kg^{-1} · min^{-1}
  Peak Respiratory Exchange Ratio: 1.15
  ECG: Sinus rhythm at rest and throughout exercise and recovery, no ST changes or dysrhythmias
  No symptoms of cardiac ischemia

Bone densitometry: 1.109 g/cm^2 with a T-score of –2.7 (> –2.5 is indicative of osteoporosis)

Body composition:
  Fat: 19.3% (skin folds)
  DEXA: 20.1% fat

Muscle strength:
  Isokinetic knee extension: 20 reps at 180°/s
  Peak torque/body weight: 41% (normal: 58-75%)

Medications: Prograf, Cellcept, Prednisone, Acyclovir, Prilosec, Dapsone, NPH, Insulin (regular)

A: 1. Deconditioning with muscle atrophy, weakness, and fatigue

  2. Status: post-liver transplantation (sclerosing cholangitis)

  3. Multiple concomitant diseases:
    Ulcerative colitis
    Diabetes mellitus
    Osteoporosis

P: 1. Complete a comprehensive rehabilitation program, including muscular strengthening, cardiovascular exercise, and gait and balance conditioning.

  2. Prescribe nutrition counseling for diabetes/cardiovascular risk.

Exercise Program
Goals:

  1. Short-term goals (1 mo):
    Be able to walk 4 laps (1 mi [1.6K]) around the track in 20 min
    Climb 1 flight of stairs 3 consecutive times
    Discontinue use of the commode
    Improve glucose regulation

  2. Long-term goals (6 mo):
    Return to work part time
    Be able to walk 3 mi (4.8K)
    Improve glucose regulation

Mode	Frequency	Duration	Intensity	Progression
Aerobic	4-5 days/wk	20 min/session	THR 98-112 contractions/min (65-75% $\dot{V}O_2$ peak) RPE 13-15/20	Add 5 min/wk to a target of 45 min Increase intensity every 2 wk to a THR of 75-85% of maximum
Strength (all major muscle groups)	3 days/wk	1 set of 10-12 reps	< 12RM	Add weight as needed to maintain comfortable resistance for 10-12 reps
Flexibility (all major muscle groups)	3 days/wk	20 s/stretch	Maintain each stretch below discomfort threshold	
Warm-up/Cool-down	Before and after each session	5-10 min	RPE 7-9/20	

Special precautions:
- Carry/wear medical alert with transplant, diabetes, and medication information.
- With incisional hernia, avoid Valsalva maneuver.
- Check blood sugars before and after exercise.
- Inject insulin into nonworking muscles.
- Carry glucose tablets.
- Keep well-hydrated and avoid exercise in hot environments.

Follow-Up

Rehabilitation was complicated by several hospitalizations for bile duct obstructions and one episode of acute organ rejection. During each hospitalization, his situation was reviewed and the exercise prescription was adapted with appropriate reductions in exercise intensity for a short period of time. The importance of adherence and safety was stressed, even for lower-intensity exercise.

Suggested Readings

Beyer, N., M. Asdahl, B. Strange, P. Kirkegaard, B.A. Hansen, T. Mohr, and M. Kjaer. 1999. Improved physical performance after orthotopic liver transplantation. *Liver Transplantation and Surgery* 5 (4): 301-9.

Green, G.A., and G.E. Moore. 1998. Exercise and organ transplantation. *Journal of Back and Musculoskeletal Rehabilitation* 10: 3-11.

Kempeneers, G.L.G., T.D. Noakes, R. Van Zyl-Smit, K.H. Myburgh, M. Lambert, B. Adams, and T. Wiggins. 1990. Skeletal muscle limits the exercise tolerance of renal transplant recipients: Effects of a graded exercise program. *American Journal of Kidney Disease* 16: 57-65.

Krasnoff, J.B. 2001. Liver disease, transplant, and exercise. *Clinical Exercise Physiology* 3 (1): 27-34.

Miller, T.D., R.W. Squires, G.T. Gau, D.M. Ilstrup, P.P. Frohnert, and S. Steriot. 1987. Graded exercise testing and training after renal transplantation: A preliminary study. *Mayo Clinic Proceedings* 62: 773-77.

Painter, P.L. 1992. Exercise following organ transplantation. *Journal of Cardiovascular Physical Therapy* 3 (1): 4-8.

Painter, P.L., M.J. Luetkemeier, G.E. Moore, S.L. Dibble, G.A. Green, J.O. Myll, and L.L. Carlson. 1997. Health-related fitness and quality of life in organ transplant recipients. *Transplantation* 64: 1795-1800.

Painter, P.L, S. Tomlanovich, L. Hector, K. Ray, P. Stock, and J. Melzer. 1998. Cardiorespiratory fitness in pancreas-kidney transplant recipients. *Transplantation Proceedings* 30: 651-52.

Van den Ham, E.C., J.P. Kooman, M.H. Christiaans, and J.P. van Hooff. 2000. Relation between steroid dose, body composition and physical activity in renal transplant patients. *Transplantation* 69 (8): 1591-98.

CHAPTER 28

Chronic Fatigue Syndrome

Stephen P. Bailey, PhD, PT, FACSM
Elon College

Overview of the Pathophysiology

Chronic fatigue syndrome (CFS) is the term currently used in the United States for a condition characterized by persistent debilitating fatigue, not relieved by rest, and not accounted for by any specifically identified medical or psychiatric condition. While a specific cause for CFS has yet to be identified, several triggers have been proposed. These conditions include, but are not limited to, viral infection, immunologic dysfunction, abnormal hypothalamic-pituitary-adrenal (HPA) axis activity, neurally mediated hypotension, nutritional deficiency, and profound psychological stress. The most current thinking is that CFS represents a common endpoint of disease resulting from multiple precipitating causes.

Consequently, CFS is defined primarily by its symptoms, which in addition to fatigue may include frequent sore throats, painful lymph nodes, headache, difficulty with concentration and memory, low-grade fever, and others. CFS and fibromyalgia share numerous symptomatic characteristics; however, individuals with fibromyalgia also experience diffuse nonarticular soft tissue pain. Fibromyalgia is discussed in more detail in chapter 29. Previously, CFS has been thought to disproportionately afflict well-educated Caucasian women. More recent evidence suggests that CFS affects all racial and ethnic groups and both sexes. It is estimated that about half a million persons in the United States have a CFS-like condition.

To provide a basis for standardizing populations used in clinical research of this condition, in 1988 the Centers for Disease Control (CDC) published a set of criteria for defining cases of CFS. In 1993, the case definition of CFS was revised. In this case definition, CFS is treated as a subset of chronic fatigue (unexplained fatigue of ≥ 6 mo duration). In turn, chronic fatigue is treated as a subset of prolonged fatigue (fatigue lasting ≥ 1 mo). Cases of unexplained chronic fatigue can be defined as CFS if they meet both of the following criteria:

- clinically evaluated, unexplained persistent or relapsing chronic fatigue of new or definite onset (i.e., not lifelong) that:

  is not the result of ongoing exertion,

  is not substantially alleviated by rest, and

  results in substantial reduction in previous levels of occupational, educational, social, or personal activities; and

- the concurrent occurrence of four or more of the following symptoms*:

  Substantial impairment in short-term memory or concentration

  Sore throat

  Tender lymph nodes

  Muscle pain

  Multijoint pain without swelling or redness

  Headaches of a new type, pattern, or severity

  Sleep that is not refreshing

  Postexertional malaise lasting more than 24 hours

*These symptoms must have persisted or recurred during six or more consecutive months of illness and must have predated the fatigue.

To diagnose a client with CFS, all other conditions that may precipitate similar symptoms must be excluded. Conditions that often exclude a CFS diagnosis are hypothyroidism, sleep apnea, hepatitis B or C, major depressive disorder with psychotic or melancholic features (including bipolar affective disorder, schizophrenia, delusional disorders, dementia, anorexia nervosa, and bulimia nervosa), alcohol or other substance abuse within two years of the onset of chronic fatigue, and severe obesity.

Because diagnosis of CFS is based on symptomology and exclusion of other conditions, there are no recommended specific laboratory tests. Laboratory tests should be directed toward confirming or excluding other possible conditions.

Effects on the Exercise Response

Exercise testing is not a routine part of establishing the diagnosis of CFS because there are no unique diagnostic findings. When tested, clients with CFS are found on average to have mild reductions in both peak oxygen consumption ($\dot{V}O_2$peak) and ventilatory threshold compared to normal, but findings in individual clients vary considerably. It is not known whether a reduction in exercise capacity may be attributed in part to CFS itself or whether it is wholly due to the deconditioning that accompanies a reduction in activity level. Although there are occasional reports to the contrary, the consensus of findings from studies of clients with CFS is that cardiac, pulmonary, muscular, metabolic, immune, and endocrine responses to acute exercise are similar to those seen in normal individuals with profound deconditioning. The symptom of fatigue is therefore viewed as being "central"

(neurological) in nature. While exercise testing does not establish a CFS diagnosis, it may be requested as part of a client's evaluation for excluding other conditions, such as cardiovascular diseases. Exercise testing may also be used for designing an individualized exercise program for clients who have a diagnosis of CFS.

Effects of Exercise Training

A common complaint among clients with CFS is that their fatigue and other symptoms are worsened in the days following any amount of physical exertion. The basis for this "push-crash" phenomenon is not understood. Attempts at exercise conditioning may be frustrated by this circumstance and a successful exercise prescription needs to respect this observation. Despite the initial aggravation of symptoms caused by exercise, some overall improvement in symptoms has been reported for clients with CFS.

Similarly, CFS clients educated on the benefits of and encouraged to participate in regular physical activity at home showed significant improvements. In most cases, the physiological and functional changes seen in CFS

Chronic Fatigue Syndrome: Exercise Testing

Methods	Measures	Endpoints*	Comments

Aerobic
Cycle
(ramp protocol 1-20 watts/
min; staged protocol 25-50
watts/3-min stage)
Treadmill
(1-2 METs/3-min stage)
	• 12-lead ECG, HR	• Serious dysrhythmias
		• >2 mm ST-segment
		  depression or elevation
		• Ischemic threshold
		• T-wave inversion with
		  significant ST change
			• Maximal aerobic power test
			  may be indicated for exclu-
			  sion of other diagnoses.

	• BP	• SBP > 250 mmHg or DBP > 115 mmHg	

	• RPE (Borg 6-20 scale)
	• METs
	• Other measures as
	  clinically indicated
			• Respired gas analysis may be
			  useful.

*Measurements of particular significance; do not always indicate test termination.

Medications	Special Considerations
The most commonly used agents (most of which will not alter physiologic responses to exercise): • Tricyclic agents • Antidepressants • Anxiolytic agents • Nonsteroidal anti-inflammatory agents • Antimicrobials • Antihistamines • Antihypotensive agents	• Clients with CFS often seek remedies for symptom relief that are available outside of the traditional medical model. • Clients may be quite deconditioned. Low work rate increments are usually appropriate. • Schedule testing for a day that the client does not have other activities scheduled.

Chronic Fatigue Syndrome: Exercise Programming

Modes	Goals	Intensity/ Frequency/Duration	Time to Goal
Aerobic •Large muscle activities (walking, rowing, cycling, swimming)	•Prevent deconditioning •Maintain functional work capacity	•RPE 9-12/20 •Intensity not main focus •3-5 days/wk •1-2 sessions/day •5 min/session, progressing to 60 min/session as tolerated	•~3 mo
Flexibility • Strength	•Maintain ROM		
Strength	•Maintain strength • Avoid muscle soreness		
Functional •Activity-specific exercise	•Increase ease of performing ADLs		

Medications	Special Considerations
•See exercise testing table. •Individual history should be obtained.	•Optimal dosing for these patients is unknown. A prudent approach is to begin with an activity that the individual is known to tolerate and build duration slowly. •Symptoms may worsen initially when exercise training begins. •Depression is associated with CFS. •Many clients will "budget" their energy reserves.

clients following exercise training are relatively modest while improvements in perceived outcomes (e.g., quality of life) can be dramatic.

Management and Medications

Because the pathogenesis of CFS is not understood, treatment is directed at reduction of symptoms rather than reversal of the underlying condition. Medications and other interventions therefore vary according to which symptoms are predominant, and may also vary with the experience and judgments of the primary physician. Medications commonly used to treat clients with CFS include tricyclic agents, antidepressants, anxiolytic agents, nonsteroidal anti-inflammatory agents, antimicrobials, antihistamines, and antihypotensive agents. CFS clients often seek relief of their symptoms through remedies that are available outside of the traditional medical model. Dietary manipulation, vitamin and mineral supplementation, herbal preparations, massage therapy, and aroma

therapy are examples of treatments that individuals with CFS may pursue without the knowledge of a physician.

Recommendations for Exercise Testing

Incremental exercise testing with monitoring of standard cardiovascular and ventilatory responses (electrocardiogram, blood pressure, heart rate, respiratory gas exchange, and ventilation) may be indicated as a screening test for clients whose diagnosis is not yet established. If a myopathic disease is suspected as an alternative diagnosis, appropriate screening for metabolic intermediates in blood or muscle samples might also be incorporated into the study. Clients with longstanding symptoms are very likely to have had a low level of exercise activity and to have undergone significant deconditioning. Work rate increments used in testing will therefore usually be low relative to the levels that would be predicted for age, size, and gender. For example, protocols initiated at work rates below 2 METs and increasing 0.5 to 1 MET per stage have been effective (see the Chronic Fatigue Syndrome: Exercise Testing table on page 187).

Recommendations for Exercise Programming

Little is known about the clinical effect of exercise training in this group of clients. Thus, general recommendations regarding exercise programming for all clients with CFS are difficult to make (see the Chronic Fatigue Syndrome: Exercise Programming table). Reports of clinical improvement resulting from exercise conditioning could reflect a systematic bias, in that clients who do not tolerate exercise may be underrepresented in such studies and therefore not be fully reflected in the outcome measurements. To date, however, there does not appear to be any evidence of adverse outcomes from prospectively studied exercise trials in clients with CFS.

For clients who wish to undertake an exercise program, the following general guidelines offer a conservative approach to exercise programming that takes into account some of the unique difficulties characteristic of this client population:

- The goal of exercise programming in this condition should be, first and foremost, to prevent further deconditioning that could compound the disability of chronic fatigue. Clients and trainers alike should resist the temptation to adopt a traditional method of training aimed at optimization of aerobic capacity and should focus instead on modest goals of preventing progressive deconditioning.

- Clients should be warned that they might feel increased fatigue in the first few weeks of an exercise program.

- Exercise should generally be initiated at very low levels, based on the client's current activity tolerance.

- Aerobic exercise should utilize a familiar activity, such as walking, that can be started at a low level.

- Flexibility exercises may be prescribed to preserve normal range of motion.

- Strength training should focus on preservation of levels of strength commensurate with daily living activities and should attempt to avoid activities and intensities that induce delayed-onset muscle soreness (DOMS).

- The progression of exercise activity should focus primarily on increasing the duration of moderate-intensity activities in preference to increasing exercise intensity. Identification of the appropriate magnitude of progression from one exercise session to the next is the most challenging aspect of exercise programming for individuals with CFS. Clients should be "coached" to not overexert themselves on days when they are feeling well and to reduce their exercise intensity when their symptoms are increased.

Special Considerations

Several psychological considerations are relevant to exercise in people with CFS:

- CFS is often accompanied by depression, although it is not clear how much of the depression is the result of the change in lifestyle resulting from persistent symptoms and how much may be inherent to CFS itself.

- Because misunderstanding abounds concerning CFS, some clients may express frustration and disillusionment with both lay and medical communities, which may have been less than sympathetic to their problems.

- A supportive and understanding environment is important in evaluating and counseling clients with CFS.

- CFS clients cope with their symptoms in part by planning their activities so as to "budget" their energy. Providing advance information about what they can anticipate when referred for exercise testing or training will help them to do so.

CASE STUDY Chronic Fatigue Syndrome

A 41-year-old Caucasian woman was referred to an exercise specialist by a psychiatrist because she had become deconditioned secondary to chronic fatigue syndrome. She stated that her fatigue started dramatically 4 years ago after her 15-year-old daughter died while attending "boot camp" for teenagers with substance abuse problems. She also had been experiencing panic attacks and was medicated for this disorder. She had a past history (8 years earlier) of alcohol abuse. She lived with her husband in a two-story home, but she rarely left her home (approximately once/wk) due to profound fatigue and fear of having a panic attack. She hoped that by participating in a regular exercise program she could "return to part of her life." Prior to quitting work 3 years earlier, she was an office manager for a group of physicians.

(continued)

CASE STUDY Chronic Fatigue Syndrome *(continued)*

S: "I used to exercise 3 to 4 times per week; now I can't do anything. I try to do chores around the house, I work for maybe 5 minutes, and then I have to stop and rest for 15. I sit down to do the bills and I can't concentrate so I give up."

O: Vitals: Height: 5'5" (1.65 m)   Weight: 157 lb (71.2 kg)   BMI: 26.2 kg/m²
                HR: 82 contractions/min   BP: 96/48 mmHg

Slightly overweight Caucasian female with normal muscle tone and bulk

Physical exam: Unremarkable

Psychiatric exam: Evidence of tangential thinking

Labs (all routine blood tests): Within normal limits

Medications: Florinef, Claritin, Zoloft, Xanax

Graded exercise test (low level; 8 min 35 s on treadmill):
  Peak work rate: 3.2 mph @ 2% grade
  Peak HR: 124 contractions/min
  Peak BP: 134/62 mmHg
  $\dot{V}O_2$peak: 17 ml · kg^{-1} · min^{-1}
  RPE: 19/20

Flexibility: Normal

Declined to perform other tests because of fatigue

A: 1. CFS

2. Aerobic exercise intolerance

3. History of axis II psychiatric problems (anxiety disorder, substance abuse)

P: 1. Continue psychiatric treatment, including trial of Florinef.

2. Prescribe an exercise program.

Exercise Program
Goals:

1. Walk on a treadmill at 3 mph @ 1% grade for 20 continuous min

2. Be able to do upper extremity strengthening exercises (3 sets of 10 reps):
   Shoulder flexion, protraction, retraction, and abduction
   Elbow flexion and extension
   Latissimus pull-down

3. Do a home exercise program twice/wk

Mode	Frequency	Duration	Intensity	Progression
Aerobic	2-3 days/wk	2 5-min sessions with 5-10 min recovery between	2-2.5 mph 0% grade	Increase until 20 min continuous at 4 wk
Strength (upper extremities)	2-3 days/wk	1 set of 10 reps	Green Theraband™	Advance to 3 sets of 10 reps in 4 wk
Flexibility	2-3 days/wk	20-60 s/stretch	As indicated	Maintain
Neuromuscular				
Functional				
Warm-up/Cool-down				

Follow-Up

The client never met any of these goals. She frequently cancelled appointments and discontinued participation after only 3 sessions.

Suggested Readings

DeBecker, P., J. Roeykens, M. Reynders, N. McGregor, and K. DeMeirleir. 2000. Exercise capacity in chronic fatigue syndrome. *Archives of Internal Medicine* 160 (21): 3270-77.

Fukada, K., S.E. Straus, I. Hickie, M.C. Sharpe, J.C. Dobbins, and A. Komaroff. 1994. The chronic fatigue syndrome: A comprehensive approach to its definition and study. International Chronic Fatigue Study Group. *Annals of Internal Medicine* 121: 953-59.

Fulcher, K., K. Claery, and P. White. 1994. A placebo controlled study of a graded exercise programme in patients with the chronic fatigue syndrome. *European Journal of Applied Physiology* 69 (supplement): S35.

Fulcher, K.Y., and P.D. White. 2000. Strength and physiological response to exercise in patients with chronic fatigue syndrome. *Journal of Neurology, Neurosurgery and Psychiatry* 69 (3): 289.

LaManca, J.J., and S.A. Sisto. 2002. Chronic fatigue syndrome. In *ACSM's resources for clinical exercise physiology: Musculoskeletal, neuromuscular, neoplastic, immunologic, and hematologic conditions.* Edited by J.N. Myers, W.G. Herbert, R. Humphrey. 219-32. Philadelphia: Lippincott Williams 7 Wilkins.

Ottenweller, J.E., S.A. Sisto, R.C. McCarty, and B.H. Natelson. 2001. Hormonal responses to exercise in chronic fatigue syndrome. *Neuropsychobiology* 43 (1): 34-41.

Powell, P., R.P. Bentall, F.J.Nye, and R.H. Edwards. 2001. Randomized controlled trial of patient education to encourage graded exercise in chronic fatigue syndrome. *British Medical Journal* 322: 387-90.

Riley, M.S., C.J. O'Brien, D.R. McClusky, N.P. Bell, and D.P. Nicholls. 1990. Aerobic work capacity in patients with chronic fatigue syndrome. *British Medical Journal* 301: 953-56.

Shafran, S.D. 1991. The chronic fatigue syndrome. *American Journal of Medicine* 90: 730-39.

Shepard, R.J. 2001. Chronic fatigue syndrome: An update. *Sports Medicine* 31 (3): 167-94.

Wilson, A., I. Hickie, A. Lloyd, and D. Wakefield. 1994. The treatment of chronic fatigue syndrome: Science and speculation. *American Journal of Medicine* 96: 544-50.

CHAPTER 29

Fibromyalgia

Barbara Meyer, PhD
University of Wisconsin-Milwaukee

Kathy Lemley, MS, PT
Milwaukee Medical Clinic

Overview of the Pathophysiology

There are approximately 6 million people in the United States diagnosed with fibromyalgia (FM), making it the third most prevalent rheumatological disorder in the country. Although the disease affects both men and women, 80% of those afflicted are women between 20 and 55 years of age. FM is a complex multidimensional condition characterized by the presence of chronic diffuse pain and tenderness at specific anatomic locations referred to as "tender points." Additional symptoms include sleep disturbance, chronic fatigue, morning stiffness, paresthesia in the extremities, enhanced perception of physical exertion, depression, and anxiety. These primary symptoms precipitate various secondary manifestations of the disease, including impaired functional ability, poor physical fitness, social isolation, low self-esteem, and poor quality of life. The etiology of FM is poorly understood and to date, no specific causal mechanism has been identified. Among those that have been discussed are muscle abnormalities (e.g., muscle microtrauma, local muscular ischemia), neuroendocrine and autonomic system regulation disorders (e.g., stage IV sleep disturbance, serotonin metabolism abnormality, hypothalamic-pituitary-adrenal [HPA] axis disturbance, diminished local muscular glucose metabolism), and genetic predisposition.

Effects on the Exercise Response

The biopsychosocial symptoms associated with FM directly and indirectly affect the acute response to exercise. Pain associated with basic aid for daily living, general fatigue, and enhanced perception of exertion contribute to the fact that individuals with FM are largely sedentary and deconditioned. Reports of morning stiffness, an exaggerated delayed-onset muscle soreness (DOMS) response with poor recovery from exercise, and difficulty with use of the arms in elevated positions may limit the timing of exercise as well as the type of activities prescribed. Specifically, eccentric muscle contractions, sustained overhead activities, and vigorous or high-impact activities are poorly tolerated.

Effects of Exercise Training

Exercise training can produce the same general benefits for individuals with FM as it does for healthy individuals (i.e., improved cardiorespiratory function, reduced coronary artery disease risk factors, decreased cardiovascular mortality and morbidity, and improved psychosocial function). However, the main goal of exercise training in this population is not to enhance cardiopulmonary fitness but rather to restore and maintain functional ability. Benefits specific to individuals with FM include:

- reduced number of tender points and decreased pain at tender points;
- decreased general pain;
- improved sleep and less fatigue;
- fewer feelings of helplessness and hopelessness;
- more frequent and meaningful social interactions; and
- lessened impact of the disease on daily activities.

Because individuals afflicted with FM tend to be unfit and fearful of the pain associated with exertion, they may be unwilling and/or unable to participate at the same level as healthy individuals. As such, they may need to begin at lower levels of intensity, duration, and frequency, and proceed in a more gradual fashion than typically prescribed.

Management and Medications

According to American College of Rheumatology (ACR) criteria, diagnosis is best made by a physician. Table 29.1 outlines the ACR criteria for FM classification, including

Table 29.1 American College of Rheumatology Criteria for Classification of FM

Widespread pain for at least three months, defined as the presence of all of the following:

- Pain on the right and left sides of the body
- Pain above and below the waist (Including shoulder and buttock pain)
- Pain in the axial skeleton (cervical, thoracic or lumbar spine, or anterior chest)
- Pain on palpation with a force of 4 kg (approx. 9 lb) in the following 11 sites (9 bilateral sites):

Occiput at the insertions of 1 or more of the following muscles:

Trapezius

Sternocleidomastoid

Splenius capitis

Semispinalis capitis

Low cervical (at the anterior aspect of the interspaces between the transverse processes of C5-C7):

Trapezius (at the midpoint of the upper border)

Supraspinatus (above the scapular spine near the medial border)

Second rib (just lateral to the second costochondral junctions)

Lateral epicondyle (2 cm distal to the lateral epicondyle)

Gluteal (at the upper outer quadrant of the buttocks, at the anterior edge of the gluteus maximus muscle)

Greater trochanter (posterior to the trochanteric prominence)

Knee (at the medial fat pad proximal to the joint line)

From Wolfe, F., H.A. Smythe, and M.B. Yunus et al. 1990. The American College of Rheumatology 1990 criteria for the classification of fibromyalgia. *Arthritis Rheumatology* 33: 160-72.

identification of the nine bilateral tender point sites. Medical personnel may guide management of the disease, but clients themselves must assume responsibility for symptom management. Evidence exists to support a variety of treatment options, including pharmacological intervention (e.g., medications for pain, sleeplessness, depression, anxiety), exercise programs, client education programs, cognitive behavioral therapy, hypnosis, and acupuncture. While there has been little control or standardization to date in the empirical study of FM treatment, multidisciplinary approaches that include some form of exercise (e.g., exercise combined with medication, cognitive behavioral therapy combined with physical activity) may be better than any single approach.

Recommendations for Exercise Testing

Individuals with FM tend to be sedentary and deconditioned, with poor ability to sustain exercise. Therefore, tests of muscular endurance (e.g., 6-min walk test; see the Fibromyalgia: Exercise Testing table on page 194) may be very useful for the prescription of an exercise program. Maximal aerobic exercise testing is usually symptom limited rather than metabolically limited in the FM population. Symptom limitations and low intrinsic motivation prompt utilization of submaximal tests, graded protocols

with smaller increments (i.e., Naughton, Balke-Ware), or ramp protocols. Walking or cycle tests are recommended, although individuals with gluteal tender points may find it difficult to tolerate cycling. Exercise testing should take place on a day when no other activities are scheduled to minimize its impact on later function.

Flexibility programs have been shown to result in short-term improvements in FM symptoms. Simple flexibility testing can identify specific areas that would benefit from routine stretching. Since individuals afflicted with the disease have a poor tolerance for eccentric movements, strength training is not a major component of their exercise program. However, a grip strength test may give some indication of functional strength.

Recommendations for Exercise Programming

Methodological inconsistencies and high attrition rates among FM clients participating in exercise programs make it difficult to identify definitive recommendations for exercise programming. However, it appears that exercise programming for individuals with FM should primarily consist of low- to moderate-intensity aerobic activities (see the Fibromyalgia: Exercise Programming table on page 195). Muscular endurance or aerobic exercise testing should be conducted prior to exercise prescription

Fibromyalgia: Exercise Testing

Methods	Measures	Endpoints*	Comments

Aerobic
Cycle
(ramp protocol 1-20 watts/
min; staged protocol 25-50
watts/3-min stage)
Treadmill
(0.5-1.0 METs/3-min stage)
	• 12- lead ECG, HR
	
	• BP
	
	• RPE (6-20)
	• METs
	• Time to exhaustion
		• Serious dysrhythmias
		• >2mm ST-segment
		  depression or elevation
		• Ischemic threshold
		• T-wave inversion with
		  significant ST change
		• SBP > 250 mmHg or
		  DBP > 115 mmHg
			• Gluteal trigger points may
			  limit usefulness of cycling.
			
			• RPE may be inaccurate.

Strength Handgrip	• MVC	• 3 attempts	• May reflect strength.
Endurance 6- and 12-min walk	• Distance	• Total distance/stops	• May be more useful than aerobic tests.
Flexibility Sit and reach Goniometry	• Length of reach • ROM	• Full flexion and extension	• Identify specific joints for stretching exercise.
Functional Lifting-specific activities			• Useful for program to maintain ADLs.

*Measurements of particular significance; do not always indicate test termination.

Medications	Special Considerations
Most commonly used agents should be unlikely to alter test results. They include the following (clients with multiple physical symptoms may take many medications): • Analgesics • Antidepressants (TCAs and SSRIs) • Anxiolytics/Benzodiazepines	• Subjects may be very deconditioned. • Perception of increased exertion may alter RPE. • Avoid early morning testing to avoid morning stiffness. • Test on a day when other activities are not scheduled. • Postexertional muscle pain may be severe 24-48 hr after testing.

so that individual programs, which may facilitate adherence, can be developed. Programs should consist of non- or low-impact activities that minimize eccentric contraction. Because the small muscles of the shoulder do not tolerate sustained overhead activities, exercise programs involving the lower body (e.g., water exercise, walking, cycling) should be utilized. While stretching may minimize muscle microtrauma and improve tolerance of aerobic exercise, few if any long-term benefits have been reported from participation in flexibility programs alone or in strength training activities.

Optimal dosing of aerobic exercise is currently unknown; however, psychophysiological responses to activity indicate the need to begin slowly and increase work rate gradually. Researchers and clinicians alike suggest that despite requests to exercise 3 times/wk, individuals with FM prefer or self-select twice/wk. It may be appropriate, therefore, to gradually increase duration of exercise from the typical 20 to 30 min/session to a 30 to 40 min/session.

Empirical and anecdotal evidence suggest poor adherence rates among individuals with FM. Thus, exercise sessions should be conducted under supervised conditions or in a group setting. Individuals with this disease should be encouraged to combine exercise with other symptom management techniques such as medication, support groups, and client education programs.

Fibromyalgia: Exercise Programming

Modes	Goals	Intensity/Frequency/Duration	Time to Goal
Aerobic • Large muscle activities (walking, cycling, aquatics)	• Restore/maintain functional ability* • Decrease pain • Decrease anxiety/depression • Increase $\dot{V}O_2$max • Decrease CAD risk • Go faster/longer • Increase time to exhaustion	• 50-60% max HR • 20-40 min • 2-3 days/wk • Monitor pace and HR • Favor duration over intensity	• Progress very gradually
Flexibility • Sit and reach • Goniometry	• Increase ROM (especially in shoulders, hips, knees, and ankles) • Decrease risk of injury	• As tolerated	• Maintain
Functional • Lifting • Individualized activities (O.T.)	• Increase ADLs • Restore work potential • Improve quality of life	• As tolerated • Avoid eccentric contractions	

*Other major goals not ascribed to specific exercises include the following:
• Reduce the number of tender points
• Reduce general pain
• Improve sleep
• Improve psychosocial well-being
• Avoid exhaustion (i.e., budget activities/exercise)

Medications	Special Considerations
• Most commonly used agents should be unlikely to alter test results. • See exercise testing table.	• Gluteal trigger points may limit usefulness of cycling. • Avoid morning exercise because of morning stiffness. • Supervision may increase adherence. • Clients may experience an increase in symptoms. • Avoid sustained overhead activities and eccentric movements.

Special Considerations

Often characterized as a "difficult" or "needy" population, individuals with FM may require more time and attention to meet compliance standards than those from a generally healthy population. FM clients are usually hesitant to exercise or increase the intensity of activity when they do exercise. Avoiding early morning exercise, eccentric movements, and repetitive overhead activities may help to minimize resultant attrition. Offering choices about the mode and timing of exercise and yielding to weather-related complaints may help to maximize participation in and adherence to the exercise program. Because symptoms may worsen initially, it is important for participants to budget exercise in conjunction with other activities and obligations. A supportive and understanding environment will also foster adherence to programs of exercise and ultimately the utilization of a comprehensive treatment program.

CASE STUDY Fibromyalgia

A 52-year-old woman complained of a having a sore right elbow and arthritis in the right knee. She complained of generalized pain and stiffness, most prominent in the neck, shoulder, legs, and feet. These symptoms were usually worse 1 to 2 days after activity, and she became easily fatigued after simple activities of daily living. She was using medication (Motrin) to get through the night. She had experienced similar symptoms since she was a teenager. She had a generally sedentary lifestyle, with the exception of using home-based stretching videos, and she wanted to try more exercise to help her symptoms.

S: "My elbow and knee are sore."

O: Vitals: Height: 5'3" (1.6 m)   Weight: 171 lb (77.6 kg)   BMI: 30.3 kg/m²
    HR: 86 contractions/min   BP: 130/80 mmHg

Middle-aged woman, flat affect; no notable joint inflammation/activity

Tender point assessment: Positive in 11 of 18 sites

Graded exercise test (modified Balke protocol):
    Completed 4 stages (12 min), terminated from fatigue
    ECG: No abnormalities
    Peak exercise capacity: 5.4 METs
    Peak HR: 149 contractions/min (89% of age-predicted)
    Normal pressor response

Questionnaires:
    Fibromyalgia impact questionnaire (FIQ): Score of 51.04/100
    Health assessment questionnaire (HAQ): Pain index score of 2.42/3.00

Medications: Motrin, Amitriptyline, Premarin, Tagamet

A: 1. Fibromyalgia with nonarticular pain
    2. Low aerobic capacity and deconditioning (decreased tolerance for ADLs resulting from pain and fatigue)

P: 1. Start a walking program.
    2. Prescribe stretching exercises as warm-up and cool-down activities.

Exercise Program
Goals:

1. Decrease myalgic pain
2. Improve ability to perform ADLs
3. Improve physical fitness

Mode	Frequency	Duration	Intensity	Progression
Aerobic	3 days/wk	12 min/session	Start at 25% of HR reserve	Slowly progress to 30 min Increase intensity 5%/wk to 50-60% of HR reserve
Strength				May want > 1 session/day
Flexibility (all major muscle groups)	3 days/wk*	As part of 10- to 15-min warm-up and cool-down Maintain each stretch 20-60 s	Maintain stretch below discomfort point	

Mode	Frequency	Duration	Intensity	Progression
Neuromuscular				
Functional				
Warm-up/Cool-down	Before and after each sesson	See Flexibility		

*May self-select 2 days/wk.

Follow-Up

At week 12, her tender points had increased to 15 out of 18, and she completed 7 stages of a modified Balke protocol (8.5 METs). Heart rate at stage IV was unchanged (148 contractions/min). Her FIQ and HAQ pain index scores, however, improved (FIQ = 40.95; HAQ pain = 2.32). After 24 weeks, she still had 14 out of 18 tender points, and her questionnaire scores showed mixed results (FIQ = 46.05; HAQ pain = 2.22). Aerobic capacity was essentially unchanged.

Suggested Readings

Burckhardt, C.S., K. Mannerkorpi, L. Hedenberg, and A. Bjelle. 1994. A randomized controlled clinical trial of education and physical training for women with fibromyalgia. *Journal of Rheumatology* 21: 714-20.

Fisher, N.M. 2002. Osteoarthritis, rheumatoid arthritis, and fibromyalgia. In *ACSM's resources for clinical exercise physiology: Musculoskeletal, neuromuscular, neoplastic, immunologic, and hematologic conditions.* Edited by J.N. Myers, W.G. Herbert, and R. Humphrey. 111-24. Philadelphia: Lippincott Williams & Wilkins.

McCain, G.A., D.A. Bell, F.M. Mai, and P.D. Halliday. 1988. A controlled study of the effects of a supervised cardiovascular fitness training program on the manifestations of primary fibromyalgia. *Arthritis Rheumatology* 31: 1135-41.

Mengshoel, A.M., H.B. Komnaes, and O. Forre. 1992. The effects of 20 weeks of physical fitness training in female patients with fibromyalgia. *Clinical Experiments in Rheumatology* 10: 345-49.

Meyer, B.B., and K.J. Lemley. 2000. Utilizing exercise to affect the symptomology of fibromyalgia: A pilot study. *Medicine and Science in Sports and Exercise* 32 (10): 1691-97.

Nichols, D.S., and T.M. Glenn. 1994. Effects of aerobic exercise on pain perception, affect, and level of disability in individuals with fibromyalgia. *Physical Therapy* 74: 327-32.

Nielens, H., V. Booisset, and E. Masquelier. 2000. Fitness and perceived exertion in patients with fibromyalgia syndrome. *Clinicians Journal of Pain* 16: 209-13.

Wigers, S.H., T.C. Stiles, and P.A Vogel. 1996. Effects of aerobic exercise versus stress management treatment in fibromyalgia. *Scandinavian Journal of Rheumatology* 25: 77-86.

Wolfe, F., H.A. Smythe, M.B. Yunus et al. 1990. The American College of Rheumatology 1990 criteria for the classification of fibromyalgia. *Arthritis Rheumatology* 33: 160-72.

CHAPTER 30

Anemia

Kirsten L. Johansen, MD
University of California, San Francisco

Overview of the Pathophysiology

Hemoglobin in red blood cells carries oxygen from the lungs to the skeletal muscle where it is needed to generate energy for physical activity. Anemia is a reduction below normal in the number of red blood cells or in the quantity of hemoglobin resulting in blood with a lower oxygen-carrying capacity. A defect in any one or more of the key components in red cell metabolism can result in anemia. Specific mechanisms of anemia and some of their causes include the following:

- reduced red blood cell production;
- marrow damage by drugs or tumor infiltration;
- failure of erythropoietin response to anemia (inflammatory disorders, renal failure);
- abnormal red blood cell precursor maturation;
- iron, B_{12}, or folate deficiency;
- thalassemia;
- drug toxicity (e.g., chemotherapeutic agents);
- increased red blood cell destruction or loss;
- hemolysis (autoimmune defects, hemoglobinopathies such as sickle cell disease); and
- blood loss (e.g., menstruation, gastrointestinal bleeding, or other source).

The signs and symptoms of anemia depend on the rapidity of development, the severity of the anemia, the age of the client, and the presence of underlying medical conditions such as atherosclerosis. The primary symptoms of anemia are easy fatigability, shortness of breath with exercise, and decreased work capacity. Anemia can also be associated with worsening of angina (chest discomfort), claudication (leg pain with exercise), or heart failure in clients suffering from these conditions. Symptoms are related primarily to the low oxygen-carrying capacity of anemic blood, but severe iron deficiency may also reduce the activity of iron-containing muscle en-zymes and impair the intrinsic ability of skeletal muscle. In the setting of rapid blood loss, symptoms may be more severe because low blood volume further reduces tissue oxygen delivery.

Effects on the Exercise Response

At rest, the anemic person compensates for low oxygen- and carbon dioxide-carrying capacity by increasing cardiac output and breathing rate. Also, there is often a rightward shift of the oxyhemoglobin dissociation curve as well as an increased percentage of oxygen extraction by the tissues. During exercise, cardiac output and muscle blood flow increase faster in anemia and remain higher, relative to the degree of exertion, for the duration of exercise. Thus, oxygen delivery to exercising muscle is preserved at near-normal levels. Heart rate and cardiac output at maximal exertion are normal in persons with anemia, but peak performance is reduced. Submaximal endurance is also reduced by anemia, and this effect may be more or less pronounced than the reduction in peak performance, depending on the severity of anemia and presence of iron deficiency.

Individuals with sickle cell anemia and thalassemia are severely limited by their low hemoglobin, but it is reported that they can exercise to exhaustion without precipitating any complications (such as sickle pain crisis). On the other hand, persons with sickle cell trait (heterogeneous hemoglobin S) are not limited because their hemoglobin levels are normal. In fact, the percentage of African-American professional athletes with sickle cell trait is about the same as in the general population. However, this does not mean that sickle cell trait is benign, as there have been numerous sudden deaths in young men with sickle cell trait. These incidents seem to have occurred after sudden increases in activity, a rapid increase in altitude, or prolonged, very high-intensity exercise. Dehydration may also have been part of these tragic deaths.

Effects of Exercise Training

While persons with chronic anemia will always have their peak aerobic performance limited by the anemia,

Anemia: Exercise Testing

Methods	Measures	Endpoints	Comments
Endurance 6-min walk	• Distance covered	• Note time and distance at rest stops	• Useful throughout exercise training program.

Special considerations

- Occult peripheral artery disease may be unmasked with increased claudication.
- Other tests (e.g., aerobic) may be used. See exercise testing table in chapter 4.
- Exercise may elicit angina in anemic persons.

Anemia: Exercise Programming

Modes	Goals	Intensity/Frequency/Duration	Time to Goal
Aerobic • Large muscle activities	• Increase $\dot{V}O_2$max, peak work rate, and endurance	• 40-70% peak HR • RPE 11-13/20 • 3-7 days/wk • 30-60 min/session • Emphasize duration over intensity	• 4-6 mo

Special Considerations

- Do not exercise if resting BP > 180/110 mmHg.
- Exercise when pressor response is controlled by medications; see chapter 12 on hypertension.
- High-intensity exercise and dehydration increase risk of sickle cell crisis.
- Exercise may elicit angina or claudication.

data gathered from animals suggest that aerobic exercise training in anemic individuals can improve exercise endurance to levels superior to those of non-anemic sedentary persons. Moreover, submaximal performance, which is largely a parameter of skeletal muscle function, can be markedly improved by endurance training.

Management and Medications

When treatment results in complete correction of anemia, exercise capacity usually returns to normal. Restoration of normal hemoglobin levels is often possible for anemia related to a deficiency state or to blood loss, but is not always possible or even desirable for clients with other conditions such as thalassemia, sickle cell disease, renal failure, or bone marrow abnormalities. Thus, individuals with these conditions may have chronic anemia and reduced exercise capacity despite appropriate treatment. Exercise limitations may persist even after normalization of hematocrit in persons with conditions that are associated with other exercise limitations, such as chronic renal failure.

Exercise capacity improves with erythropoietin treatment in clients with renal failure, but not as much as would be expected based on observed increases in hematocrit, and normal exercise capacity is not achieved. This has led investigators to conclude that renal failure causes muscle abnormalities that also limit exercise capacity. Similarly, clients with underlying heart failure, lung disease, or other conditions may have exercise limitations that are not related to anemia. However, since anemia can exacerbate the exercise intolerance associated with all of these conditions, treatment is usually associated with improvement.

Recommendations for Exercise Testing

The exaggerated heart rate response to exercise and limited peak performance in persons with anemia suggest that aerobic exercise tests will be likely to end sooner than predicted by age and gender. Thus, one should consider choosing a low-level exercise protocol. Submaximal endurance testing may also be helpful in monitoring the response to training or to treatment of anemia (see the Anemia: Exercise Testing table on page 199).

Recommendations for Exercise Programming

The main goal of the exercise program is to improve endurance. Any form of large muscle exercise is acceptable (see the Anemia: Exercise Programming table on page 199), although intensity of exercise should be moderate. The optimal frequency and duration of training sessions are not known. Adaptability is not known, but the time course of improvement in performance is presumably normal after anemia is corrected.

Special Considerations

Special precautions may be necessary in the exercise testing and training of persons with specific medical conditions.

• Sickle cell anemia or trait: High-intensity exercise and dehydration may increase the risk of sickle cell crisis. Therefore, moderate exercise and liberal fluid intake is especially recommended for these individuals.

• Known or suspected coronary artery disease: Vigorous exercise, especially in combination with anemia, may cause angina (chest discomfort). For this reason, exercise testing and training should be carefully monitored until the cause of anemia has been identified and treated or until tolerance of the exercise program has been established.

CASE STUDY Anemia

A 65-year-old man complained of chest pressure and dyspnea with exertion, which had been present for a couple of weeks. Symptoms resolved rapidly with rest, and he reported no symptoms at rest. He had a history of end-stage renal disease, and the resulting anemia was managed with intravenous erythropoietin and iron. His hematocrit was typically 34 to 39% over the past 6 months. He also had a history of myocardial infarction 4 years ago, with a left ventricular ejection fraction of 20%.

S: "I get short of breath when I walk."

O: Vitals: HR: 80 contractions/min   BP: 130/80 mmHg
      Regular HR with 2/6 systolic murmur and no peripheral edema

Lungs: Clear

Lab: Endoscopy positive for GI bleeding

Medications: Digoxin, angiotensin-converting inhibitor, calcium-channel blocker, aspirin daily, erythropoietin, iron, multivitamin, phosphorus binders

A: 1. Acute anemia secondary to gastrointestinal bleeding

2. End-stage renal failure

3. Prior MI

P: 1. Stabilize bleeding and find/treat the underlying cause.

2. Transfuse 2 units of red blood cells.

3. Increase erythropoietin/iron.

4. Better control angina with beta blocker.

5. Cardiac stress test to determine the extent of CAD.

Exercise Program
Goal:
   No dyspnea/chest pressure

Mode	Frequency	Duration	Intensity	Progression
Aerobic	3-5 days/wk	30 min/session	RPE 11-14/20	
Strength				
Neuromuscular				
Functional				
Warm-up/Cool-down	Before and after each sesson	10-15 min	RPE <10/20	Maintain

Follow-Up

He had complete resolution of symptoms after transfusion. Thallium stress testing revealed reversible defects in the inferolateral and anterior walls, which were managed medically. He had no further symptoms with a hematocrit of 33 to 36%.

Suggested Readings

Gozal, D., P. Thiriet, E. Mbala, D. Wouassi, H. Galas, A. Geyssant, and J. Lacour. 1992. Effect of different modalities of exercise and recovery on exercise performance in subjects with sickle cell trait. *Medicine and Science in Sports and Exercise* 24: 1325-31.

Gregg, S.G., W.T. Willis, and G.A. Brooks. 1989. Interactive effects of anemia and muscle oxidative capacity on exercise endurance. *Journal of Applied Physiology* 67: 765-70.

Jones, S., R. Binder, and E. Donowho. 1970. Sudden death in sickle cell trait. *New England Journal of Medicine* 282: 323-25.

Koskolou, M.D., R.C. Roach, J.A. Calbet, G. Radegran, and B. Saltin. 1997. Cardiovascular responses to dynamic exercise with acute anemia in humans. *American Journal of Physiology* 273: H1787-93.

McConnell, M., S. Daniels, J. Lobel, F. James, and S. Kaplan. 1989. Hemodynamic responses to exercise in patients with sickle cell anemia. *Pediatric Cardiology* 10: 141-44.

Sproule, B., J.H. Mitchell, and W. Miller. 1960. Cardiopulmonary physiological responses to heavy exercise in patients with anemia. *Journal of Clinical Investigation* 39: 378-88.

CHAPTER 31

Bleeding and Clotting Disorders

Geoffrey E. Moore, MD, FACSM
McGill University

Peter H. Brubaker, PhD, FACSM
Wake Forest University

Overview of the Pathophysiology

Activities of daily living inevitably involve physical and chemical trauma to vascular structures, so the circulatory system includes a blood hemostatic system that serves to minimize blood loss and to maintain blood flow to body tissues. Hemostasis involves a complex balance of blood clotting (coagulation) and clot dissolution (fibrinolysis). Clot formation also involves plugging of blood vessel defects by platelet aggregation. Coagulation, fibrinolysis, and platelet aggregation involve many proteins and enzymes, and all three processes continually work to maintain the integrity of the vascular system. In addition to these processes, the inflammatory response is an essential component of initiation and resolution of hemostasis. All of these processes are intimately involved in the development of a number of vascular diseases such as atherosclerosis, although in this chapter we will mainly be concerned with bleeding and clotting disorders.

The ability of the body to control bleeding after trauma requires the intricate coordination of coagulation and platelet aggregation. When a vessel is torn or cut, the open ends spasm, reducing blood flow and allowing blood platelets to aggregate at the site of injury. Substances released from the damaged tissues initiate a series of reactions known as the extrinsic pathway of the coagulation cascade. The combination of platelet plugging and coagulation produces a durable clot at the site of injury. As the injured tissues heal, the degradation of the clot involves the destruction of fibrin, which is a key proteinaceous component of blood clots, so fibrinolysis is essential to counteract coagulation. Diseases of hemostasis, therefore, have two main forms of disorder: too much bleeding (hemorrhage), or too much clotting (thrombosis).

Abnormalities of platelet function can produce inappropriate bleeding or inappropriate clotting. The most common platelet disorder that causes bleeding is thrombocytopenia, which is an insufficient number of platelets. The hemorrhages of thrombocytopenia, petechiae, are pinpoint-sized red spots, too small to feel, that look like a rash. Normal platelet counts range from 120,000 to 600,000/mm^3. The most common disorder associated with activated platelet aggregation is probably atherosclerosis, since platelet aggregation disorders alone rarely cause clinically meaningful obstruction of blood flow.

Abnormalities of the coagulation pathway generally cause excess bleeding. The coagulation cascade consists of proteins (factors) that are suspended in blood and form a web-like tangle of precipitated proteins when activated. Bleeding disorders from factor deficiencies can be congenital or acquired. The most common congenital bleeding disorders are factor VIII deficiency (classic hemophilia), factor IX deficiency (Christmas disease), and von Willebrand's disease. Acquired factor deficiencies can be caused by autoimmune illnesses, but these illnesses are rare. Also, many people have medically induced factor deficiencies because they take anticoagulant drugs such as warfarin. Fortunately, medical anticoagulation very rarely causes spontaneous bleeding, although there is increased risk of bleeding after an injury.

Abnormalities in the fibrinolytic cascade generally cause problems with excessive clotting. Common congenital deficiencies of this system include deficiency of protein S or protein C. Again, autoimmune illnesses can cause acquired forms of thrombotic disorders. These diseases generally cause clotting disorders because coagulation is ineffectively counteracted by fibrinolysis.

General clinical manifestations of bleeding disorders include the following:

- trombocytopenia: petechial bleeding;
- hemophilia: hemarthrosis (bleeding into joints) with subsequent contractures; retroperitoneal bleeding;

- von Willebrand's disease: prolonged bleeding after minor trauma; gastrointestinal bleeding; and

- medical anticoagulation: easy bruising ability; gastrointestinal bleeding,

General clinical manifestations of clotting disorders include the following:

- thrombocytosis: deep venous thrombosis (DVT); and

- fibrinolytic deficiencies: arterial occlusion and tissue infarction; deep venous thrombosis.

Effects on the Exercise Response

Disorders of bleeding and clotting have little effect on the exercise response, but exercise markedly alters the thrombotic and fibrinolytic pathways. During exercise, activity of both systems is increased, but the thrombotic pathway activity remains increased long after the fibrinolytic activity has returned to baseline. This is consistent with the fact that myocardial infarction is increased in the hours shortly after physical activity, but the correlation between these two phenomena is not certain. The clinical effect of changes in the thrombotic and fibrinolytic pathways caused by a single exercise session is not known. Moreover, for purposes of this text, there is virtually no data available on how exercise affects bleeding and/or clotting in persons with disorders in these pathways.

The major risks for exercise in persons with low platelet counts or coagulation factor deficiencies are bleeding from trauma or from high blood pressure associated with exercise. In sedentary persons, bleeding from a low platelet count is rarely a problem unless the count is well below 100,000/mm^3. Occasionally, intracranial (inside the skull) bleeds occur spontaneously when the platelet count is markedly low (< 20,000/mm^3). There are no controlled data on exercise in clients with low platelets, but vigorous exercise is probably contraindicated when platelet counts are below 50,000/mm^3. Use of elastic bands, stationary cycles, range of motion exercises, and ambulation should be encouraged in persons with platelet counts between 20,000 and 50,000/mm^3.

A few circumstances deserve special mention. First, since lifting heavy weights dramatically increases blood and intracranial pressures, the risk of an intracranial bleed probably outweighs the benefits in persons with platelets between 50,000 and 100,000/mm^3. Second, in persons with hemophilia or von Willebrand's disease, the mode of testing should minimize joint trauma and weight bearing. Additional limitations may be imposed by preexisting joint contractures from prior bleeds. Of course, these contractures may be good targets for flexibility testing and stretching exercises.

Effects of Exercise Training

The effects of exercise training on the blood hemostasis system are complex and not well understood. It is well known that regular exercise is protective against myocardial infarction and sudden cardiac death during physical activity, but this does not mean that clotting is causally related to this observation. Exercise training studies examining the balance of thrombosis and fibrinolysis have not given consistent results, so it is not clear how exercise training affects blood hemostasis. As mentioned above, inflammation is an important aspect of atherosclerosis, and recent data suggest that C-reactive protein (a marker of inflammation) is increased in coronary artery disease. Exercise training often reduces blood pressure and may reduce C-reactive protein, so the compound effects of exercise training on all the factors that influence hemostasis are extremely complex. The effects of exercise training on the thrombotic and fibrinolytic cascades in persons with disorders of these cascades are not researched.

Persons with hemophilia benefit from regular exercise but consequently are at some risk of bleeding into joints and developing joint contractures. Neither aerobic nor strength training alters the underlying disorder of hemophilia, but non-weight-bearing aerobic exercise, as well as strength and flexibility training, can be of immense functional and psychological benefit.

Recently, a number of case reports have been published on deep venous thrombosis (DVT) in athletes. DVTs are potentially life threatening because of their potential to break loose and create a pulmonary embolus. For this reason, continued training is contraindicated in an athlete who has developed a DVT. The duration of convalescence prior to resumption of sporting activities has not been objectively studied, but most sources advise an extended layoff of six months or more, until the thrombus has clearly resolved on vascular imaging studies.

Management and Medications

The management of bleeding disorders is determined by whether the problem predisposes to bleeding or to clotting and also by the cause of the disease. Anticoagulants are used much more commonly than natural and recombinant biologic factors because these latter medications are extraordinarily expensive. Persons with platelet disorders, then those with coagulation factor disorders, and finally those with prosthetic heart valves will be considered in turn.

In persons with low platelets caused by an overly rapid destruction of platelets (most often by the immune system), the treatment is to decrease the rate of platelet

Bleeding and Clotting Disorders: Exercise Testing

Methods	Measures	Endpoints	Comments
Strength Free weights Weight machines Elastic bands		•MVC or 1 RM	
Flexibility Goniometry		•Asymmetrical or limited ROM	•Assess effect of hemarthrosis or surgery on walking ability.
Functional Gait analysis		•Symmetric gait	•Assess effect of hemarthrosis or surgery on walking ability.

Medications	Special Considerations
•Minor risk of hemarthrosis in clients on anticoagulant therapy. •Asprin and other nonsteroidal anti-inflammatory drugs (e.g., ibuprofen): Contraindicated.	•Clients with hemophilia or von Willebrand's disease may have decreased ROM and secondary atrophy of shoulders, elbows, wrists, hips, knees, and ankles secondary to old hemarthroses. •If considered at risk for CAD, see exercise testing tables in chapters 4, 5, and 6.

destruction. This is done with immunosuppressive medicines, such as prednisone, and sometimes through removal of the spleen. Replacing platelets by transfusion works only for a very short while and is therefore limited to hospitalized persons. In people with high platelets resulting from overproduction of platelets, the treatment is to decrease the rate of platelet formation. This is usually achieved by chemotherapy.

In persons with coagulation factor deficiencies, a variety of medicines can be used to raise factor concentrations. Purified factor transfusions are available for some factor deficiencies. Mild von Willebrand's disease can be treated to increase the level of von Willebrand's factor. Unfortunately, as with platelet disorders, treatment for coagulation factor deficiencies is temporary.

Persons at risk for inappropriate clot formation because of mechanical heart valves, dilated hearts, or DVT require some form of anticoagulation. These inappropriate clots are highly dangerous because they can either grow in place and block blood flow or break off and lodge downstream in blood vessels critical to vital organs such as the brain or lungs. For this reason, such individuals are given anticoagulants, usually either warfarin or heparin.

Aspirin is commonly used for prophylaxis against stroke and myocardial infarction. The antiplatelet effects of aspirin at rest are, however, acutely overwhelmed by the pro-thrombotic effects of exercise. The longer-term interaction of aspirin and exercise, including postexercise recovery, is not known.

There have been some recommendations on the use of medications in athletes who have had a clotting disorder, such as DVT caused by protein C and/or protein S deficiencies. Persons with such deficiencies who are genetically heterozygous are usually not detected unless a thorough family history is known, or until they present with a clot. Since such cases seem to be relatively rare despite these deficiencies being common in the general population, prophylaxis with anticoagulants has not been recommended. Treatment for an acute case of DVT and prophylaxis against future episodes are commonly recommended for individuals who have had a clot. Persons with homozygous factor deficiencies should be treated with the appropriate factor replacement or anticoagulant (e.g., warfarin or heparin).

Recommendations for Exercise Testing

When exercise testing a person with bleeding or clotting disorders, adhere to the following recommendations (also see the Bleeding and Clotting Disorders: Exercise Testing table):

- Persons with hemophilia should avoid weight-bearing exercise.

Bleeding and Clotting Disorders: Exercise Programming

Modes	Goals	Intensity/Frequency/Duration	Time to Goal
Aerobic	• Improve endurance	• Program should follow ACSM guidelines for normal sedentary persons • Exercise training contraindicated in persons with recent DVT	
Strength • Circuit training	• Reverse secondary atrophy	• Mix of high reps/low resistance and low reps/high resistance	• 4-6 mo
Flexibility • Stretching	• Normalize ROM in hemarthritic joints	• 20 s/stretch	

Medications	Special Considerations
• Aspirin and other non-steroidal anti-inflammatory analgesics are contraindicated.	• Avoid high-impact activities. • See exercise testing table. • Avoid high resistance in persons with platelets < 50,000/mm³ and bleeding disorders.

- Range-of-motion (ROM) testing will help in managing flexibility exercises for persons with hemophilia.
- No high-resistance strength testing should be performed by persons with low platelet counts (risks intracranial bleed).
- Presence of a DVT is a contraindication to exercise.

Recommendations for Exercise Programming

The goal of exercise training is to improve endurance, strength, and flexibility. Swimming or stationary cycling is recommended for persons with hemophilia. Outdoor cycling is a non-weight-bearing activity on joints but risks trauma and subsequent bleeding in a crash (sooner or later, virtually every cyclist falls). Flexibility exercises may help restore joint mobility in persons with hemophilia who are affected with contractures. The optimal frequency and duration of training are not known. Adaptability is not known but is presumably normal (see the Bleeding and Clotting Disorders: Exercise Programming table).

Exercise training should be curtailed in individuals who have had a DVT. The necessary duration of exercise restriction has not been studied, but close follow-up with vascular studies should detect resolution of the thrombus. Resumption of training should occur some time afterward, so 3 to 9 months of reduced activity seems a likely figure.

Special Considerations

- Aspirin and other nonsteroidal anti-inflammatory drugs (e.g., ibuprofen) render platelets inactive, and their use is dangerous in individuals who have concomitant bleeding or platelet disorders.
- Persons who have any bleeding disorder or who are receiving medical anticoagulation should avoid contact sports (e.g., football, hockey, basketball).
- Persons with low platelet counts should avoid high-resistance strength training.
- Lower resistance should not be a risk.
- Nonsteroidal anti-inflammatory drugs should not be used either as analgesics or as thrombosis prophylaxis.

CASE STUDY Deep Venous Thrombosis

A 20-year-old female track athlete presented to the emergency department after 5 to 6 days of swelling and tightness in the left thigh and calf. She had a history of a synovial sarcoma in the left hip 3 1/2 years prior to admission, which was surgically excised and treated with 6 months of radiation therapy. A CT scan 3 weeks prior to admission showed no recurrence of cancer. She did not use tobacco or oral contraceptives, and did not recall a recent injury. She denied family history of bleeding or clotting disorders. Venous ultrasound revealed a DVT extending from the iliac vein to the popliteal vein.

S: "My leg is swollen."

O: Vitals: HR: 53 contractions/min   BP: 110/62 mmHg   Temp: 99.1° F (37.3° C)

Left leg/thigh: Warm, red

2+ non-pitting edema

Good posterior tibial pulses

Neurological: Intact in both lower extremities

Doppler ultrasound: DVT from iliac to popliteal vein in left leg

A: 1. DVT in a track athlete

2. History of synovial sarcoma with surgical excision, lymph node dissection, radiation therapy

P: 1. Lovenox and Coumadin

2. Lovenox

3. No running or other forms of heavy exertion.

4. Advise on the bleeding risks of Coumadin therapy.

Follow-Up

Six days later, she had improved symptoms and no bleeding. Coagulation studies were followed weekly to biweekly. Repeat Doppler ultrasound revealed that the DVT had resolved. The plan:

1. Continue Coumadin.

2. Monitor coagulation status (via INR).

3. Evaluate for etiology of DVT prior to resuming sports. Consider the following:
   Vascular injury secondary to treatment for cancer, Factor V Lyden, protein C, protein S, lupus anticoagulant, etc.

After diagnosis and stable prophylaxis for recurrent DVT, gradually resume activity over next 6 months, progressing from non-weight-bearing activities (i.e., cycling, pool exercise) to slow jogging.

Suggested Readings

Burke, L., and R. Parisotto. 2002. Hematologic disorders. In *ACSM's resources for clinical exercise physiology: Musculoskeletal, neuromuscular, neoplastic, immunologic, and hematologic conditions.* Edited by J.N. Myers, W.G. Herbert, and R. Humphrey. 233-41. Philadelphia: Lippincott Williams & Wilkins.

El-Sayed, M. 1996. Effects of exercise on blood coagulation, fibrinolysis, and platelet aggregation. *Sports Medicine* 22 (5): 282-98.

Gilbert, M., J. Schorr, T. Holbrook, and D. Tiberio. 1985. *Hemophilia and sports.* New York: National Hemophilia Foundation.

Hilberg, T., G. Moessmer, M. Hartard, and D. Jeschke. 1998. APC resistance in an elite female athlete. *Medicine and Science in Sports and Exercise* 30 (2): 183-84.

Li, N., N.H. Wallén, and P. Hjemdahl. 1999. Evidence for prothrombotic effects of exercise and limited protection by aspirin. *Circulation* 100: 1374-79.

Lin, X., M.S. El-Sayed, J. Waterhouse, and T. Reilly. 1999. Activation and disturbance of blood haemostasis following strenuous exercise. *International Journal of Sports Medicine* 20: 149-53.

Mattusch, F., B. Dufaux, O. Heine, I. Mertens, and R. Rost. 1999. Reduction of the plasma concentration of C-reactive protein following nine months of endurance training. *International Journal of Sports Medicine* 20: 21-24.

Mittleman, M.A., M. Maclure, G.H. Tofler, J.B. Sherwood, R.J. Goldberg, and J.E. Muller. 1993. Triggering of acute myocardial infarction by heavy physical exertion-protection against triggering by regular exertion. *New England Journal of Medicine* 329: 1677-83.

Willich, S.N., M. Lewis, H. Lowel, H.R. Arntz, F. Schubert, and R. Schroder. 1993. Physical exertion as a trigger of acute myocardial infarction. *New England Journal of Medicine* 329: 1684-90.

Wong, C., and M. Bracker. 1993. Coagulopathy presenting as calf pain in a racquetball player. *Journal of Family Practice* 37 (4): 390-93.

SECTION VI

Orthopedic Diseases and Disabilities

Kenneth H. Pitetti, PhD, FACSM

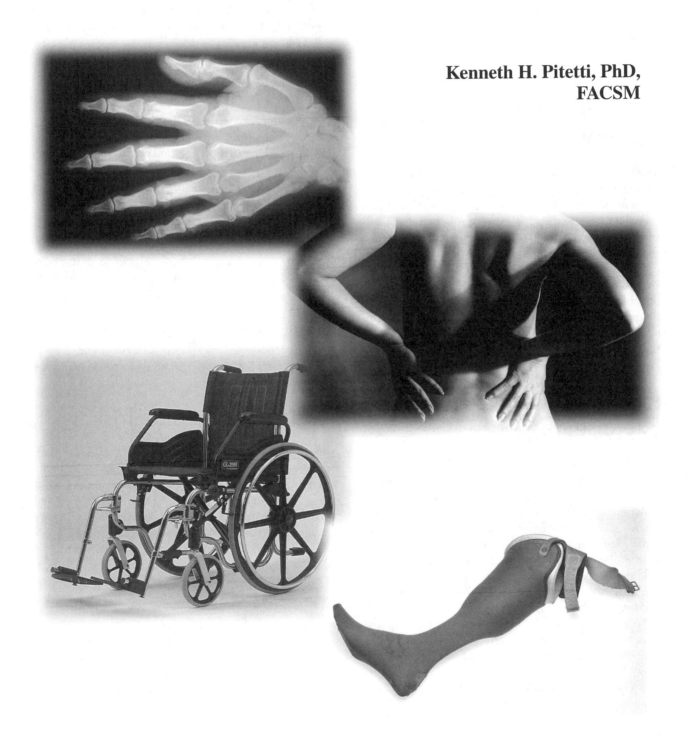

CHAPTER 32

Arthritis

Marian A. Minor, PhD, PT
Missouri Arthritis Rehabilitation Research and Training Center

Donald R. Kay, MD
University of Missouri Health Sciences Center

Overview of the Pathophysiology

There are more than 100 rheumatologic diseases, each having varying degrees of articular and systemic involvement. (See table 32.1 for the most common rheumatologic diseases.) The two most common conditions are osteoarthritis (degenerative joint disease) and rheumatoid arthritis (an inflammatory, multijoint, multisystem disease). Degenerative joint disease is localized to the affected joint or joints and appears first as deficits in articular cartilage. Rheumatoid arthritis is an inflammatory disease arising from pathological activity of the immune system against joint tissue. The inflammatory response may affect many joints and other organ systems.

Effects on the Exercise Response

Inflammatory rheumatic diseases can affect cardiac and pulmonary function, as well as cause widespread vasculitis, so this must be considered before anyone with a systemic rheumatic disease performs vigorous exercise. Vigorous exercise is contraindicated in the presence of acute joint inflammation (red, hot, swollen, painful) or uncontrolled systemic disease. However, the more common presentation of a person with inflammatory rheumatic disease is subacute or chronic joint symptoms combined with possible sequelae of previous systemic inflammation. In the absence of acute flare-ups in persons with systemic forms of arthritis (e.g., rheumatoid, lupus), the degenerative and inflammatory joint diseases have similar effects on exercise tests, whether musculoskeletal, biomechanical, or cardiovascular. There are few differences among the various systemic forms

of arthritis in terms of effects on the response to moderate exercise. In persons having an acute flare-up of systemic illness, the exercise response can be quite blunted.

- Persons with joint involvement tend to be less active and less fit (cardiovascular and musculoskeletal) than their unaffected peers.

- Resting energy expenditure may be elevated in persons with systemic inflammatory disease, even when the disease clinically appears inactive or under control.

- Pain, stiffness, biomechanical inefficiency, and gait abnormalities can increase the metabolic cost of physical activity by as much as 50%.

- Joint range of motion may be restricted by stiffness, swelling, pain, bony changes, fibrosis, and ankylosis.

- Inability to perform rapid, repetitive movements may affect exercise performance in terms of walking speed and cycle revolutions/min.

- Site and severity of joint involvement determine exercise mode for aerobic and strength tests.

- Deconditioned and poorly supported joints are at high risk for injury from high-intensity exercise or poorly controlled movement.

Effects of Exercise Training

Persons with either inflammatory or degenerative joint disease are able to participate in regular, conditioning exercise to improve cardiovascular status, muscular fitness, flexibility, and general health status. Improved aerobic capacity, endurance, strength, and flexibility are associated with improved function, decreased joint swelling and pain, increased social and physical activity in daily life, and reduced depression and anxiety. Disease-specific patterns of joint involvement should be considered during exercise prescription, monitoring, and follow-up assessments.

The most immediate benefit of conditioning exercise in this population may be to diminish effects of inactivity. Loss of flexibility, muscle atrophy, weakness, osteoporosis, elevated pain threshold, depression, and fatigue, which are problems common to both inflammatory and degenerative conditions, respond favorably to a low to

Table 32.1 Most Common Rheumatologic Diseases With Joint Involvement

Diagnosis	Disease type	Commonly affected joints	Features related to exercise
Osteoarthritis	Local degeneration	Hands, spine, hips, knees	Joint pain, stiffness Osteophyte Cartilage destruction
Rheumatoid arthritis	Inflammatory, systemic	Wrists, hands, knees, feet, cervical spine	Morning stiffness > 30 min Acute and chronic inflammation Chronic pain and loss of joint integrity
Ankylosing spondylitis Lupus Psoriatic arthritis	Inflammatory, systemic	Hands, knees, elbows, feet, spine	Arthralgia Fatigue
Gout Pseudogout	Crystal deposition	Great toe, ankles, knees, wrists	Acute joint inflammation Pain Tophi

moderate, gradually progressed exercise program. The potential for conditioning exercise to have a therapeutic effect on the disease process itself has yet to be determined.

Management and Medications

Joint protection, exercise, and education for self-management are essential components of comprehensive management. The goals are to decrease impairment, maintain or restore function, protect joint structures from further damage, and maintain healthful levels of physical activity. Ideally, care is coordinated in a multidisciplinary setting that offers preventive and rehabilitative care as well as medical management. To meet individual needs in an integrated program, the exercise component should incorporate joint protection and therapeutic exercise as needed. Health, safety, and successful exercise experiences for persons with joint disease can best be achieved by ongoing consultation with health care providers experienced in rheumatologic care and rehabilitation.

The major therapeutic goal in treatment of inflammatory rheumatologic disease is to control the destructive inflammatory process. Medications prescribed to achieve this goal range from aspirin and other nonsteroidal anti-inflammatory drugs (NSAIDs) to disease-modifying drugs (DMARDs) and biologic response modifiers (BRMs), which are designed to target specific immune processes believed to cause inflammation and tissue damage. Oral corticosteroids may be used when other drugs do not control inflammation. Combination therapy with two or more slower-acting DMARDs is commonly used to pro-

vide maximum inflammation and disease suppression. Drug therapy is usually continued indefinitely except when all signs of disease activity/progression disappear. In osteoarthritis, NSAIDs or acetaminophen is prescribed to manage symptoms of pain and stiffness. Local corticosteroid injections may be effective in both inflammatory and noninflammatory diseases to alleviate inflammation within specific joints or at other specific sites. Intraarticular injections should be given no more often than every 4 to 6 months because frequent injections can cause tissue destruction. The need to restrict activity following an injection is debated; however, vigorous weight-bearing activities are probably best avoided for at least one week.

Recommendations for Exercise Testing

In spite of the challenges presented by joint pain and dysfunction in arthritis, safe and clinically meaningful exercise testing can be performed. Submaximal and subjective symptom-limited treadmill tests requiring less than 3 mph walking speed and common cycle ergometer protocols are well tolerated and informative of aerobic capacity. Early-onset muscle fatigue may limit information regarding cardiopulmonary disease, so if a client is suspected of having coronary artery disease, the recommendations outlined in chapter 4 should be followed. Range-of-motion measurements (goniometry) are useful for persons who have limited flexibility and need stretching programs. Gait analysis may be necessary for people who have severe disease, altered biomechanics, and a need for orthotics (see the Arthritis: Exercise Testing table on page 212).

Arthritis: Exercise Testing

Methods	Measures	Endpoints*	Comments
Strength Isokinetic machines (90-120°/s) Isometric knee extension		• Ability to exceed 20-30% body weight for knee extension • 70 kg force	• Method depends on specific joint involvement and pain.
Endurance 6-min walk	• HR, RPE (6-20) • Time to exhaustion: 75% of maximal voluntary contradiction/ peak torque	• 6 min • Fatigue	• Method depends on specific joint involvement and pain.
Flexibility Goniometry	• Assess asymmetry		• Physical/occupational therapist consultation may help clarify goals.
Neuromuscular Gait analysis Balance			• Useful if client has antalgic gait.
Functional 50 ft (15.2-m) walk Sit to stand Arthritis impact measurement Scale/Health assessment questionnaire	• Walk: Observe for symmetry • Stands: Use if patient is weak and/or unstable		• Assess vocational potential.

*Measurements of particular significance; do not always indicate test termination.

Medications	Special Considerations
• Nonsteroidal anti-inflammatory drugs: May cause anemia from GI bleeding. • Rheumatoid arthritis remitting drugs: May cause secondary organ disease, including myopathy. • Oral corticosteroids: May cause skeletal myopathy, truncal obesity, osteoporosis, and anemia from GI bleeding.	• Pain/swelling may reduce performance. • Vigorous, highly repetitive exercise should not be performed with unstable joints. • Some arthritides involve cardiopulmonary systems, which may decrease performance. • Spinal involvement may cause radiculopathy. • Avoid morning exercise in clients with rheumatoid arthritis because of morning stiffness. • Variable-speed protocols should be available. Cycle ergometers should have loose-fitting toe straps to accommodate genu valgum. • If at risk for CAD, see chapter 4 exercise testing table.

Recommendations for Exercise Programming

The major impact of joint disease on exercise programming is the need for joint protection. Thus, the following recommendations apply:

- select low-impact activities;
- avoid stair climbing, contact sports, and activities requiring prolonged one-legged stance or rapid stop-and-go actions in persons with symptomatic hip or knee involvement;
- condition muscles prior to increasing exercise intensity;

Arthritis: Exercise Programming

Modes	Goals	Intensity/ Frequency/Duration	Time to Goal
Aerobic • Large muscle activities (walking, cycling, rowing, swimming, water aerobics, dance)	• Increase $\dot{V}O_2$max, peak work, and endurance	• 60-80% peak HR or 40-60% $\dot{V}O_2$max • RPE 11-16/20 • 3-5 days/wk • 5 min/session building to 30 min/session • Emphasize progression of duration over intensity	• 4-6 mo
Strength • Circuit training with free weights • Weight machines • Isometric exercises • Elastic bands	• Increase MVC, peak torque, or power	• Use pain tolerance to set %MVC • 2-3 reps initially, build to 10-12 reps • 2-3 days/wk	
Flexibility • Stretching	• Increase/maintain pain-free ROM • Decrease stiffness	• 1-2 sessions/day	
Neuromuscular • Exercises individualized to client	• Improve gait and balance		
Functional • Activity-specific exercise	• Increase/maintain ADLs • Return to work • Improve quality of life		

Medications	Special Considerations
• Steroids: Predispose to stress fractures. • See exercise testing table.	• Avoid overstretching unstable joints; avoid medial/lateral forces. • High-repetition, high-resistance, and high-impact exercise not recommended. • Depression may be an obstacle to lifestyle change.

• include flexibility and joint range of motion as key exercise components;

• avoid overstretching and hypermobility;

• if pain or swelling appears or persists, reduce load on joint (reduce exercise duration or intensity, exercise in a pool, cycle or row);

• select shoes and insoles for maximum shock attenuation during weight-bearing activities; and

• if hip or knee pain occurs with weight bearing, evaluate for rigid/semirigid orthotics.

One should also design programs with an individualized progression of intensity and duration (see the Arthritis: Exercise Programming table on page 213):

• use low intensity and duration during initial phase of programming;

• if necessary, accumulate exercise dose during several sessions throughout the day;

• recommend alternate exercise modes and interval or cross-training methods to allow for changes in disease status;

- set time goals, rather than distance goals, to encourage self-management to pace activity; and

- choose an appropriate exercise/fitness goal, and recommend that the person not exceed intensity, duration, and frequency guidelines for training.

Encourage exercise as a component of a fitness routine that is part of self-management:

- stretching/warm-up should be used daily, even on days when the disease flares and vigorous activity is undesirable;

- use aerobic activities that incorporate alternative forms of exercise (weight-bearing, partial weight-bearing, and non-weight-bearing) to allow for migrating joint symptoms and changes in disease activity;

- recommend that the person learn a strengthening routine;

- avoid activities that cause increased joint pain; and

- some postexercise soft tissue discomfort may be expected.

See table 32.2 for complications related to exercise programming for people with various forms of arthritis.

Table 32.2 Complications in Exercise Programming

Osteoarthritis	
Spinal stenosis	Localized and radiating back pain; spinal cord compression; neurologic deficits; claudication-like symptoms; worsens with spinal extension and weight bearing
Spondylosis	Localized and/or radiating back pain
Rheumatoid	
Cervical spine subluxation	Cervical instability; spinal cord compression; neurologic deficits (numbness, tingling, weakness) Life threatening
Foot disease	Metatarsalgia; subluxation of metatarsal heads; mid-foot pain/instability; calcaneal valgus; overpronation on weight bearing; gait deviation
Wrist/hand disease	Joint pain/instability; loss of grip strength Avoid power grip; ulnar deviation; joint stress at wrist
Systemic lupus erythematosus	
Necrosis of femoral head	Hip pain (also associated with long-term corticosteroid use)
Ankylosing and psoriatic spondylitis	
Enthesopathy	Acute and chronic plantar fasciitis; Achilles tendinitis costochondritis

CASE STUDY Arthritis

A 52-year-old woman referred herself to an exercise program complaining of knee pain and difficulty controlling her weight. Pain interfered with her ability to stand or sit, exercise, and engage in recreational and social activities, and it severely limited her ability to work as an elementary school teacher. She took extra strength Tylenol as needed for relief.

She was in a car accident 15 years ago and spent several months in the hospital. She had a steel rod placed in her left femur, a full cast on her right leg, was in traction for two months, and was told she would never be able to dance or play sports again. Since then, she had had pain in her knees and hips and had been very inactive. Six years ago, her doctor diagnosed osteoarthritis and told her she was not to do any kind of weight-bearing exercise, that aquatic exercise was the only thing she should do. So she started taking an "Aquacize" class 3 days/wk. She was once referred to physical therapy, which resulted in a home program for knee strengthening.

S: "I hurt every time the weather changes, and when I even run the vacuum I want to lie in bed afterward because my knees hurt so badly."

O: Vitals: Height: 5'6" (1.7 m)   Weight: 156 lb (70.9 kg)   BMI: 25.2 kg/m²
          HR: 74 contractions/min   BP: 120/80 mmHg

Tender knees, bilaterally, with notable crepitus; hip joint motions normal

Decreased range of knee flexion, full extension motion

X rays: Some narrowing of the medial joint space bilaterally; no osteophytes or bony deformities observed

Graded exercise test:
$\dot{V}O_2$peak: 26.3 ml $\cdot$ kg^{-1} $\cdot$ min^{-1}
50-ft (15.2-m) walk: 7.7 s (normal for age)
Grip strength: Right = 51 lb (23.1 kg); left = 45 lb (20.4 kg) (slightly below average for age)
Calf strength: Right = 55 lb (25 kg); left = 55 lb (25 kg) (normal for age)
Sit-to-stand test: 31.3 s (age-predicted: 15.9 s)
Sit-and-reach: 20.8 in (52.8 cm) (normal for age)

A: 1. Physical activity limited by knee pain

2. Low cardiovascular fitness

3. Lower extremity weakness

P: 1. Manage pain with the following:
Heat and cold
Joint-protection techniques (wear athletic shoes/shock-absorbing insoles)
Limited standing, walking, or sitting with knees flexed ($\leq$ 1 hr)
Pain evaluation (0-10 visual analog scale)

2. Strengthen lower extremities with exercises.

3. Prescribe an aerobic exercise program.

Exercise Program

Goals:

1. Increase functional capacity for ADLs

2. Supplement pain-coping skills

Mode	Frequency	Duration	Intensity	Progression
Aerobic (walking, cycling, aquatics)	3 days/wk	3 10-min sessions allow for full recovery	THR (102-128 contractions/min)	Increase to 30-min continuous, 4-5 days/wk in 1-2 mo, as tolerated
Strength (lower extremity)	3 days/wk supervised			Progress to circuit resistance training as tolerated
Flexibility (all major muscle groups)	3 days/wk	Stretch glutei, thighs, calves for $\leq$ 60 s/stretch	Maintain stretch below discomfort point	
Neuromuscular				
Functional				
Warm-up/Cool-down	Before and after each session	See Flexibility		

Strength program is as follows:
- Isometric knee extension at 90°: 4 sets of 6 reps, 6 s/rep; 2-min rest between sets
- Isotonic knee extension, free weights: 70% 1RM; 90-0° 1 min
- Stationary cycle: 2 min, no resistance
- Functional exercises, 1 min: sit to stand; step-ups, step-downs

Suggested Readings

Coleman, E.A., D.M. Buchner, M.E. Cress, B.K.S. Chan, and B.J. de Lateur. 1996. The relationship of joint symptoms with exercise performance in older adults. *Journal of the American Geriatrics Society* 44: 14-21.

Ettinger, W.H., R. Burns, S.P. Messier et al. 1997. A randomized trial comparing aerobic exercise and resistance exercise with a health education program in older adults with knee osteoarthritis. *Journal of the American Medical Association* 277: 25-31.

Fisher, N.M. 2002. Osteoarthritis, rheumatoid arthritis, and fibromyalgia. In *ACSM's resources for clinical exercise physiology: Musculoskeletal, neuromuscular, neoplastic, immunologic, and hematologic conditions.* Edited by J.N. Myers, W.G. Herbert, and R. Humphrey. 111-24. Philadelphia: Lippincott Williams & Wilkins.

Hurley, M.V., and D.L. Scott. 1990. Improvements in quadriceps sensorimotor function and disability of patients with knee osteoarthritis following a clinically practicable exercise regime. *British Journal of Rheumatology* 37: 1181-87.

Minor, M.A., J.E. Hewett, R.R. Webel et al. 1988. Exercise tolerance and disease related measures in patients with rheumatoid arthritis and osteoarthritis. *Journal of Rheumatology* 15: 905-11.

Minor, M.A., J.E. Hewett, R.R. Webel, S.K. Anderson, and D.R. Kay. 1989. Efficacy of physical conditioning exercise in patients with rheumatoid arthritis or osteoarthritis. *Arthritis Rheumatology* 32: 1397-1405.

Philbin, E.F., G.D. Groff, M.D. Ries et al. 1990. Cardiovascular fitness and health in patients with end-stage osteoarthritis. *Arthritis Rheumatology* 38: 799-805.

Rall, L.C., S.N. Meydani, J.J. Kehayias, B. Dawson-Hughes, and R. Roubenoff. 1996. The effect of progressive resistance training in rheumatoid arthritis. *Arthritis Rheumatology* 39: 415-26.

Stenström, C.H. 1994. Therapeutic exercise in rheumatoid arthritis. *Arthritis Care and Research* 7: 190-97.

van Baar, M.E., W.J.J. Assendelft, J. Dekker, R.A.B. Oostenforp, and J.W.J. Bijlsma. 1999. Effectiveness of exercise therapy in patients with osteoarthritis of the hip or knee. *Arthritis Rheumatology* 42: 1361-89.

van den Ende, C.H.M., T.P.M. Vliet-Vlieland, M. Munneke, and J.M.W. Hazes. 1999. Dynamic exercise therapy for rheumatoid arthritis (Cochrane Review). In *The Cochrane library.* Issue 2. Oxford: Update Software.

CHAPTER 33

Lower Back Pain Syndrome

Maureen J. Simmonds, PhD, PT, MCSP
Texas Women's University

Thomas E. Dreisinger, PhD, FACSM, RCEP
Progressive Spine Care and Rehabilitation

Overview of the Pathophysiology

Lower back pain (LBP) is one of the most widely experienced health-related problems in the world. This condition may occur suddenly and be unclear in onset; result from major trauma or multiple episodes of microtrauma; have muscular and joint pain; involve single or multiple sites; and persist for weeks, months, or a lifetime. The lifetime prevalence of LBP is between 58 and 70% of the population in industrial countries and the yearly prevalence rate is between 15 and 37%.

An extensive network of intersecting nerve fibers supplies the lower spine, the surrounding facet joints, soft tissues (muscle and ligaments), and the neurovascular tissues. This network is the reason why the source of pain is frequently difficult to determine. Any innervated structure of the lower back can trigger a nociceptor (receptors that detect painful stimuli) signal, and most structures in the lower back are well innervated, relatively small, and in close proximity to each other. The sensation of pain (resulting from the nociceptor signal), evoked within the central nervous system, is more complex. It is a combination of an unpleasant and emotional experience, usually associated with actual or potential tissue injury. Indeed, tissue injury, nociception, and pain are not synonymous and the relationship between them may be trivial, especially in chronic pain, because nociceptive signals can persist even after the tissue has healed. Moreover, the nociceptive signal is modified during its transmission from peripheral nerves to neurons in the spinal cord and then up to the sensory centers in the brain. Therefore, the interpretation of the signal can be influenced by myriad psychological (e.g.,

past experience, mood) and social (e.g., work, leisure activity) factors.

In summary, LBP is a multidimensional experience. It has sensory, emotional, cognitive, and behavioral components. The relative magnitude of each component helps to determine how the individual's problem should be managed. Managing LBP can involve:

- modifying sensory input by medications and/or therapeutic modalities (e.g., thermotherapy, biofeedback, mobilization, manipulations, postural retraining, various types of exercise); and
- addressing misunderstandings about the meaning of the pain, the relationship of pain to the injury, or anxieties about pain and its relationship to activity.

Effects on the Exercise Response

In and of itself, LBP will not have an effect on the exercise response. However, standing or sitting positions may exacerbate pain and prevent the individual from reaching his or her best effort or may contribute to a variation in effort. Therefore, individuals with LBP should be allowed to practice different exercise modalities in different positions, and limiting factors should be identified.

Effects of Exercise Training

Individual beliefs about LBP will influence the approach to exercise. Some individuals will consider LBP minor or inconvenient, ignore it, and go about performing their usual exercise regimen. Others will stop their daily activities immediately and seek professional advice. If pain is aggravated by certain exercise activities, some individuals with LBP may avoid their activities or even avoid those activities they anticipate will cause pain. Therefore, the ability to exercise may be greatly compromised by the degree to which individuals respond to LBP based on their beliefs.

Lower Back Pain Syndrome: Exercise Testing

Methods	Measures	Endpoints	Comments
Aerobic Maximal and submaximal testing unnecessary			• Testing may by warranted if risk factors/symptoms of CAD are present.
Strength Isometric trunk testing			• Measure isometric strength in multiple positions to find true peak torque.
Flexibility Straight leg stretch Iclinometry	• Angle to elicit pain/ radiarlor symptoms		

Medications	Special Considerations
	• Testing is not helpful during the first 4 wk following acute LBP.

Lower Back Pain Syndrome: Exercise Programming

Modes	Goals	Intensity/ Frequency/Duration	Time to Goal
Strength • Resistance abdominal strengthening • Back extensions	• Increase abdominal strength • Increase lumbar extensor strength	• > age 50: 10-15 reps/day • < age 50: 8-12 reps/day • ≥ 2 days/wk	• 2-4 wk
Flexibility • Any standard flexibility exercises that do not increase LBP	• Increase trunk and hip flexor and extensor ROM	• 2 min/muscle group; hold position for 3 reps, 10 s/stretch	
Functional • 5-min walk • 1-min chair sit and stand	• Increase/maintain ADLs	• Brisk walk, 3-5 days/wk • Chair sit and stand, 2-3 days/wk	• 2-4 wk

Medications	Special Considerations
• NSAIDs, acetaminophen, and occasionally narcotics for severe pain. • Muscle relaxants (e.g., Robaxin) • In chronic pain, tricyclic antidepressants and neurotin may be used in combination.	• Avoid high-impact exercises such as running. • On the basis of the Quebec Task Force report (1987) and the AHCPR (Agency for Health Care Policy and Research) Clinical Practice Guidelines (1994), there is little evidence to suggest that exercise has any direct impact on reducing LBP. However, proponents of exercise suggest that factors such as increased submaximal endurance, improved strength, and greater flexibility and ROM may be beneficial to the general health of some individuals with LBP. Whether these will potentially result in increased ADLs, prevent physical deterioration, or restore ability to work is unclear. • Low-stress aerobic activities can be safely started in the first 2 wk following onset of LBP symptoms. Trunk exercises should be delayed at least 2 wk.

For significant acute LBP (< 3 mo in duration), where pain and injury are related, it is reasonable to reduce exercise, treat the pain (with analgesics or a physical modality such as ice), and be guided by pain intensity and duration as normal exercise is resumed (1-2 days). However, the period of inactivity should be limited by time, not pain. An early return to normal exercise activities should be encouraged. Any advice to rest for a period of time longer than a week must be accompanied by advice about exact time for exercise resumption.

The acute LBP approach is inappropriate for chronic or recurrent LBP (>3 mo in duration). Pain associated with chronic and recurrent LBP is not indicative of ongoing tissue injury because the LBP will most likely persist and, therefore, cannot be used as a guide to adjust exercise management. This does not imply that practitioners should focus on pain and pain behavior, but that they should address the misconception or fears about chronic pain (e.g., it is not indicative of ongoing tissue injury) and motivate the individual to resume appropriate exercise activity.

Management and Medications

Nonsteroidal anti-inflammatory medications (e.g., aspirin, ibuprofen, indomethacin, nabumetone) and/or nonnarcotic analgesics (acetaminophen, tramadol) are commonly used by individuals with LBP. These medications should have no effect on the individual's exercise capacity. Muscle relaxants and antidepressants are sometimes used and may cause drowsiness. Opiates and oral steroids are occasionally used for short-term management (1-3 wk) of acute back pain. Short-term use (1-3 wk) of oral steroids should have no adverse effect on exercise capacity. Exercise should be curtailed when using opiates.

Recommendations for Exercise Testing

Individuals with LBP should be able to perform all seven families of exercise tests (i.e., aerobic, anaerobic, endur-ance, strength, flexibility, coordination, and functional) recommended by ACSM Guidelines (2000), although use of all seven families is usually not necessary. However, individuals may be limited in exercise test performance from an actual or anticipated increase in pain. Therefore, (1) allowing practice time on different test modalities in order to select the best modality is essential; and (2) the limiting factor (i.e., pain or fatigue) should be identified so that the data can be interpreted correctly (see the Lower Back Pain Syndrome: Exercise Testing table).

Recommendations for Exercise Programming

The failure to report clients' natural histories of LBP condition and the many methodological differences among research studies makes it difficult to identify specific exercise regimens that have been scientifically validated to improve LBP. In addition, the role exercise plays in the prevention of lower back injuries is also unclear because of poorly designed studies. For more background on this topic, see Suggested Readings at the end of this chapter, specifically Simmonds (2002). Exercise guidelines for individuals with LBP are, therefore, similar to the guidelines set forth by ACSM (2000) for the general, nondisabled population, with appropriate adjustments for individuals with LBP.

The goals for exercise programming are to prevent debilitation caused by inactivity and to improve exercise tolerance and muscular strength. Exercise modalities of the seven families of exercise (i.e., aerobic, anaerobic, endurance, strength, flexibility, coordination, and functional), which minimize stress to the lower back, can and should be started during the first two weeks of acute LBP. If the client has other health problems, the reader is referred to that specific chapter (e.g., see chapter 4 for coronary artery disease). During the acute stage of LBP, exercises for hip and back muscles should be delayed at least two weeks and the intensity should be very low with gradual increases in intensity and duration (see the Lower Back Pain Syndrome: Exercise Programming table).

CASE STUDY Low Back Pain

A 32-year-old male presented with a 2-year history of frequent episodic LBP. The onset of the recent symptoms occurred 2 weeks prior to examination. Over the 2 years, he had seen several different health care providers (family physician, orthopedic surgeon, physical therapist, chiropractor, and massage therapist). He had been treated with home exercise, passive stretching, supervised exercise, manipulations, medications (NSAIDs and muscle relaxants), and pool therapy. None of these treatments provided more than temporary symptomatic relief. X rays, magnetic resonance imaging (MRI), and CAT scans had all reported negative findings.

(continued)

CASE STUDY Low Back Pain (continued)

S: "I have pain in my left leg, and I'm numb below the knee."

O: Adult male, in no acute distress

Spine: Normal lordosis, low lumbar tenderness, pain with percussion

Neurological: Reflexes normal, motor strength normal

Straight leg raise (SLR): Limited on the symptomatic side by back pain

Back flexion: Caused symptoms to move further down his leg

Back extension: Relieved the leg symptoms

Gait: Antalgic (i.e., decreased time of weight bearing on left leg)

Heel and toe walking: Done with some difficulty

Inclinometer: Greatly decreased lumbar

Isokinetic lumbar spine function:
  Strength: 100 ft-lb (13.83 kg-m) (65% of predicted)
  ROM: 39° (normal: 72°)

A: 1. Low back pain

2. Osteoarthritis of the lumbar spine

P: 1. Prescribe a strengthening/retraining program.

2. Instruct on postural training exercises.

3. Learn self-management.

Exercise Program

Goals:

1. Reduced pain

2. Increased strength and flexibility

3. Improved posture/gait

4. Ability to self-manage future episodes

Mode	Frequency	Duration	Intensity	Progression
Aerobic				
Strength (multifidus erector spinae, latissimus dorsi, rhomboids)	Daily	1-2 sets of 10-20 reps	Antigravity	Increase to 2 sets of 10-20 reps, as tolerated
Flexibility	Daily			Incorporated into strength and postural exercises
Neuromuscular	Daily	1-2 sets of 10-20 reps		
Functional				
Warm-up/Cool-down				

Follow-Up

Following 8 weeks of rehabilitation, his symptoms were completely abolished. His lumbar strength had increased to 211 foot-pounds (29.18 kg-m) with an ROM of 72°. He had also become well educated in self-treatment during flare-ups of LBP.

Suggested Readings

Abenhaim, L., M. Rossignol, J.P. Valat, M. Nordin, B. Avouac et al. 2000. The role of activity in the therapeutic management of back pain. Report of the International Paris Task Force on Back Pain. *Spine* 25 (supplement 4): S1-33.

American College of Sports Medicine. 2000. *ACSM's guidelines for exercise testing and prescription.* Edited by B.A. Franklin, M.H. Whaley, and E.T. Howley. 6th ed. Philadelphia: Lippincott Williams & Wilkins.

Frost, H., S.E. Lamb, J.A. Klaber-Moffett, J.C.T. Fairbank, and J.S. Moser. 1998. A fitness programme for patients with chronic low back pain: 2-year follow-up of a randomized controlled trial. *Pain* 75: 273-79.

Leggett, S., V. Mooney, L. Matheson, B. Nelson, T. Dreisinger, J. Van Zytveld, and L. Vic. 1999. Restorative exercise for clinical low back pain: A prospective two-center study with 1-year follow-up. *Spine* 24: 889-98.

Malmivaara, A., U. Hakkinen, T. Aro, M.L. Heinrichs, L. Kosskenneimi, E. Kuosma et al. 1995. The treatment of acute low back pain: Bed-rest, exercises, or ordinary activity? *New England Journal of Medicine* 332: 351-55.

Mannion, A.F., M. Muntener, S. Taimela, and J. Dvorak. 1999. A randomized clinical trial of three active therapies for chronic low back pain. *Spine* 24: 2435-48.

Protas, E.J. 1999. Physical activity and low back pain. In *Pain 1999: An update review*, edited by M. Max, 145-52. Seattle, WA: IASP Press Seattle.

Protas, E.J. 1996. Aerobic exercise in the rehabilitation of individuals with chronic low back pain: A review. *Critical Reviews in Physical and Rehabilitation Medicine* 8: 283-95.

Quebec Task Force on Spinal Disorders. 1987. Scientific approach to the assessment and management of activity-related spinal disorders. A monograph for clinicians. *Spine* 12 (7 supplement): S1-59.

Simmonds, M.J. 2002. Exercise and activity for persons with non-specific back pain. In *ACSM's resources for clinical exercise physiology: Musculoskeletal, neuromuscular, neoplastic, immunologic, and hematologic conditions.* Edited by J.N. Myers, W.G. Herbert, and R. Humphrey, 125-38. 3rd ed. Philadelphia: Lippincott Williams & Wilkins.

Simmonds, M.J., and Claveau, Y. 1997. Psychometric characteristics and clinical usefulness of physical performance tests in patients with low back pain. *Spine* 23: 2412-21.

CHAPTER 34

Osteoporosis

Susan A. Bloomfield, PhD, FACSM
Texas A & M University

Susan S. Smith, PhD, FACSM
Texas Women's University

Overview of the Pathophysiology

Because of declining activity of bone-forming cells after age 35, all humans incur some minute loss of bone mass every year. This phenomenon has been observed in multiple races, geographical locations, and historical epochs. Dietary habits and physical activity patterns over the life span may alter the timing or rate of bone loss, but nearly all elderly men and women in industrialized countries have some degree of osteopenia, or lowered bone mass. This is of concern because bone strength and resistance to fracture, key functional attributes of bone, are determined in large part by bone mass. Bone status for most individuals over age 60 is somewhere on the continuum between benign age-related osteopenia and bone loss severe enough to make fracture imminent.

Textbooks and medical dictionaries show little difference in the meanings of *osteoporosis* and *osteopenia*, but their current use is a semantic issue. The World Health Organization (WHO) standards for defining osteopenia (bone mineral density [BMD] >1 standard deviation below young-normal values) and osteoporosis (BMD values >2.5 standard deviations below young-normal values) are now widely utilized by clinicians to establish these diagnoses. Current data estimate that over 18 million Americans have osteopenia; 10 million more have osteoporosis. Indeed, 1 in 2 women and 1 in 8 men now over age 50 will likely have an osteoporotic fracture in their lifetime. Women tend to start losing bone early in life and may experience a 3- to 5-year acceleration of bone loss after menopause because the effects of estrogen withdrawal are temporarily superimposed on age-related loss. This fact, in addition to a lower peak bone mass in young adulthood, largely explains the greater incidence of osteoporotic fractures in women as compared to men.

The presumed mechanism for so-called type I osteoporosis, often first diagnosed in women aged 50 to 75, is estrogen deficiency. This endocrine change at menopause results in increased activity of bone-resorbing cells and an acceleration of bone resorption, which exceeds bone formation rates. Men less frequently experience clinically significant bone loss before the age of 70, but various diseases, medications (e.g., chronic glucocorticoid therapy), or lifestyle factors (e.g., alcoholism) can produce early loss of bone mass and strength. Type II osteoporosis is thought to be related to vitamin D deficiency and secondary hyperparathyroidism, and is commonly diagnosed in individuals over 70 years of age. The severe bone loss observed in this group and the resulting high risk for hip fractures make it less likely that these individuals can safely engage in vigorous or high-impact exercise routines.

Most of the commonly cited risk factors for osteoporosis are related either to estrogen deficiency or the other exogenous factors affecting bone metabolism:

- female gender;
- advanced age;
- caucasian/Asian race;
- family history of osteoporosis;
- low body weight for height;
- premature menopause;
- prolonged premenopausal amenorrhea;
- low testosterone levels in men;
- lack of physical activity;
- chronic smoking;
- excessive alcohol consumption;
- low dietary calcium intake; and
- chronic use of medications causing bone loss (e.g., glucocorticoids, anticonvulsants).

Compression or wedge fractures of the vertebrae are common in older individuals with osteoporosis. Several may accumulate without obvious symptoms before they are detected, often as a chance finding with a chest X ray done for other purposes. A significant functional limitation imposed by multiple vertebral fractures is the severe kyphosis that can result. In extreme cases, this spinal deformity can impede normal ventilatory function by altering respiratory muscle function and decreasing vital capacity. It can also produce a forward shift in the center of gravity, increasing the risk of falls. About one-third of individuals with vertebral fractures experience significant back pain in the acute phase of recovery. If pain persists for a longer period, weakness of the back extensor muscles may be a causative factor.

Far more serious are hip fractures, which are actually fractures (most often) of the femoral neck. These fractures are ominous: About 25% of hip fracture patients over age 50 die in the first year after that fracture. Many others lose functional ambulatory ability and require nursing home care. The risk of hip fracture for an average American woman is equivalent to her combined risk of developing breast, uterine, and ovarian cancer. It should be noted that the loss of lean body mass over the decades with chronic inactivity may be a strong contributor to the development of osteoporosis; individuals with low muscle mass and strength are more likely to have lower bone mass.

Effects on the Exercise Response

The primary consideration relative to this clinical group is the degree of orthopedic limitation imposed by bony fractures, if they have occurred, or to coexisting conditions such as osteoarthritis. Some individuals will have limited locomotor abilities after hip fracture, which directly impacts their ability to perform exercise testing. The primary clinical goals for this group tend to be appropriate physical therapy to maximize mobility and prevent further falls. Exercise testing can proceed as usual for individuals with diagnosed vertebral fractures (once physician approval has been obtained) unless severe kyphosis is present. For those clients whose only complication thus far is severe osteopenia, exercise testing can proceed as usual, with careful attention to minimizing risk of falls during the test. In many cases, the fear of falling often leads to reduced physical activity in elderly populations, which exacerbates the risk of developing coronary artery disease (CAD). ECG monitoring for ischemic responses to exercise is advised during aerobic exercise tests in almost all persons with osteoporosis.

Effects of Exercise Training

There are two primary interactions of established osteoporosis with exercise training effects. First, many of these individuals are likely to be more unfit than the average population because of the decreased mobility common in persons with diagnosed osteoporosis, mandating a low-intensity program at the outset. Second, orthopedic limitations may slow progress or mandate the use of additional supports during walking. There is no evidence in the literature that osteoporosis, in and of itself, should alter the usual beneficial cardiovascular and skeletal muscle adaptations with chronic exercise. One exception might be the mechanical limitations imposed on respiratory muscle function in individuals with severe kyphosis. Whether regular participation in physical activity by itself can produce significant increases in bone mass in older adults appears doubtful.

There is no support for the concept that exercise can provide an effective alternative to hormone replacement therapy (HRT) in preventing bone loss in the early menopausal years. Better evidence suggests that regular exercise can significantly slow the age-related decline in bone mass and thereby delay the point at which osteopenia progresses to clinically significant osteoporosis. However, increasing bone mineral density and therefore bone strength is only part of the equation in reducing fragility fractures. What exercise training can provide that HRT or other medications cannot are improvements in muscle strength, posture, and balance, all of which have been shown to minimize risk of falling and therefore of fractures.

Management and Medications

Once osteoporosis has been diagnosed, with confirmation of low bone mineral density and fractures incurred with little or no trauma, the primary form of treatment is the use of medications to slow bone resorption or, more rarely, to increase bone formation. Should significant spinal deformities develop, bracing of the torso may be recommended to prevent worsening of the deformity, along with appropriate physical therapy to symptomatically treat back pain and improve back extensor and abdominal muscle strength. Independently, hip and knee extensor strength may be poor, requiring focused exercise/physical therapy regimens.

HRT is the most commonly prescribed of all medical regimens for bone loss in postmenopausal women. Common trade names are Premarin, Ogen, Estrace, Estraderm, Estratab, and Prempro, among others. Estrogens with or without progestogen components are prescribed in relatively low doses in an effort to replace the endogenous hormone levels lost at menopause or after surgical removal of the ovaries. It relieves menopausal symptoms (e.g., hot flashes) if present. Estrogen's benefits for bone health derive from its inhibitory effect on bone remodeling; HRT has been shown to increase bone mineral density and to reduce fracture risk, even if initiated after the age of 70. If engaging in exercise training while on

HRT, a postmenopausal woman is more likely to experience absolute gains in bone mass.

Other medications currently used to treat osteoporosis include the following:

• Raloxifene (trade name Evista) is a relatively new FDA-approved option, being one of the selective estrogen receptor modulators (SERMs) that produce small increases in bone mineral density with few to none of the undesirable side effects of HRT (e.g., uterine cancer). Risk of spine fractures can be significantly reduced. Like HRT, raloxifene produces positive changes in the lipid profile, lowering risk of CAD.

• Bisphosphonates inhibit bone resorption, resulting in absolute increases in bone mineral density and

reduced fracture risk. Side effects are uncommon and include nausea, irritation of the esophagus, and diarrhea. Alendronate (trade name Fosamax) and risedronate (trade name Actonel) are the two bisphosphonates currently approved for treatment of osteoporosis in men and women.

• Calcitonin (trade name Miacalcin) inhibits bone resorption at cancellous bone sites (e.g., spine); its effects on cortical bone are uncertain. It is usually prescribed for women at least five years past menopause and may have a unique analgesic effect in relieving pain associated with bone fractures. Because it is a peptide, calcitonin must be administered via subcutaneous injection or as a nasal spray.

• Sodium fluoride, vitamin D, and parathyroid hormone (PTH) all promote bone formation when given in

Osteoporosis: Exercise Testing

Methods	Measures	Endpoints*	Comments
Aerobic Cycle (ramp protocol 5-20 watts/min; staged protocol 25-50 watts/3-min stage) Treadmill (1-2 METs/stage)	• 12-lead ECG, HR	• Serious dysrhythmias • >2 mm ST-segment depression or elevation • Moderate to severe angina • T-wave inversion with significant ST change	• Most clients will be at a high risk for CAD.
	• BP	• SBP > 250 mmHg or DBP > 115 mmHg, or failure of SBP to rise	• Helpful to check for hyper- or hypotensive response.
	• RPE (6-20)		• Useful for clients who have difficulty with HR measurements.
	• METs	• Volitional fatigue	• Helpful in determining exercise intensity.
Strength Weight machines Free weights Handheld dynamometer	• 3-10 reps		• Helpful in determining resistance training intensity. • Decline in muscle strength is common in those with osteoporosis.
Neuromuscular Gait analysis Balance	• By observation or instrumentation • Timed or forced		• Especially useful for severely symptomatic clients.
Functional 6-m walk Tandem gait speed Sit to stand ADL/functional performance tests Posture	• Distance • Speed • Try to perform without use of arms • Flexicurve		• Sit-to-stand test provides good practical evaluation of strength. If arms are required to stand, it indicates weak hip/knee extensors. • Useful to document kyphotic curve.

*Measurements of particular significance; do not always indicate test termination.

Medications	Special Considerations
• HRT or Raloxifene, bisphosphonates, calcitonin, or flouride • Also see exercise testing table in chapter 24.	• Neuromuscular and functional capacity testing is best performed by skilled physical therapists familiar with standardized procedures. • Orthopedic: Extreme kyphosis in advanced cases alters center of gravity and can affect gait and balance. • Pulmonary: Severe kyphosis may result in increased fatigability due to impaired pulmonary function (e.g., decreased maximal ventilatory capacity). • Sensory: Severe kyphosis may make seeing the front of the treadmill difficult. • Muscular: Chronic back pain with multiple vertebral fractures is an issue in some individuals; may be muscular in origin due to extensive weakness of the back and hip extensors. • Psychological: Anxiety about falling during a treadmill test may be an impediment to testing and, therefore, the method of choice is a cycle ergometer.

appropriate doses and have been shown to increase bone mass in some cases, but these are not yet FDA approved. Fluoride therapy may promote the rapid formation of mechanically weak bone at some sites, which could account for the increased fracture incidence reported in some studies.

Recommendations for Exercise Testing

The usual exercise testing protocols employed with older individuals at risk for CAD are appropriate for people with diagnosed osteoporosis. If there are co-existing conditions (e.g., osteoarthritis with joint pain), testing must be modified to accommodate those additional limitations. For those clients with severe kyphosis, treadmill exercise is likely to be unsafe if forward vision is limited or if the neck is affected; a significant shift in the center of gravity may occur that could affect balance. Stationary cycle ergometry, if it does not compress the anterior aspect of the spine, provides a safer alternative.

Additional testing beyond the standard graded exercise test would be extremely beneficial for this population (see the Osteoporosis: Exercise Testing table). Assessment of muscle strength, to identify particularly weak muscle groups, would also assist in exercise prescription. Tests of neuromuscular function such as dynamic balance, assessed by a timed backward walk over 20 feet (6.1 m), are appropriate, as are functional tests such as time to rise from a chair without use of the arms. A qualitative

assessment of gait biomechanics may be appropriate in some cases.

Recommendations for Exercise Programming

Definitive training studies have yet to be done, but currently experts believe that a well-balanced exercise program focusing on both aerobic and strength training activities should be emphasized for the person with osteoporosis. The individual's physician, ideally in consultation with a physical therapist experienced with the limitations of persons with osteoporosis, needs to make the initial judgment about the safety of the proposed exercise program. There is little information in the literature about the safety of various forms of exercise for individuals with osteoporosis.

In general, aerobic weight-bearing activity (4 sessions/wk) and resistance training (2-3 sessions/wk) are recommended, with the more vigorous, impact-oriented activities reserved for those not yet classified as severely osteoporotic (see the Osteoporosis: Exercise Programming table on page 226). Specific exercises focusing on improving balance and modifying activities of daily living can also be helpful in individual cases. Improving muscle strength helps to conserve bone mass and improve dynamic balance. Best results are obtained when clients can progress to using relatively high intensities (> 75% of 10RM) and fewer repetitions. Adaptations in bone are site specific to the limbs used; any program should include exercise for upper

Osteoporosis: Exercise Programming

Modes	Goals	Intensity/ Frequency/Duration	Time to Goal
Aerobic • Large muscle activities (walking, cycling, swimming, water walking)	• Improve/maintain work capacity • Maintain bone mass	• 40-70% peak HR, METs • 3-5 days/wk • 20-30 min/session	• 2-6 mo • 9-12 mo to see effect on BMD
Strength • Dumbbell • Weight machines • Cuff weights • Floor calisthenics	• Improve strength of arms, shoulders, legs, and hips; emphasis on hip flexors/ extensors, back extensors, and lower abdominals • Improve posture; emphasis on postural muscle strength	• 75% of 1RM, 3-10 reps • 2 sets of 8-10 reps • 2-3 days/wk for 20-40 min	• ≥ 6 mo to reach maximum
Flexibility • Stretching • Chair exercises	• Increase/maintain ROM, especially in pectoral muscles	• 5-7 days/wk	
Functional • Activity-specific exercises • Brisk walk • Chair sit and stand	• Increase/maintain ADLs • Balance exercises • Decrease fall risk	• 3-5 days/wk • 2-3 days/wk	• 2-4 wk

Medications	Special Considerations
• Estrogen and bisphosphonates: Will affect exercise only if nausea or diarrhea is experienced; can interfere with motivation to exercise. • Calcitonin is commonly used if the client has bone pain.	• Aerobic power: All modes of exercise (e.g., walking, cycling, swimming) are possible as long as forward flexion and twisting is minimized. • Role of impact: Those classified as osteopenic should incorporate impact loading (e.g., jogging, heel drops, aerobics) into exercise. Clients with severe osteoporosis should avoid impact (see Overview of the Pathophysiology for definitions). • Time frame: Any long-term effect on conservation of bone mass will require ≥ 9-12 mo of effort before change (or lack thereof) can be ascertained. • Orthopedic: Clients with extreme kyphosis will be limited to stationary equipment or walking with support. Avoid flexion/ twisting of spine and stooping with forward flexion, which can increase incidence of vertebral fractures. Many clients will not be able to lie prone; standing or sitting exercise is easier. • Cardiac: Since most individuals with osteoporosis are > age 50, many have latent or overt CAD. Thus, staff must be alert to signs of myocardial ischemia (see chapters 4, 5, and 6). • Muscular: Many individuals with vertebral fractures are likely to have reduced strength of the back extensor muscles and must start with low work rates and progress slowly. • Psychological: Assure a safe exercise environment with minimal floor obstacles to reduce anxiety and the possibility of falling. Avoid unguarded exercises on unstable surfaces (e.g., trampolines, gymnastics balls).

and lower body and trunk muscles, particularly the extensors.

Floor calisthenics and some lifting activities need to be modified to avoid forward flexion and twisting of the spine, particularly in combination with stooping. Regular performance of flexion exercises increases the risk of causing new vertebral fractures in the person with established osteoporosis. If multiple vertebral fractures, severe osteopenia, or back pain limit an individual's participation in weight-bearing exercise, it is recommended that the client shift to swimming, walking in the water, water aerobics programs, or chair exercises. Although not as optimal for bone impact as strength training, these programs are likely to improve muscle strength and balance and contribute to a lowered risk of CAD.

Special Considerations

One special consideration that exercise professionals must be aware of in working with clients with osteoporosis relates to the justifiable anxiety many may have about falling. Careful attention must be paid to make the exercise environment free of hazards such as loose floor tiles or mats and exercise equipment strewn over the floor. Wall railings in exercise areas would be helpful for exercises done while standing. Close monitoring by staff, particularly if balance training is used (e.g., heel-to-toe walks, balancing on a single foot), should help prevent unintended injuries during exercise sessions.

CASE STUDY Osteoporosis

An 82-year-old woman presented with a 25-year history of back/hip pain. She complained that her pain had increased over the past 2 years, to a rating of 6/10, and said it was aggravated with standing or walking but eased with lying or sitting. She drove and performed most ADLs independently but had help with bathing and cooking. She lived in a 1-story house with steps to the garage, and walked independently at home but used a walker when out. She needed 2 pillows to lie prone or supine. She had been participating in water walking up to 3 times/wk until she had problems with the increasing pain.

She had many concerns, including her loss of mobility, lack of motivation, decreased activity, posture, weight control, falling, and loss in height. She stated her previous height was 5'7" (1.70 m). Her goals were to relieve pain and to improve activity level as well as her overall function, balance, posture, and bone health.

S: "I want to be able to do daily activities."

O: Vitals: Height: 5' 2.5" (1.58 m)   Weight: 154.9 lb (70.3 kg)   BMI: 24.3 kg/m^2

Elderly woman with thoracolumbar scoliosis and forward head posture

Past history:
  Fractures of left shoulder (10 yr earlier) and L1 (7 yr earlier) after falls
  Hypertension
  Congestive heart failure
  Diabetes
  Osteoarthritis
  Stress incontinence

DEXA: Hips - 2.8 SD below young-adult T-Score

Spinal postural curve measurements (Flexicurve):
  Thoracic: Width 6.2 cm (increased kyphosis); length 44.5 cm
  Lumbar: Width: 0 cm (decreased lordosis); length: 0 cm

Functional reach (standing; yardstick): 5.0 in (12.7 cm)

Muscle performance/strength (dynamometer):

	Left	Right	
Hip flexors	18.2	24.1	(N-m)
Hip extensors	17.3	17.8	(N-m)
Hip abductors	11.6	19.4	(N-m)
Knee extensors	38.6	30.4	(N-m)
Ankle dorsiflexors	1.5	2.5	(N-m)
Ankle plantar flexors	0	0	(reps)

(continued)

CASE STUDY Osteoporosis (continued)

Flexibility (goniometer):

	Left	Right	
Rectus femoris	91	94	(°)
Hamstrings	49	45	(°)
Gastrocnemius	5	4	(°)

Postural stability (force plate):

	Left	Right	
1-leg, eyes open	0	0	(s)

A:
1. Hip/back pain
2. Kyphotic posture
3. Decreased stability/balance
4. Decreased leg and trunk strength
5. Decreased flexibility
6. Difficulty with ADL
7. Loss of stature/height
8. General deconditioning

P:
1. Prescribe exercise (in center/home based).
2. Education sessions are necessary.

Exercise Program

Goals (1-yr outcomes at estimated 50% adherence rate):
1. Pain reduced to 3/10
2. Decreased thoracic curve width to 4.7 cm, increased lumbar curve width to 0.5 cm
3. Stability of 10 s in 1-leg stance
4. Trunk and leg strength to 65% age-norm referenced data
5. Flexibility to 70% normative values
6. Independent management of personal ADLs
7. Increase height by 1 in (2.5 cm)
8. Walking speed of 3.3 ft/s (1 m/s) without a walker
9. No falls

Mode	Frequency	Duration	Intensity	Progression
Aerobic (water walking)	1 day/wk	30 min	Self-selected	Increase to 2 days/wk 30 min
Strength (back laterals: standing hip flexion, abduction, extension; partial squats; and heel raises) (abdomen: 1-leg lowering, bent-over rows, and upright rows)	2 days/wk	10 min	5 reps/exercise using 1 lb (0.5 kg)	Increase to 2 days/wk, 15 min using 2 lb (0.9 kg), 10 reps/ exercise

Mode	Frequency	Duration	Intensity	Progression
Flexibility (hamstrings, pectorals, trunk flexors)	2 days/wk	2 min/muscle group	3 reps, hold for 10 s/stretch	Increase to 2 days/wk, 1 rep, holding 30 s/stretch Advance trunk flexors to lying prone on elbows 1 min, 2 days/wk
Neuromuscular (static stork stand)	2 days/wk	10 s/leg	5 tries/leg	Goal of 1 rep, 10 s/leg
Functional (walking without walker, showering)	Daily trials	Self-selected	Self-selected	Goal of walking without walker in safe areas
Warm-up/Cool-down (sitting arm circles)	Before each sesson	15 s	10 reps	Advance to standing arm circles, 20 reps in 30 s

Follow-Up

After 4 months (by her 10th visit), with moderate adherence, she reported increased mobility and the ability to shower independently. She had restarted her water-walking program, was able to lie prone and supine with only one pillow, and had had no falls. Her hip/back pain was rated 3 to 4/10, but episodes of pain were still a problem.

Suggested Readings

American College of Sports Medicine. 1995. ACSM's position stand on osteoporosis and exercise. *Medicine and Science in Sports and Exercise* 27 (4): i-vii.

Bloomfield, S.A. 1995. Bone, ligament, and tendon. In *Perspectives in exercise science and sports medicine, exercise in older adults,* edited by C.V. Gisolfi, E.R. Nadel, and D.R. Lamb, 175-227. Vol. 8. Carmel, IN: Cooper Publishing.

Bonnick, S.L. 2001. *The osteoporosis handbook.* 3rd ed. Dallas, TX: Taylor.

Dalsky, G.P. 1990. Effect of exercise on bone: Permissive influence of estrogen and calcium. *Medicine and Science in Sports and Exercise* 22 (3): 281-85.

Kanis, J.A., L.J. Melton III, C. Christiansen, C.C. Johnston, and N. Khaltaev. 1994. Perspective: The diagnosis of osteoporosis. *Journal of Bone Mineral Research.* 9: 1137-41.

Kelley, G.A. 1998. Aerobic exercise and bone density at the hip in postmenopausal women: A meta-analysis. *Preventive Medicine* 27: 798-807.

Layne, J.E., and M.E. Nelson. 1999. The effects of progressive resistance training on bone density: A review. *Medicine and Science in Sports and Exercise* 31(1): 25-30.

McClung, M.R. 1994. Nonpharmacologic management of osteoporosis. In *Osteoporosis,* edited by R. Marcus, 336-53. Boston: Blackwell Scientific.

National Institutes of Health, Osteoporosis and Related Bone Diseases National Resource Center. Web site: **www.osteo.org**.

National Osteoporosis Foundation. Web site: **www.nof.org**.

Nichols, D.L., M. Horea, and L. Trudelle-Jackson. 2002. Osteoporosis. In *ACSM's resources for clinical exercise physiology: Musculoskeletal, neuromuscular, neoplastic, immunologic, and hematologic conditions.* Edited by J.N. Myers, W.G. Herbert, and R. Humphrey. 3-15. Philadelphia: Lippincott Williams & Wilkins.

CHAPTER 35

Lower-Limb Amputation

Kenneth H. Pitetti, PhD, FACSM
Wichita State University

Mark H. Pedrotty, PhD
Carrie Tingley Hospital

Overview of the Pathophysiology

The main causes of lower-limb (LL) amputation are:

- vascular and circulatory diseases caused by either type 2 diabetes or peripheral vascular disease, 70%;

- trauma (e.g., traumatic amputation; massively crushed limbs; massive fractures causing ischemia and irreparable vasculature; thermal, chemical, and electrical burns; and frostbite), 23%;

- curative treatment of tumors (e.g., a malignant osteogenic sarcoma that has not yet metastasized), 4%; and

- congenital deformities (i.e., a prosthetic limb replaces the amputated deformed limb to allow for improved ambulation), 3%.

The majority of individuals requiring LL amputation are older than 55 years of age, and their amputations result primarily from neuropathies and peripheral vascular disease secondary to either type 2 diabetes or atherosclerosis. These amputees are classified in this chapter as vascular amputees. Individuals with LL amputation from trauma, tumors, or congenital deformities are usually below the age of 50 (e.g., children, adolescents, and young adults), classified in this chapter as nonvascular amputees.

It is important to determine the specific classification for an LL amputee because the purpose of exercise differs between these classifications. The main purpose of exercise management for vascular amputees is to preclude or abate the pathogenesis of diabetes and/or atherosclerosis. On the other hand, exercise management for nonvascular LL amputees is similar to that for non-disabled persons. That is, it focuses on risk reduction for developing secondary disabilities such as cardiovascular disease, diabetes, high blood pressure, and obesity. In fact, LL amputees have a higher risk for developing secondary cardiovascular-related disabilities than non-disabled individuals because of the LL amputee's predisposition of living a sedentary lifestyle.

Classification of LL amputees:

- Symes (amputation of the forefoot or midfoot, usually leaving the heel bones intact and, therefore, allows full weight bearing onto the heel of the foot)

- Transtibial (below-knee amputation)

- Transfemoral (above-knee amputation)

- Hip disarticulation (removal of the leg at the femoral hip joint)

- Unilateral amputation (involves only one leg, as in a unilateral below-knee or unilateral above-knee)

- Bilateral amputation (involves both legs, as in one leg amputated below the knee and the other above the knee)

Effects on the Exercise Response

The appropriate exercise modality for nonvascular unilateral above- or below-knee, unilateral hip disarticulation, bilateral below-knee (both legs are amputated below the knee), or bilateral above- and below-knee (one leg amputated above the knee, the other below the knee) should incorporate a sufficient amount of muscle mass (e.g., for aerobic and anaerobic testing) to elicit exercise responses similar to non-disabled individuals. However, for bilateral above-knee (both legs amputated above the knee), or bilateral hip disarticulation, individual responses will be limited by the muscle mass and work capacity of their upper body musculature (e.g., arms, shoulders, chest, and trunk), similar to persons with paraplegia lesions below L-1. The same precepts hold true for vascular amputees but are further complicated by their medications and the extent of their primary disease (e.g., type 2 diabetes).

Effects on Exercise Training

The effect of exercise training is dependent on the modality used and amount of musculature involved for LL amputees. For instance, a unilateral below-knee, above-knee, or hip disarticulation amputee will involve enough muscle mass exercising on a sitting arm-leg ergometer (e.g., Schwinn Air-Dyne™ ergometer) to improve cardiovascular fitness in a magnitude similar to a non-disabled person on that same modality. However, a bilateral above-knee amputee, limited to modalities such as arm ergometry or swimming, which incorporates a smaller muscle mass, will elicit cardiovascular improvements but of a smaller magnitude obtained by the unilateral amputee exercising on an arm-leg ergometer.

In addition, the modalities of walking or jogging are not viable or feasible long-term exercise regimens for many LL amputees for the following reasons:

• Energy expenditure (i.e., physical effort) of walking is higher for LL amputees compared to non-disabled individuals and is directly related to the level of amputation (i.e., energy cost for a unilateral above-knee amputee is greater than for a unilateral below-knee amputee).

• The potential painful consequences of skin breakdowns or infections can further exacerbate a disability, acutely limiting all exercise, recreational activities, work-related activities, or activities of daily living.

• Any additional trauma and painful consequences to the amputated limb(s) as well as noninvolved limb (e.g., overuse injuries) will impair the ability to walk or jog.

The combination of additional energy expenditure, the painful consequences of skin breakdown or infections, and the high risk of overuse injuries precludes walking or jogging as a physical activity pattern that can be maintained or easily integrated into the daily activities of most LL amputees.

Management and Medications

A large majority of LL amputations are the direct result of peripheral vascular disease and diabetes (see chapters 13 and 21), which require specific medications. The type of medications specific to these conditions and their exercise effects is covered in other chapters within this book.

Most amputees experience the so-called phantom pain phenomenon (i.e., pain that seems to come from the amputated body part). Phantom pain can range from mild to severe. When severe in nature, relief is often obtained

Lower-Limb Amputation: Exercise Testing

Methods	Measures	Endpoints	Comments
Aerobic Submaximal Maximal (for athletes)	• HR • BP • Work rate • RPE (6-20)	• RPE 16/20 • Volitional exhaustion (athletes)	• Use measure to prescribe exercise intensity.
Strength Weight machines	• 1RM		• Use 1RM to prescribe exercise intensity (e.g., 60% 1RM).
Flexibility Goniometer	• Abduction, adduction, flexion, extension of available ankle, knee, hip joints		• Over time, loss of flexibility suggests reassessing stretching program.
Functional 100- to 600-yd (91.4- to 548.6-m) walk	• Time (in s) • Number of steps		• Walk at a "comfortable" walking speed; should not be a race.

(continued)

Lower-Limb Amputation: Exercise Testing *(continued)*

Medications	Special Considerations
• See chapters 13 and 21.	Aerobic testing using arm-leg ergometer • Vascular amputees or nonvascular amputees >40 yr should begin at 25 watts for 2 min, with incremental increases of 12.5 or 25 watts every 2 min until endpoint is reached. • Nonvascular amputees < 40 yr should begin at 50 watts, with incremental increases of 25-50 watts every 2 min until endpoint is reached. • Nonvascular athletic amputees (i.e., Paralympics) should begin at 50 watts, with incremental increases of 50 watts every 2 min. • For all tests, HR should be monitored and recorded every min, BP taken after the 1st min of each work level, and RPE recorded at the end of the 2nd min of each work level. Aerobic testing using arm crank ergometer • Sedentary amputees or amputees > 40 yr should begin at 5 watts for 2 min at a constant cadence of 50 rpm, with incremental increases of 5 watts every 2 min until endpoint is reached. • Active or exercising amputees or amputees < 40 yr should begin at 5 watts for 2 min, with incremental increases of 10-20 watts every 2 min until endpoint is reached. • An intermittent protocol should be used for all tests using arm crank ergometer, with 1-min rest periods between each intermittent increase in order to (1) allow for clear ECG tracings if electrocardiographic responses are being followed; (2) allow time for accurate BP measurement; and (3) avoid early fatigue. Strength assessment • For safety purposes, prior to starting 1RM tests, (1) amputees should perform an initial warm-up (i.e., 5 min on an arm-leg ergometer or arm ergometer at low intensities followed by stretching); (2) sufficient practice time should be allowed before actual weight is selected (i.e., performing the weight lifting movement at low to moderate work rates). • Because of advanced age and/or poor health and physical condition, rest periods of 5-10 min between 1RM tests may be appropriate; or the battery of 1RM tests may need to be spread over 2-3 days to prevent muscle discomfort or muscle soreness from affecting the motivation of the LL amputee.

from drugs that are also given to counteract epilepsy or depression and are thought to have little or no exercise effect. Some amputees find that their phantom pain is eased by a combination of antidepressants and narcotics (e.g., methadone). Antidepressants can cause drowsiness. Amputees using narcotics for their phantom pain should consult their physician before continuing an exercise program.

Recommendations for Exercise Testing

In the aerobic and anaerobic methods of exercise testing, unilateral above- or below-knee amputees, bilateral below-knee amputees, and bilateral amputees having one below-knee and one above-knee amputation should use an arm-leg

Lower-Limb Amputation: Exercise Programming

Modes	Goals	Intensity/ Frequency/Duration	Time to Goal
Aerobic • Ergometers: Sitting arm-leg Arm Rowing Cycle Standing arm/leg • Swimming	• Increase cardiovascular fitness and endurance of uninvolved and involved limbs • Increase efficiency of ADLs and ambulation	• RPE 11-15/20 • 3-5 days/wk • 30-60 min/session	• Duration should be 10-20 min initially, with a goal of 30-60 min
Strength • Weight machines	• Increase strength of trunk, hip, and involved and uninvolved leg • Increase efficiency of ADLs and ambulation	• 1-2 sets @ 60-80% 1RM or a weight that allows for 8 reps • 2-3 days/wk • Perform ≥ 5 separate exercises/ session	• Initial weight used until 12 reps can be performed, then increase weight 5-10 lb (2.3-4.5 kg) and return to 8 reps • Do not lift 2 days in a row • 2 upper body, 1 trunk, and 2 lower body exercises/ session
Flexibility • Stretching (target trunk, hip, and available lower limb joints)	• Maintain ROM		

Medications	Special Considerations
• See chapters 13 and 21.	• See exercise testing table.

ergometer such as the Schwinn Air-Dyne™ or SciFit™ Pro II Power Trainer™. LL amputees who are unable to involve their lower extremities when using an arm-leg ergometer (e.g., bilateral above-knee amputees) should be tested with either an arm crank ergometer (e.g., Monark Rehab Trainer™ Model 881), Cybex upper body ergometer (UBE), or the arm mechanism of an arm-leg ergometer.

For safety purposes, weight machines rather than free weights should be used in testing for muscle strength and endurance. Trunk (e.g., sit-ups, back extension) and upper body strength (e.g., sitting military press, bench press, biceps curl) tests can be performed using the same protocols as non-disabled individuals. Lower body strength and endurance testing should involve both the noninvolved limb (if unilateral) and the muscles of the amputated leg.

For instance, an above-knee amputee may not be able to perform knee extension and flexion with the amputated limb but could perform hip extension and flexion. Appraising flexibility, especially the joints of the lower extremities (e.g., hip, knee) of both involved and noninvolved legs, is also recommended (see the Lower-Limb Amputation: Exercise Testing table on page 231).

The most important functional evaluation for LL amputees is walking capacity (i.e., time to walk a certain distance) because it has been established that exercise programs improve the walking efficiency of LL amputees. The distance of the walk test will depend on the level of amputation and the physical condition of the individual. For instance, a physically fit unilateral above- or below-knee amputee should be tested in distances of 500 to 600 yards (457.2 to 548.6 m), whereas distances of 100 to 200 yards (91.4 to 182.9 m) would be appropriate for deconditioned unilateral and bilateral amputees or amputees with a hip disarticulation. Walking tests should be performed on gymnasium floors, indoor tracks, tennis courts, or any smooth, level surface.

Recommendations for Exercise Programming

For aerobic exercise, LL amputees should use a mode of exercise that (1) incorporates enough muscle mass to produce improvements in cardiovascular fitness, and (2) will not cause overuse injuries, skin breakdowns, and joint pain/inflammation to the non-amputated or amputated limbs. Based on the level of amputation, the following modalities are recommended (see the Lower-Limb Amputation: Exercise Programming table on page 233):

- Sitting arm-leg ergometer (e.g., Schwinn Air-Dyne™), arm ergometer, swimming, and rowing ergometer for all amputees

- Cycle ergometer, reclined or sitting, for all amputees except bilateral below-knee (may not incorporate sufficient muscle mass) and bilateral above-knee (will most likely be unable to perform) amputees

- Standing arm-leg ergometers (e.g., Reebok Body Trec™) for unilateral below-knee amputees, although unilateral above-knee and bilateral below-knee amputees may be capable of performing

Strength and stretching regimens as well as exercise progression (i.e., frequency, duration, and intensity) would follow the same guidelines as non-disabled individuals or individuals with only type 2 diabetes or cardiovascular disease.

CASE STUDY   Lower Extremity Amputation

A 14-year-old female had her left leg amputated (Symes amputation), because of a congenital deformity (5-in [12.7-cm] discrepancy between her lower left and right leg), at the age of four. She also had congenital short femurs, hip dysplasia, and proximal femur focus deficiency, and had undergone an osteotomy of the right hip at age 8. She was referred for a multidisciplinary weight-loss program involving diet, exercise, and psychiatric evaluation and counseling. She expressed a desire to lose weight and be involved in an activity program that would help her ambulate on her prosthetic leg (she was restricted to a wheelchair). She also wanted to discuss the circumstances and her feelings about her amputation. Her parents agreed to participate.

S: "I wish I could get around like everyone else."

O: Vitals: Height: 5'1" (1.55 m)   Weight: 235 lb (106.6 kg)   BMI: 44.4 kg/m²

Morbidly obese young woman, flat affect, in wheelchair

Left leg amputation below the knee

Psychological evaluation: Axis I (major depression)

Poor ambulation; hip in the involved side unable to support weight for more than a few steps

A: 1. Left leg amputation below the knee

2. Major depression

3. Morbid obesity

P: 1. Orthopedic evaluation (prosthetic/surgical modification) is necessary.

2. Medically manage weight loss and depression.

3. Individual psychotherapy (cognitive behavioral therapy/increase self-esteem) is needed.

4. Group counseling on the family culture that produced her situation would be helpful.

5. Prescribe a weight-loss diet (1500 kcal/day).

6. Formulate an exercise program.

Exercise Program

Goals:

1. Ambulation without crutches

2. 25 lb (11 kg) weight loss

3. Improved ADLs

Mode	Frequency	Duration	Intensity	Progression
Aerobic	3 days/wk	10-20 min	RPE 12/20	Increase to 30-60 min as tolerated
Strength (upper and lower body)	3 days/wk	1 set of 8-12 reps	Versus gravity	Increase to 2 sets Full recovery between sets
Flexibility (upper and lower body)	3 days/wk	20-60 s/stretch	Maintain stretch below discomfort point	
Neuromuscular				
Functional				
Warm-up/Cool-down	3 days/wk	5 min on arm-leg ergometer	As tolerated/low	

Follow-Up

By 6 months, she had lost 17.5 lb (7.9 kg). Psychotherapy was slowly progressing with her many issues. She was ready to focus medically on lifestyle changes specific to exercise and diet. She had begun ambulating at school without crutches, using the crutches only as a backup for muscle/stump fatigue. She participating in an adapted physical education program focused on improving walking capacity.

Suggested Readings

Lockette, K.F., and A.M. Keyes. 2000. *Conditioning with physical disabilities*. Champaign, IL: Human Kinetics.

Pitetti, K.H., and R.C. Manske. (in print). Lower limb amputation. In *Clinical exercise physiology: Application and physiological principles*, edited by L. LaMura and S. von Duvillard. Baltimore: Lippincott Williams & Wilkins.

Pitetti, K.H., and R.C. Manske. (2002). Amputation. In *ACSM's resources for clinical exercise physiology: Musculoskeletal, neuromuscular, neoplastic, immunologic, and hematologic conditions*. Edited by J.N. Myers, W.G. Herbert, and R. Humphrey. 170-178. Philadelphia: Lippincott Williams & Wilkins.

Pitetti, K.H., P.G. Snell, J. Stray-Gunderson, and F.A. Gottschalk. 1987. Aerobic training exercise for individuals who had amputation of the lower limb. *Journal of Bone Joint Surgery* 69A: 914-21.

SECTION VII

Neuromuscular Disorders

Stephen F. Figoni, PhD, RKT, FACSM

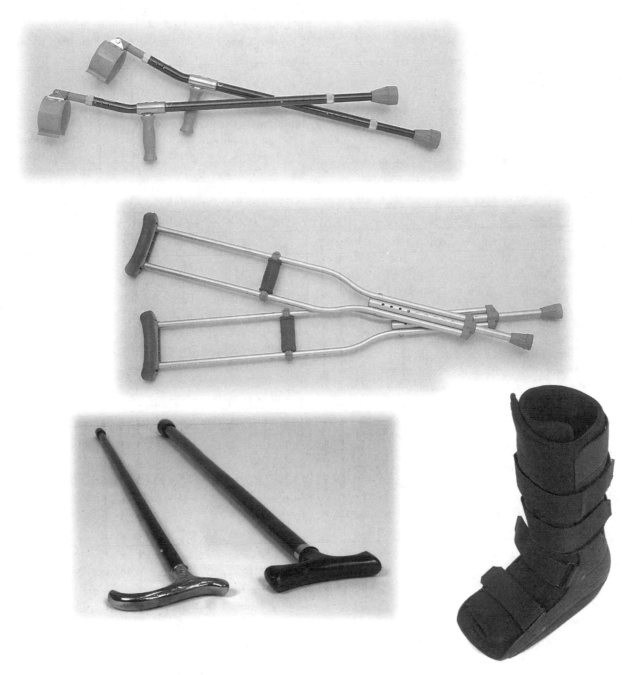

CHAPTER 36

Stroke and Brain Injury

Karen Palmer-McLean, PhD, PT
University of Wisconsin-La Crosse

Kimberly B. Harbst, PhD, PT
University of Wisconsin-La Crosse

Overview of the Pathophysiology

A cerebrovascular accident (CVA), a stroke or brain attack, occurs secondary to vascular insufficiency in the brain. Common causes include thrombosis, embolism, or hemorrhage secondary to aneurysm. Cell death follows and results in an impairment of central nervous system function. Recent studies estimate that each year 750,000 individuals in the United States experience a CVA with approximately a 66% survival rate. The majority of strokes affect the elderly, mostly in their 60s, 70s, and 80s, although 20% of strokes occur in individuals younger than 65. Of those who have a stroke, approximately 30% have a history of previous stroke.

In North America, the following factors put one at risk of developing a CVA: systolic and diastolic hypertension, diabetes mellitus, cigarette smoking, alcoholism, and coronary artery disease. Other factors may also increase the risk of stroke, but their roles are less well defined, including obesity, platelet hyperaggregability, and elevated blood lipid levels.

The resulting neurological impairment depends on both the size and the location of the ischemic area, as well as the availability of collateral blood flow. Following a CVA, persons may present with the following:

- impairment of motor and sensory function in the upper or lower extremity, or in both extremities, on the involved side;
- visual field deficits;
- expressive and receptive aphasia (impaired ability to communicate through speech);
- mental confusion; and
- apraxia (impaired sequencing of voluntary movements).

Traumatic brain injuries (TBI) occur at the rate of approximately 1.5 million new cases/yr in the United States, with about 85,000 of these individuals experiencing long-term disability. The typical age of TBI onset is bimodal with peaks at the 15 to 24 and 75+ age groups. Injuries sustained in the 75+ age group are most often a consequence of a fall and are associated with a high mortality rate. Motor vehicle accidents are the most frequent cause of TBI within the 15 to 24 year age group.

Traumatic brain injury can result in both primary and secondary insults. Primary insults comprise the structural brain injury that occurs at the time of injury, while secondary insults include events such as edema, ischemia, and metabolic derangements that may be superimposed on the initial trauma. These secondary insults may increase the extent of permanent brain damage. In contrast to the brain damage associated with CVA, which tends to be fairly localized, TBI often results in diffuse injury to the brain and impairments throughout the body.

Physical disabilities are prominent after moderate to severe brain injuries. However, the primary factors limiting a person's return to independence following any brain injury, even those classified as mild, are behavioral and cognitive disturbances. Agitation, confusion, impulsiveness, inattention, memory disturbances, apathy, and learning deficits may all occur as acute or long-term deficits following brain injury.

Effects on the Exercise Response

The ability to exercise depends on the severity of neurological involvement and existing co-morbidities. The following are some examples of potential effects of neurological deficits on exercise.

- Muscle weakness, limited range of motion, and impaired sensation may preclude independent ambulation or ability to exercise in the standing position.
- Lack of adequate balance may interfere with the ability to perform sitting arm crank or leg cycle ergometry.
- Weakness and/or limited range of motion of the arm or leg may also interfere with a person's ability to maintain crank rates during ergometry.

- Receptive aphasia, mental confusion, and/or apraxia may interfere with the ability to understand and follow directions during exercise testing or training sessions.

Cognitive and behavioral sequelae may influence compliance with and retention in an exercise program. Involvement of the frontal lobe can result in lack of initiation, apathy, easy frustration, loss of inhibition, and impaired cognitive and executive functions. Lesions in the temporal lobe may cause difficulties with new learning, memory deficits, and possible outbursts of aggression. Involvement of the areas of the brain mediating perception and arousal may lead to difficulty screening out irrelevant sensory input in the environment and focusing on important cues.

Since the majority of strokes occur in elderly individuals, participation in aerobic exercise may be further complicated by the arthritic, orthopedic, and cardiovascular problems common in elderly populations. While most individuals with brain injuries are young, their general physical capacities and endurance may be severely limited secondary to orthopedic and other injuries incurred at the time of the accident. Seizures are another co-morbidity associated with brain injury that may pose a safety concern during exercise.

Lack of motor function may interfere with exercise performance. In previous studies, only 20 to 34% of individuals with stroke were able to achieve 85% of age-predicted maximal heart rate. Because of the physical impairments associated with TBI, clients with this diagnosis typically exhibit aerobic capacities 67 to 74% below predicted levels based on height and age. These clients will also have much higher submaximal heart rates during cycle ergometry relative to age-matched controls without physical impairments.

Effects of Exercise Training

Exercise training may have differential impact on people who have experienced a stroke and those who have sustained a brain injury. Most individuals with a recent history of CVA are very deconditioned, exhibiting a peak oxygen consumption ($\dot{V}O_2$peak) that is about half that achieved by age-matched individuals without CVA. This deconditioned state leaves tremendous room for improvement. If a person with CVA recovers enough motor function to take part in a leg cycle exercise program, the few aerobic training studies that have included persons with stroke suggest that 60% increases in $\dot{V}O_2$peak might be expected. Endurance training not only has the potential to increase aerobic capacity but may also:

- increase self-selected walking speed;

- decrease reliance on assistive devices during ambulation; and
- increase functional mobility scores.

Clients who sustain a brain injury will also have very low oxidative capacities and fatigue at a rate 2.6 times faster than their unimpaired counterparts. Exercise training programs can significantly improve $\dot{V}O_2$peak, endurance, and muscle strength. As a result, clients can become more independent in their daily activities, more efficient in their locomotion, and more employable. In addition, clients post-TBI who exercise are typically less depressed and report fewer cognitive symptoms relative to individuals who do not exercise after a TBI.

Management and Medications

Medical management for people after CVA depends on the type of stroke, the degree of neurologic deficit, and the condition of the individual. Medical treatment for persons who have experienced CVA may include the following:

- short-term use of anticoagulants and long-term use of platelet-inhibiting agents;
- vasodilators if vasospasm of the cerebral arteries is suspected; and
- antihypertensive medication for those with hemorrhagic stroke requiring strict control of blood pressure.

It is unusual for persons with a brain injury to require intensive medical management after the acute treatment of their injury. Many, however, may have a tendency toward seizures and may require long-term anticonvulsant medication. Posttraumatic epilepsy may be addressed prophylactically with medications such as phenytoin or phenobarbital. However, clients may experience cognitive slowing as a side effect of these drugs. The balance between adequate seizure control and adequate arousal for function is often very sensitive and difficult to achieve. Carbamazepine is an alternative drug that may be used with fewer cognitive side effects. These medications may be withdrawn after one or more seizure-free years.

Hypertonia may significantly impair movement in individuals experiencing either a CVA or TBI. Oral medications (e.g., baclofen, diazepam, tizanidine) may reduce hypertonia but may produce intolerable side effects, including diminished arousal and cognitive capabilities. An alternative to oral medications includes implantation of an intrathecal pump to deliver baclofen directly into the spinal canal or a variety of injections that block local motor activity. The use of some medications may affect acute physiologic response during graded exercise tests.

- Individuals on vasodilators will require a longer cool-down period after a single session of exercise to prevent postexercise hypotension.

Stroke and Brain Injury: Exercise Testing

Methods	Measures	Endpoints*	Comments
Aerobic Cycle ergometer (5-10 watts/min using ramp protocol or 20 watts/stage) Treadmill (0.5-2 METs/stage) Combination arm/leg ergometer Seated stepper Arm ergometer	• 12-lead ECG, HR • BP, rate pressure product • RPE • $\dot{V}O_2$peak	• Serious dysrhythmias • >2mm ST-segment depression • T-wave inversion with significant ST change • SBP > 250 mmHg or DBP > 115 mmHg • Ischemic threshold • Volitional fatigue	• CAD is a major risk factor for CVA. • Hypertension is a major risk factor for CVA. • Useful in prescribing exercise intensity. • Necessary only if conducting research.
Endurance 6- or 12-min walk Leg cycle ergometer (or combination arm/leg ergometer)	• Distance walked • Time of exercise at 60% peak power	• Note time, distance, symptoms at rest stops	• Use with ambulatory clients (with/without assistive devices). • Use with clients who cannot ambulate long distances.
Strength Manual muscle test with/without handheld dynamometer Computerized dynamometer (e.g., isotonic, isokinetic, isometric)	• Force generated on dynamometer • Peak torque normalized to body weight • Total work normalized to body weight	• lb, kg, number of repetitions • Max torque	• Valid only if client can isolate movement.
Flexibility Handheld goniometer	• ROM in shoulder, elbow, wrist, knee, ankle, and other joints of affected limbs	• Degrees of full flexion/extension • Total arc	
Neuromuscular Gait analysis Berg balance Functional reach Tinetti (Performance-Oriented Mobility Assessment)	• Gait speed • Symmetry of movement		• Useful in assessing safety and efficiency of movement.
Functional Duke mobility Functional independence measure (FIM) Individualized criterion-referenced tests			• Useful in overall progress in ADLs.

*Measurements of particular significance; do not always indicate test termination.

Medications	Special Considerations
• A large percentage of clients who have had a CVA are on hypertension and cardiovascular medications. See appendixes A, B, and C. • Anticonvulsants: Usually indicated for seizure-prone clients. • Clients with hypertonia may use medications to reduce muscle tone.	• Arthritis, particularly osteoarthritis, of shoulder, hip, and knee is common in clients with CVA. • Reduced motor control of limb may necessitate using only the uninvolved limb in arm, leg, or arm/leg ergometry. • Exercise device may need to be modified (e.g., using hand mitts on arm ergometer, adding toe clips to bicycle ergometer). • Clients who have had a CVA are also at risk for CAD, so close monitoring of ECG is essential. • Sensation may be impaired, so careful observation is necessary to prevent injury. • Clients who have had a CVA may also have peripheral arterial disease, which may impair their ability to ambulate or cycle.

- Lower peak heart rates will be achieved by persons receiving medication that limits cardiac output by reducing heart rate.
- Use of diuretics to reduce fluid volume may alter electrolyte balance, causing dysrhythmias.

Recommendations for Exercise Testing

Because most strokes occur secondary to atherosclerotic lesions, many persons who experience CVA either have coexisting coronary artery disease or are at risk for developing coronary artery disease. Thus, exercise tests of clients with stroke should be supervised by a physician and clients should be monitored with a 12-lead ECG. The mode of exercise testing depends on the severity of neurological involvement (see the Stroke and Brain Injury: Exercise Testing table).

Exercise testing in individuals with focal neurologic deficits can be more challenging than in able-bodied persons. For this reason, extra emphasis will be given to instructions on specific test methods.

Leg Cycle Ergometry

A standard leg cycle ergometer could be used if the individual can safely maintain sitting balance on the cycle. The affected lower extremity may have to be secured on the pedal with straps if the person is unable to keep it secure independently. Test protocols may have to be individually determined on the basis of the person's strength. A pedaling rate of 50 rpm and a starting power output of 20 watts, with 20-watt increments per stage, are suggested as general guidelines.

Treadmill

Treadmill testing may be appropriate in individuals with minimal motor impairment who have good standing balance and are able to ambulate independently without the use of an assistive device such as a cane or walker. Many individuals with minimal physical impairment can complete progressive exercise tests using a treadmill protocol, such as the Balke. Treadmills should be equipped with a "zero start" feature to avoid an abrupt change in speed that might result in a fall. Individuals with sensorimotor impairments that result in weakness, loss of movement, or balance deficits may be unsafe on a treadmill. Treadmill testing could still be conducted using a partial body weight support harness system. In cases of severe weakness, the harness could be used to partially support some body weight during treadmill testing. For other individuals, the harness system could be used simply as a safety measure to prevent a fall in the event of a missed step or a loss of balance.

Preferred walking speeds will be much slower, and energy expenditure at a specific work rate will be about 55 to 64% greater than in the individual without a stroke. Exercise protocols with a very gradual increase in exercise intensity, such as the Naughton-Balke or modified Balke, should be used. The treadmill speed in these protocols may have to be decreased to accommodate the slower walking speeds in this population.

Combined Arm and Leg Ergometry

If spasticity or muscle weakness in the affected extremity interferes with the ability to maintain pedal cadence during leg-cycle testing, the subject should use only the unaffected lower extremity. However, it is very difficult to achieve a work rate that can stress the heart when using only one extremity. In such cases, a combination arm/leg ergometer, such as the Schwinn Air-Dyne™, is particularly useful. Subjects can use just the unaffected upper and lower extremity or can assist with the affected upper and/or lower extremity if spasticity or weakness does not interfere with cadence. Because of muscle fatigue of the upper extremities, an intermittent protocol is suggested.

The exercise physiologist should consider the client's motor abilities when selecting an appropriate exercise device. For example, impaired sitting balance may preclude the use of some particular upright ergometers that do not include a backrest. Therefore, a recumbent device may be more appropriate. In addition, seatbelts and/or chest straps could be used for additional trunk stability. Some ergometers may need to be further adapted to allow the individual with motor impairment to use them effectively. A strap or a mitt may be used to secure the hand of an individual who has difficulty using the handgrip on an arm ergometer or a combination arm/leg ergometer. Similarly, the individual who cannot maintain the foot on the pedal of a cycle ergometer may need the foot secured with a strap or wrap. Many products are commercially available to customize the exercise devices to the client's unique needs. Clients should be closely supervised if a strap is used to secure an extremity on a handle or pedal because the individual will be unable to stop a fall by extending the arm or leg. Finally, a step stool may be required for an individual to get on and off a cycle ergometer. The client should step up onto the stool with the unaffected leg and step down with the affected leg.

Seated Steppers

Another commercially available exercise mode that combines both arm and leg exercise is the seated stepper (Nu-Step™) with reciprocating levers that allow arm exercise. Some of these types of devices include a seat with back support and the option of a seatbelt that would provide additional trunk stability for the client with poor sitting balance. For the client with significant mobility impairment, the seat can swivel and has flip-up armrests, facilitating transfer onto the device. In contrast to most of the other arm and combination arm/leg ergometers where the client grasps the device in a pronated position, these types of devices allow the client to grip the handle in a position midway between pronation and supination. This neutral position is usually easier for clients with limited range of motion and encourages a more upright trunk position. Finally, as opposed to the traditional bike pedal found on most leg ergometers, the foot plate on this device supports the entire sole of the foot and has raised lateral and posterior borders to maintain the heel in the proper position. Foot straps are optional.

Muscle Strength Tests

Muscle strength can be measured using a variety of computerized dynamometers (e.g., Cybex™, Biodex™). A handheld dynamometer can also be used to measure the amount of resistance that can be applied as the individual attempts to maintain a manual muscle testing position. It should be noted that strength testing can be problematic in a population with brain injury. Strength can only be reliably tested when an individual can isolate joint movement.

Flexibility Tests

Flexibility is a particularly important component of fitness that should be tested in both the post-CVA and post-TBI populations. As noted earlier, 80% of stroke patients will be in their 60s, 70s, and 80s, a time when arthritic complaints are much more common. Following TBI, an individual is more likely to demonstrate limited joint range of motion caused by the multiple joint trauma that may have accompanied the TBI, reduced mobility during the acute phase of recovery, and the increased risk of heterotopic ossification in this population. Brain injury that results in muscle weakness or hypertonia also has the potential to limit joint range. Joint range of motion can be measured with a handheld goniometer.

Recommendations for Exercise Programming

As indicated earlier, hypertension is one of the primary risk factors for stroke. Exercise training programs for individuals with stroke should be aimed not only at increasing the level of physical fitness but also at reducing risk factors such as hypertension. Theoretically, a reduction of risk factors should decrease the incidence of secondary strokes. An aerobic conditioning program can alter several of the risk factors associated with the incidence of CVA, including reduced hypertension, enhanced glucose regulation, improved blood lipid profile, and reduced body fat. Depression and apathy are also common and might interfere with long-term adherence to an endurance training program (see the Stroke and Brain Injury: Exercise Programming table).

Clients who survive traumatic brain injury are at risk for sustaining permanent cognitive and behavioral sequelae that might interfere with their ability to follow directions for exercise testing and training. Cognitive deficits might include memory loss and decreased rate of information processing, while behavioral problems might include loss of impulse control, increased agitation, and mood lability. It should be noted that many of these deficits can be addressed using cognitive retraining, behavioral management, and medication.

Stroke and Brain Injury: Exercise Programming

Modes	Goals	Intensity/Frequency/Duration	Time to Goal
Aerobic • Upper and lower body ergometer • Cycle ergometer • Treadmill • Arm ergometer • Seated stepper	• Increase independence in ADLs • Increase walking speed • Decrease risk of cardio-vascular disease	• 40-70% $\dot{V}O_2$peak*; RPE 13/20 • 3-5 days/wk • 20-60 min/session (or multiple 10-min sessions)	• 2-4 mo
Strength • Isometric exercise • Weight machine • Free weights	• Increase independence in ADLs	• 3 sets of 8-12 reps • 2 days/wk	• 2-4 mo
Flexibility • Stretching	• Increase ROM of involved extremities • Prevent contractures	• 2 days/wk (before or after Aerobic or Strength activities)	• 2-4 mo
Neuromuscular • Coordination and balance activities	• Improve level of safety during ADLs	• 2 days/wk (consider performing on same day as strength activities)	• 2-4 mo

* $\dot{V}O_2$max is undefined in stroke, brain injury, and many other neurological pathologies.

Medications	Special Considerations
• See exercise testing table.	• See exercise testing table. • Deconditioned individuals may need to start at very low intensity. • May need to do resistance exercises in seated positions. • Psycho-cognitive and emotional effects of brain injury may require a more isolated environment to avoid distraction.

Aerobic Training

Training mode depends on the individual's ability, but the various modes described for exercise testing could also be employed for exercise training. Suggested frequency is 3 to 5 sessions/wk. Exercise intensity should be based on the initial fitness level of the subject. The very deconditioned individual may have to begin at exercise intensities equivalent to 40 to 50% $\dot{V}O_2$peak. Duration of training sessions also depends on the subject's initial level of fitness. Intermittent training protocols may be needed during the initial weeks of training because of the extremely deconditioned level of many clients after a CVA or a TBI. Exercise managers should aim for at least a 20-min duration (or two 10-min exertion sessions). Once an individual can comfortably complete a 20-min aerobic exercise session, the duration should be gradually increased until the individual can complete an exercise session equivalent to a caloric expenditure of 300 kcal.

This can be achieved with a shorter exercise session at a higher intensity or a longer exercise session at a lower intensity.

Strength Training

Previously it was thought resistance exercise resulted in further increases in muscle tone in those individuals demonstrating hypertonia. Therefore, resistance exercise training programs were often not included in the rehabilitation programs of many individuals following TBI or CVA. These fears appear to be unfounded. Resistance exercises should be prescribed to address any muscle weakness identified during the fitness assessment.

Individuals with neurological impairments may have difficulty with preparatory postural adjustments and recruiting strength quickly enough to combat the loss of balance. Thus, some of the positions typically used for weight training may need to be modified. For example, many individuals perform dumbbell exercises while standing to increase upper body strength. A person who has difficulty maintaining standing balance should perform these exercises unilaterally while holding onto a bar or other stationary object. They could also perform these exercises from a seated position.

Exercise Environment

Behavioral factors (e.g., impulsivity, a tendency to display outward aggression, lack of judgment, misunder-

standing directions) exhibited by a client following TBI should be considered when selecting the most appropriate environment for exercise. A client who lacks judgment may need closer supervision during exercise, while the individual who displays outward aggression may not succeed in certain group exercise settings. A client who is easily agitated/frustrated or highly distractible might be scheduled to exercise at a facility during a quieter time of the day or work out in an area with fewer distractions. The client who lacks initiative might be more successful in a group setting.

CASE STUDY Cerebrovascular Accident

Two years ago, a 73-year-old retired salesman had a hemorrhagic CVA of the right middle cerebral artery, which caused severe sensory and motor losses in the left arm and leg. He was hospitalized for six weeks and received extensive physical and occupational therapy as an outpatient. He stopped making functional gains and had residual sensory impairment and weakness on the left side. He was independent in bed mobility, and could walk short distances in the home, but needed a wide-based quad cane and a short leg brace on the left foot. He could propel a manual wheelchair, although someone usually pushed the chair for him. He also had a history of emphysema but quit smoking seven years prior to his stroke. He was referred for an exercise program to attempt further gains in performance, or at least preserve his level of function.

S: "I can't climb stairs, and I want to walk without using my cane."

O: Hemiplegic elderly male

Medications: Albuterol, Atrovent, Ibuprofen

Graded exercise test (Schwinn Air-Dyne™):
  Limited by dyspnea; no ECG abnormalities
  Functional capacity: 4.5 METs
  $\dot{V}O_2$peak: 15 ml·kg^{-1}·min^{-1}
  Peak HR: 135 contractions/min
  Peak BP: 180/82 mmHg

Strength: Not tested due to inability to isolate movement

Flexibility:
  Hip internal rotation: Right 10°; left 5°
  Ankle dorsiflexion: Right 10°; left 0°
  Shoulder elevation: Right 175°; left 155°
  Finger extension (wrist neutral): Right 180°; left 110°

Active movement of the left arm about 30% of total range

Passive movement of the left shoulder about 75% of contralateral shoulder

Considerable tightness of the left finger flexors 65% of normal range

Neuromuscular:
  Gait: Walks using left ankle-foot orthosis (AFO) and right wide-based quad cane with weight primarily borne over right foot; stumbled when changing direction
  Trunk kyphotic during gait, hips flexed during stance
  Gait speed: 0.2 m/s
  Single-limb stance: Right leg 4 s; left leg 1 s
  Sit-and-reach test: 4 in (10.2 cm)

Functional performance (Duke mobility scale): 14/26

Major limitations:
Cannot ascend/descend stairs independently
Cannot step over an obstacle in walking path
Cannot come to an abrupt stop without stumbling or grabbing
Cannot turn while walking without staggering or falling

A: 1. Low aerobic capacity due to inactivity, CVA, and emphysema
2. Weak left arm and leg
3. Poor balance
4. Decreased ROM on left
5. Slow gait speed precludes functional ambulation
6. Not independent in many ADLs

P: 1. Exercise to increase strength and speed of gait.
2. Adapt devices to facilitate exercise/independent function.

Exercise Program
Goals:

1. Increase speed and safety of gait
2. Be able to climb stairs independently

Mode	Frequency	Duration	Intensity	Progression
Aerobic (Schwinn Air-Dyne™)	3 days/wk	10 min continuous	60% of peak HR RPE ~13/20	Increase to 20 min continuous, over 2-4 mo
Strength				
Flexibility (all major muscle groups)	3 days/wk	20-60 s/stretch	Maintain stretch below discomfort point	
Neuromuscular				
Functional				
Warm-up/Cool-down				

Follow-Up
He began an 8-week program in a community-based cardiac rehabilitation program. Initially, he could cycle for only 10 min and required frequent rest periods to relieve dyspnea. By 8 weeks, he could complete 20 min of exercise with only three 15-s rest periods. His gait speed had increased to 0.3 m/s, but he still required an assistive device to walk. He also improved his score on the Duke mobility scale to 16/26, reflecting new abilities to ascend and descend stairs with a railing and to turn while walking without stumbling or falling.

Suggested Readings

Gordon, N.F. 1993. *Stroke: Your complete exercise guide.* Champaign, IL: Human Kinetics.

Gordon, W.A., M. Sliwinski, J. Echo, M. McLouglin, M.S. Sheerer, and T.E. Meili. 1998. The benefits of exercise in individuals with traumatic brain injury: A retrospective study. *Journal of Head Trauma Rehabilitation* 134: 58-67.

Gresham G.E, P.W. Duncan, H.P. Adams, A.M. Adelman, D.N. Alexander, D.S. Bishop, L. Diller, N.E, Donaldson, C.V. Granger, A.L. Holland, M. Kelley-Hayes, F.H. McDowell, L. Myers, M.A. Phipps, E.J. Roth, H.C. Siebens, G.A. Tarvin, and C.A. Trombly. 1995. *Clinical practice guideline number 16: Post-stroke rehabilitation.* Rockville, MD: U.S. Department of Health and Human Services. Public Health Service. Agency for Health Care Policy and Research. AHCPR Publication No. 95-0662.

Halar, E.M. 1999. Management of stroke risk factors during the process of rehabilitation: Secondary stroke prevention. *Physical Medicine and Rehabilitation Clinics of North America* 10 (4): 839-56.

Hunter, M., J. Tomberlin, C. Kirkikis, and S.T Kuna. 1990. Progressive exercise testing in closed head-injured subjects: Comparison of exercise apparatus in assessment of a physical conditioning program. *Physical Therapy* 70: 363-71.

Jankowski, L.W., and S.J. Sullivan. 1990. Aerobic and neuromuscular training: Effect on the capacity, efficiency, and fatigability of patients with traumatic brain injury. *Archives of Physical Medicine and Rehabilitation* 71: 500-504.

Monga, T.N., D.A. Deforge, J. Williams, and L.A. Wolfe. 1988. Cardiovascular responses to acute exercise in patients with cerebrovascular accidents. *Archives of Physical Medicine and Rehabilitation* 69: 937-40.

NINDS. 2001. *NINDS post-stroke rehabilitation fact sheet.* [Online]. Available: **www.ninds.nih.gov/health-and-medical/pubs/poststrokerehab.htm** [17 January 2001].

O'Sullivan, S.B., and T.J. Schmitz. 2001. *Physical rehabilitation assessment and treatment.* 4th ed. Philadelphia: F.A. Davis.

Rimmer, J., and T.L. Nicola. 2002. Stroke. In *ACSM's resources for clinical exercise physiology: Musculoskeletal, neuromuscular, neoplastic, immunologic, and hematologic conditions.* Edited by J.N. Myers, W.G. Herbert, R. Humphrey. 3-15. Philadelphia: Lippincott Williams & Wilkins.

Rimmer, J.H., B. Riley, T. Creviston, and T. Nicola. 2000. Exercise training in a group of predominately African-American group of stroke survivors. *Medicine and Science in Sports and Exercise* 32 (12): 1990-96.

Vitale, A.E., S.J. Sullivan, L.W. Jankowski, J. Fleury, C. LeFrancois, and E. LeBouthillier. 1995. Screening of health risk factors prior to exercise or a fitness evaluation of adults with traumatic brain injury: A consensus by rehabilitation professionals. *Brain Injury* 10: 367-75.

CHAPTER 37

Spinal Cord Disabilities: Paraplegia and Tetraplegia

Stephen F. Figoni, PhD, RKT, FACSM
VA Palo Alto Health Care System

Overview of the Pathophysiology

Spinal cord disabilities frequently result in paraplegia or tetraplegia, with segmental neuromuscular, autonomic, and physiologic impairment of the legs, arms, and/or trunk. The majority of people with spinal cord disabilities acquire their disability during adolescence or early-middle adulthood from traumatic injuries to the spinal cord. Most traumatic spinal cord injuries (SCIs) result from motor vehicle accidents and falls, with fewer caused by sports/diving, violence, infection/ tumor of the spinal cord, and surgical complications. Fewer traumatic SCIs occur during childhood and old age from similar causes. In the United States, the incidence of new traumatic SCI is about 32/million population, producing 8,000 new SCIs/year and 75,000 total SCI survivors.

Additionally, about 1 out of every 1,000 live births in the United States results in spina bifida (SB), the congenital developmental form of spinal cord disability. Therefore, about 4,000 infants are born with this condition each year. SB is a defect due to neural tube abnormalities that usually becomes evident during prenatal sonogram or at birth. It involves incomplete development and closure of the vertebral arch and results in spinal cord damage. It is usually of the myelomeningocele-type affecting the lumbosacral neural segments and causing low-level paraplegia.

Congenital and acquired/traumatic spinal cord disability can both result in the same sensorimotor, autonomic, physiological, and locomotor impairments. However, in adolescents and adults with SB, secondary conditions tend to accumulate across the entire life span. Therefore, beware of complicated medical and psychosocial histories that frequently include hydrocephalus, implanted cerebral shunts, multiple orthopedic and plastic surgery, skin ulceration, tendinitis, gastrointestinal disorders, obesity, impaired mobility, latex allergy, learning disability, low self-esteem, depression, social immaturity, and hygiene and sexual issues.

Spinal cord disability from any etiology results in impairment or loss of sensorimotor and other functions in the trunk and/or extremities caused by damage to the neural elements within the spinal canal. Injury to the cervical segments (C1-C8) or the highest thoracic segment (T1) causes tetraplegia (formerly quadriplegia), with impairment of the arms, trunk, legs, and pelvic organs (bladder, bowels, and sexual organs). Injury to thoracic segments T2 to T12 causes paraplegia, with impairment to the trunk, legs, and/or pelvic organs. Injury to the lumbar or sacral segments of the cauda equina (L1-L5, S1-S4) results in impairment to the legs or pelvic organs, or both. The neurological level and completeness of injury determine the degree of impairment.

Physiological impairment may include extensive muscular paralysis and sympathetic nervous system impairment. These frequently result in two major exercise-related problems:

- reduced ability to voluntarily perform large muscle group aerobic exercise (i.e., without electrical stimulation of paralyzed muscles), and
- inability to stimulate the cardiovascular system to support higher rates of aerobic metabolism.

Therefore, catecholamine production by the adrenal medullae, skeletal muscle venous pump, and thermo-regulation may be impaired, restricting exercise cardiac output to subnormal levels. Common secondary complications during exercise, especially in persons with tetraplegia, may include limited positive cardiac chronotropic and inotropic states, excessive venous pooling, orthostatic and exercise hypotension, exercise intolerance, autonomic dysreflexia (a syndrome resulting from mass activation of autonomic reflexes causing extreme hypertension [BP >200/110 mmHg]), headache, bradycardia, flushing, gooseflesh, unusual sweating, shivering, and nasal congestion.

Effects on the Exercise Response

In persons with paraplegia, the primary pathologic effects are usually limited to paralysis of the lower body, precluding exercise modes such as walking, running, and voluntary leg cycling. Therefore, the upper body must be used for all voluntary activities of daily living and exercise: arm cranking, wheelchair propulsion, and/or ambulation with orthotic devices and crutches. The proportionally smaller active upper body muscle mass typically restricts peak values of power output, oxygen consumption ($\dot{V}O_2$), and cardiac output to approximately one-half of those expected for maximal leg exercise in individuals without SCI.

In persons with tetraplegia, the pathologic effects are more extensive than with paraplegia. The active upper body muscle mass will be partially paralyzed, and the sympathetic nervous system may be completely separated from control by the brain. Upper body power output and $\dot{V}O_2$, as well as cardiac output, are typically reduced to approximately one-half to one-third of the levels seen in individuals with paraplegia. Furthermore, strenuous exercise may not be tolerated because of orthostatic and exercise hypotension, which may produce symptoms of dizziness, nausea, and others. Peak heart rates for persons with tetraplegia typically do not exceed 130 contractions/min.

Effects of Exercise Training

Arm exercise training adaptations are believed to be primarily peripheral (muscular) in nature and may include increased muscular strength and endurance of the arm musculature in the exercise modes used. These may result in 10 to 20% improvements in peak power output and peak oxygen consumption ($\dot{V}O_2$peak), as well as enhanced sense of well-being. Central cardiovascular adaptations to exercise training, such as increased maximal stroke volume or cardiac output, have not yet been documented.

Management and Medications

Management of persons with paraplegia or tetraplegia is complex because of the multitude of associated complications.

• **Skin.** People with spinal cord disability should avoid sitting for long periods without pressure relief; avoid abrasion/bumping of bony weight-bearing areas of hips, especially ischial tuberosities, sacrum, and coccyx; and sit on a cushion.

• **Bones.** Those working with spinal cord disability patients should avoid dropping during transfers or allowing the person to fall (e.g., from a wheelchair or exercise equipment). These persons have an increased risk for fractures secondary to osteoporosis.

• **Stabilization.** If trunk control and balance are impaired, sufficient strapping and seatbelts should be used during upright exercise.

• **Handgrip or foot placement.** The hands or feet of persons with weak/absent handgrip or impaired foot control should be secured to ergometer and exercise equipment handle/pedals with elastic bandages, gloves with Velcro straps, toe clips, tape, and the like.

• **Bladder.** Persons should empty their bladder or leg bag just before exercise testing to avoid bladder overdistension or overfilling of the leg bag during exercise, as this may induce autonomic dysreflexia (with hypertension) in persons with paraplegia above T6 or with tetraplegia.

• **Bowels.** A regular bowel-maintenance program is useful to avoid autonomic dysreflexic symptoms in persons with tetraplegia or accidental bowel movement during exercise.

• **Illness.** Postpone exercise if the person is ill (e.g., has such conditions as bladder infection, pressure ulcer, cold, flu, allergy, unusual spasticity, autonomic dysreflexia, constipation).

• **Hypotension.** If resting blood pressure before the test is below 80/50 mmHg, the person should wear elastic support stockings and an abdominal binder, or both, to elevate resting blood pressure. Exercise should be avoided within three hours of eating a large meal because food intake may induce hypotension. Regularly monitor blood pressure and symptoms of hypotension (e.g., dizziness, lightheadedness, nausea, pallor, cyanosis, extreme or sudden weakness, mental confusion, visual disturbances, inability to respond to questions or instructions).

• **Hypertension.** Autonomic dysreflexia is possible in persons with paraplegia above T6 or tetraplegia. Preventive measures include proper bowel and bladder management. Monitor blood pressure regularly, and check for dysreflex-

Spinal Cord Disabilities: Exercise Testing

Methods	Measures	Endpoints*	Comments
Aerobic Arm ergometer Wheelchair ergometer Wheelchair treadmill Wheeling on track or treadmill	• Peak HR, METs, or $\dot{V}O_2$peak • BP • RPE (6-20)	• Serious dysrhythmias • > 2 mm ST-segment depression or elevation • Ischemic threshold • T-wave inversion with significant ST change	• Adjust incremental power levels to subject's capacity. • Peak HR will be low (110-130 contractions/min) in tetraplegia (above T-1) due to sympathetic impairment. • Persons with tetraplegia will need gloves or hand wrappings.** • Give rest periods between stages (i.e., stop exercise). • Watch for hypertension from autonomic dysreflexia or hypotension caused by orthostasis and exertion. • Indicates basic exercise tolerance and effort.
Flexibility Goniometer Stretching tests	• Flexibility of shoulders, elbow, wrist, hip, and knee		• Helpful in preventing contractures and injury.

*Measurements of particular significance; do not always indicate test termination.

Special Considerations

- Osteoporosis may exist in leg bones; possible contractures.
- Persons with tetraplegia will usually display bradycardia and have peak HR limited to approximately 120 contractions/min. They do not adapt acutely to stressors such as heat or cold (e.g., blood shunting, shivering, and sweating may be profoundly impaired or abolished) or to exercise because of sympathetic dysfunction, including vasomotor paralysis, cardiac sympathetic blockade, and adrenal denervation. Orthostatic and exercise hypotension is common; persons with quadriplegia are also at risk for deep venous thrombosis leading to pulmonary embolism.
- Depending on level of injury, forced expiration can be limited or absent.
- Skeletal muscle paralysis depends on the level and completeness of injury, with upper motor neuron injury producing spastic paralysis and lower motor neuron injury producing flaccid paralysis. Spastic paralyzed muscles can be electrically stimulated to produce movements for functional or therapeutic purposes; flaccid paralyzed muscles do not respond to electrical stimulation techniques. Paralyzed leg muscles are also aggravated by venous pooling secondary to loss of the venous muscle pump.
- Sensory loss depends on level and completeness of injury according to dermatome maps. Insensate weight-bearing areas are at risk for pressure ulceration and need periodic pressure relief.
- In some settings, electrically stimulated muscle contractions can recruit sufficient muscle mass to significantly increase $\dot{V}O_2$peak.
- $\dot{V}O_2$peak depends on total active muscle mass.
- Each subject has his/her own bladder program. Be sure bladder is empty prior to exercise.
- Voluntary anal sphincter control is often lost along with abdominal muscle denervation, necessitating a special bowel care program.
- Hypotension is common, and may necessitate use of support stockings and abdominal binder.
- Never leave a person with tetraplegia exercising unsupervised.
- Keep exercise environment thermally neutral.

ic signs and symptoms. Discourage "boosting" (i.e., induction of autonomic dysreflexia to improve exercise tolerance).

• **Pain.** Discontinue arm exercise that aggravates chronic shoulder joint pain. Overuse syndromes are common in people who use their arms to transfer and propel wheelchairs.

• **Orthopedic.** Bone or joint swelling, discomfort, or deformity may indicate fracture or sprain.

Allow the person to take normal prescription medications. However, beware of medications/drugs that either induce hypotension (e.g., Ditropan/oxybutinin chloride, Dibenzyline/phenoxybenzamine hydrochloride) or induce diuresis (e.g., alcohol, diuretics).

Recommendations for Exercise Testing

When exercise testing a person with a spinal cord disability, the following recommendations should be considered (see the Spinal Cord Disabilities: Exercise Testing table on page 249).

• For clinical cardiovascular exercise testing, consult a medical or allied health professional with specific training in exercise testing of persons with paraplegia or tetraplegia. Utilize any reproducible exercise mode that is not contraindicated, such as arm and/or leg cycle ergometry (with or without electrical stimulation of paralyzed muscles), wheelchair ergometry, and rowing.

• For general fitness testing, consult Winnick and Short (1999). Tests can be adapted for adults.

• Consider functional mobility testing with timed wheeling/walking (6 to 12 min) or a custom-designed mobility obstacle course including potential environmental barriers such as ramps, stairs, curbs, doorways, soft/uneven surfaces, turns, transfers, lifting, carrying, and manipulation of objects on shelves.

• Adapt the exercise equipment as needed, and provide for special needs in terms of trunk stabilization (straps), securing hands on crank handles (holding gloves),

Spinal Cord Disabilities: Exercise Programming

Modes	Goals	Intensity/Frequency/Duration	Time to Goal
Aerobic •Arm ergometer •Wheelchair ergometer •Wheelchair treadmill •Free wheeling •Arm cycling •Seated aerobics •Swimming •Wheelchair sports •Electrical stimulation leg cycle ergometry, with/without arm ergometry	•Increase active muscle mass and strength •Maximize overall strength for functional independence •Improve efficiency of manual wheelchair propulsion	•50-80% peak HR •3-5 days/wk •20-60 min/session	•4-6 mo
Flexibility •Stretching	•Avoid joint contracture	•Before aerobic or strength activities	•4-6 mo
Strength •Weight machines or dumbbells •Wrist weights	•Increase active muscle mass and strength •Maximize overall strength for functional independence •Improve efficiency of manual wheelchair propulsion	•2-3 sets of 8-12 reps •2-4 days/wk	•4-6 mo

Special Considerations

• See exercise testing table.

skin protection (seat cushion and padding), prevention of bladder overdistension (i.e., emptying bladder or using urinary collection device immediately before test), and vascular support to help maintain blood pressure and improve exercise tolerance (elastic stockings and abdominal binder).

• Use an environmentally controlled thermoneutral or cool laboratory or clinic to compensate for impaired thermoregulation.

• Design a discontinuous incremental testing protocol that allows monitoring of heart rate, blood pressure, rating of perceived exertion, symptoms, and exercise tolerance at each stage. Power output increments may range from 5 to 20 watts depending on exercise mode, level and completeness of paraplegia or tetraplegia, and activity/training status.

• Expect peak power outputs for persons with tetraplegia to range from 0 to 50 watts and from 50 to 120 watts for persons with paraplegia. Treat postexercise hypotension and exhaustion with recumbency, leg elevation, rest, and fluid ingestion.

Recommendations for Exercise Programming

Exercise training can provide a variety of health-related benefits for the person with a spinal cord disability. In developing an exercise program, the following recommendations should be considered (also see the Spinal Cord Disabilities: Exercise Programming table).

• Cardiopulmonary training modes may include arm cranking, wheelchair ergometry, wheelchair propulsion on treadmill or rollers, and free wheeling; swimming; vigorous sports such as wheelchair basketball, quad rugby, and racing; arm-powered cycling, vigorous activities of daily living such as ambulation with crutches and braces; seated aerobic exercises; and electrically stimulated leg cycle exercise (ESLCE), or ESLCE combined with arm cranking.

• To prevent upper extremity overuse syndromes, (1) vary exercise modes from week to week; (2) strengthen muscles of the upper back and posterior shoulder, especially external shoulder rotators; and (3) stretch muscles of anterior shoulder and chest.

• Use an environmentally controlled, thermoneutral gym, laboratory, or clinic for persons with tetraplegia. Individuals with thermoregulatory abilities can exercise outdoors if provisions are made for extreme conditions. Emptying the bladder or urinary collection device immediately before exercise may prevent dysreflexic symptoms during exercise. The person should drink plenty of fluids after exercise.

• The greater the exercising muscle mass, the greater the expected improvements in all physiologic and performance parameters. Arm training will probably induce training effects in the arm muscles only; combined arm and leg exercise may induce both muscular and cardiopulmonary training effects.

• Remember such training principles as specificity, overload, progression, and regularity.

Special Considerations

There are many special considerations in persons with SCIs.

• Depression is common among people with paraplegia or tetraplegia. Be supportive and set realistic goals.

• Cognitive impairment and learning disability is common among people with SB.

• Expect small but progressive improvements in fitness ($<5\%$/wk). Progress may be interrupted periodically due to chronic secondary health conditions.

• Always supervise persons with tetraplegia. If they are not exercising in their own wheelchair, two assistants may be needed for manual transfer of large individuals to and from exercise equipment. Monitor blood pressure and symptoms regularly during exposure to orthostatic or exercise stress. To achieve good program adherence, provide supportive structure and motivation for those who need it.

• Follow the precautions outlined earlier (see Management and Medications) concerning skin, bones, stabilization, handgrip, bladder, bowels, illness, hypotension, hypertension, pain, orthopedic complications, and medications. If necessary, hypotensive individuals should use supine posture and wear support stockings and abdominal binder to help maintain blood pressure. Avoid contacting persons with SB with latex products (e.g., coating on equipment, stretch bands, latex gloves)

• Consult the physician and appropriate allied health personnel to answer specific questions concerning medical complications to which the person may be susceptible.

• For persons with tetraplegia and high-level paraplegia, exercise should take place only in thermally neutral environments, such as a laboratory or clinic with air conditioning to control temperature and humidity.

• In many conditions, little research is available to support specific guidelines. Thus, for some conditions the exercise professional may want to suggest some innovative recommendations.

CASE STUDY Spinal Cord Injury

A 22-year-old male was in a car accident 5 years prior to evaluation and survived a cervical spinal cord injury resulting in a complete C7 tetraplegia. He had marked spasticity in the hip and knee flexors and ankle plantar flexors. The muscle strength of his shoulders, elbow flexors, and wrist extensors was normal, but his elbow extensors, wrist flexors, and finger muscles were weak. His latissimus dorsi, pectoralis major, and triceps brachii muscles were all partially innervated. He had gained 50 lb (22.7 kg) over the previous 5 years since his discharge from rehabilitation. He lived independently without assistance, but transferred independently with great difficulty using a sliding board. He pushed a manual wheelchair independently in the community and drove an adapted van.

S: "My arms get tired, I have shoulder pain, and I get short of breath pushing my wheelchair up inclines."

O: Vitals: Height: 5'9" (1.75 m)   Weight: 220 lb (99.8 kg)   BMI: 32.6 kg/m²
Supine HR: 50 contractions/min   Supine BP: 110/75 mmHg
Upright HR: 60 contractions/min   Upright BP: 90/55 mmHg

Young, obese, tetraplegic male

Posture is kyphotic with rounded shoulders and forward head

Triceps skin fold: 25 mm

Standard 4-m (13-ft) ramp test (12:1 slope): 20 s

6-min push test (dense-carpeted surface): 600 m (0.4 mi)

Graded exercise test (arm crank):
  Peak power: 40 watts
  Peak HR: 130 contractions/min
  Termination secondary to arm muscle fatigue (RPE 8/10)

Medications: Baclofen, Bactrim, Mandelamine, Vitamin C, Dulcolax, Dibenzyline

A: 1. Weakness from complete C7 tetraplegia
2. Deconditioning
3. Obesity

P: 1. Exercise to increase physical fitness.
2. Dietary counseling is necessary.
3. Consult physician/physical therapist re: shoulder pain.

Exercise Program
Goals:

1. Pain-free ADLs using normal wheelchair
2. Increase triceps and shoulder depressor strength
3. Increase shoulder strength, endurance, and overall muscle balance
4. Lose 20 kg (44 lb)
5. Exercise at an accessible fitness facility/clinic 3 times/wk

Mode	Frequency	Duration	Intensity	Progression
Aerobic (arm crank)	3 days/wk	To fatigue forward and backward	1 day: 25 W 2 days: 5 1-min intervals @ 35 W	Increase as tolerated to 30-60 min/session Advance to supervised swimming 2 days/wk
Strength (rickshaw, lat pull-downs, rowing, incline, bench press)	2 days/wk	2 sets of 10 reps	80% of 10RM	Increase weight Reassess every 2 wk
Flexibility (anterior chest and deltoids)	3 days/wk	Maintain stretch for 20 s or below discomfort point		
Neuromuscular (shoulder extension, rotators, scapular retractors)	3 days/wk			
Functional				
Warm-up/Cool-down	Before and after each session	10-15 min	Light	

Suggested Readings

Davis, G., and R. Glaser. 1990. Cardiorespiratory fitness following spinal cord injury. In *Key issues in neurological physiotherapy*, edited by L. Ada and C. Canning, 155-96. London: Butterworth-Heinemann.

Davis, G.M. 1993. Exercise capacity of individuals with paraplegia. *Medicine and Science in Sports and Exercise* 25: 423-32.

Ditunno, J.F., W. Young, W.H. Donovan, and G. Creasey. 1994. The international standards booklet for neurological and functional classification of spinal injury patients. *Paraplegia* 32: 70-80.

Figoni, S.F., B.J. Kiratli, and R. Sasaki. 2002. Spinal cord dysfunction. In *ACSM's resources for clinical exercise physiology: Musculoskeletal, neuromuscular, neoplastic, immunologic and hematologic conditions*. Edited by J.N. Myers, W.G. Herbert, and R. Humphrey. 48-67. Philadelphia: Lippincott Williams & Wilkins.

Figoni, S.F. 1993. Exercise responses and quadriplegia. *Medicine and Science in Sports and Exercise* 25: 433-41.

Glaser, R.M. 1987. Exercise and locomotion for the spinal cord injured. *Exercise and Sport Sciences Reviews* 13: 263-303.

Glaser, R.M., and G.M. Davis. 1989. Wheelchair-dependent individuals. In *Exercise in modern medicine*, edited by B.A. Franklin, S. Gordon, and G.C. Timmis, 237-67. Baltimore: Williams & Wilkins.

Hoffman, M.D. 1986. Cardiorespiratory fitness and training in quadriplegics and paraplegics. *Sports Medicine* 3: 312-30.

Lutkenhoff, M., and S. Oppenheimer, eds. 1997. *SPIN abilities: A young person's guide to spina bifida*. Bethesda, MD: Woodbine House.

Miller, P. 1994. *Fitness programming and physical disability*. Champaign, IL: Human Kinetics.

Rimmer, J.H. 1994. *Fitness and rehabilitation programs for special populations*. Madison, WI: Brown.

Shephard, R.J. 1990. *Fitness in special populations*. Champaign, IL: Human Kinetics.

Winnick, J.P., and F.X. Short. 1999. *The Brockport physical fitness test manual*. Champaign, IL: Human Kinetics.

CHAPTER 38

Muscular Dystrophy

Mark A. Tarnopolsky, MD, PhD
McMaster University Medical Center

Overview of the Pathophysiology

The muscular dystrophies (MDs) are a group of hereditary disorders of skeletal muscle structure. These result in the progressive destruction of muscle cells and their replacement with connective tissue. As a consequence of this process, there is a progressive loss of strength that leads to a loss of functional capacity. In the past 15 years, there has been an explosion of knowledge regarding the fundamental genetic bases for these conditions and the cellular consequences (necrosis and/or apoptosis of muscle cells). The more common MDs include the dystrophinopathies (Becker MD [BMD] and Duchenne MD [DMD]), facioscapulohumeral (FSHD), limb girdle (LGMD), myotonic (MD), and Emery-Driefuss (EDMD). Only the MDs will be considered here, not the other myopathies (e.g., channelopathy, metabolic, endocrine, congenital, and inflammatory) or congenital MD.

DMD and the milder BMD are both X-linked recessive genetic disorders affecting the dystrophin gene. This leads to complete (DMD) or partial (BMD) absence of the dystrophin protein (this is involved in linking the contractile proteins to the sarcolemma). DMD has the highest incidence of the dystrophies presenting in childhood (~1 in 3500 live male births). In general, these children have proximal muscle weakness presenting at about age 4 that is associated with calf muscle hypertrophy and a very high plasma creatine kinase (CK) activity. DMD progresses to involve distal muscles, at which time ambulation becomes more difficult. By about age 10, most children are wheelchair bound and scoliosis often ensues. The course of BMD is less aggressive and most children remain ambulatory beyond age 12. In both DMD and BMD, there can be an associated cardiomyopathy. Some children with DMD will also have cognitive developmental delays.

The limb girdle MDs (LGMDs) are broadly divided into autosomal recessive disorder (25% of carrier parents can have an affected child) and autosomal dominant (one parent has the disorder, so there is a 50% chance of passing this on to the offspring). In general, the autosomal recessive form has an earlier onset and a more rapid progression (often as severe as that seen in DMD). The LGMDs are usually caused by mutations in genes encoding for cytoskeletal proteins (e.g., sarcoglycans). Some clients with LGMD may have cardiac involvement.

FSHD is an autosomal dominant condition that is named after the muscles that are most affected. Recently, the genetic cause was found to be related to a deletion in chromosome 4. The majority of clients will notice some facial weakness and periscapular weakness by the late teens. This will slowly progress to involve the biceps, tibialis anterior, and thigh muscles. Most clients remain ambulatory well into their 50s and 60s; however, there are rare cases of a more severe phenotype with infantile onset and cognitive delays.

EDMD is usually an X-linked recessive condition, although some are autosomal dominant. The X-linked form of EDMD is caused by a mutation in the emerin gene that codes for a nuclear protein, while the autosomal dominant form is caused by a mutation in the lamin gene (which likely interacts with emerin). This condition is characterized by the development of elbow, Achilles tendon, and cervical spine contractures, followed by atrophy and weakness of the upper arms and peroneal muscles. This disorder is often associated with conduction blocks and atrial paralysis.

Myotonic MD is the most common MD presenting in adulthood. It is an autosomal dominant disorder caused by a mutation (trinucleotide [CTG] expansion) in the region of the myotonin kinase gene. The size of the CTG expansion is reasonably well correlated with the severity of the phenotype. On average, this condition results in slowly progressive atrophy, weakness, and myotonia noted in the teens. In more severe cases, children can present with a congenital form with severe life-threatening weakness and cognitive delays, while in milder cases the disease may go unnoticed aside from cataracts. In addition to the muscle problems, these clients may have balding, cataracts, swallowing problems, cardiac conduction block, gastrointestinal dysmotility, and diabetes.

Effects on the Exercise Response

Isometric and isokinetic strength may be within normal limits early in the course of a dystrophy. For example, children with DMD often have normal strength until age 3 to 4, when progressive proximal weakness begins. It is also important to understand the underlying disease process and patterns of weakness. For example, clients with FSHD may have completely normal handgrip strength and yet be unable to raise their arms above their head. The

Muscular Dystrophy: Exercise Testing

Methods	Measures	Endpoints*	Comments

Aerobic
Cycle
(ramp protocol 5 watts/
2 min; stage protocol 5-10
watts/min)
	• 12-lead ECG, HR
	
	• BP
	
	• RPE (6-20 Borg scale)
		• Serious dysrhythmia
		• > 2 mm ST-segment
		  depression
		• Chest pain
		• T-wave inversion
		• Hypotensive response
		• SBP > 250 mmHg or
		  DBP > 110 mmHg
		• Volitional exhaustion
			• 12-lead initially for DMD,
			  BMD, EDMD, or any patient
			  over age 40.

**Muscular endurance
and power**
Wingate test
 	
Isokinetic fatigue test
	• Peak and mean power
	
	• Mean power in 1st 5
	  and last 5 contractions
		• 30s or voluntary
		  termination
		• 50 contractions
			• Not possible in moderate to
			  severe cases.

Strength
Grip strength
Knee extension
Weight machine
 	
Spirometry
	• Isokinetic torque at 30
	  and 180 rad/sec
	• Isometric
	• Peak strength
	
	• FVC, FEV$_1$
		• Peak strength
		• Peak value
		• Best RM
		• Best of 3 attempts
			• 3 measurements.
			• 2-min rest between speeds.
			• Measure 1 proximal + 1 distal
			  muscle in upper and lower
			  extremities.

Flexibility
Goniometry
	• ROM	• Maximal range (3
		  attempts)
			• Ankle, knee, and hip are
			  important.

Neuromuscular Gait/Balance analysis	• Foot drop • Trendelenburg gait • Antalgic gait		• Requires sophisticated equipment to semiquantitate.

Functional capacity
Lifestyle-specific tests:
• Put on a T-shirt
• 4-stair climb
 	
• Square (1 in² [2.54 cm²])
  cut art
 	
• Supine to stand
 	
• Walk/Run 20 in
  (50.8 cm)
	• Time
	• Time up and down
	
	• Time to cut square (from
	  standard 4 ft² [1.2 m²]
	  paper)
	• Time to get up (feet
	  together)
	• Time from tape
			• Indicate with/without hand-
			  rail.
			• Use plastic (children's)
			  scissors.
			
			• Wheelchair if not ambulatory.

*Measurements of particular significance; do not always indicate test termination.

Special Considerations

- Use arm ergometry if legs are too weak.
- Test every yr in slowly progressive dystrophies and every 3 mo if more rapidly progressive.
- Tests are very helpful to assess the efficacy of an intervention (e.g., surgery, braces/orthotics [ambulation], prednisone, and so on).
- An ergometer that will go to < 10 watts is often required if patient is very weak.
- A reclining cycle ergometer is often helpful for patients who have balance problems or are too weak to use a regular ergometer.
- A familiarization trial should be done before recording initial values.
- If possible, use the same evaluation to minimize test-retest variance.
- Stretching and standard warm-up should be done before testing.

Muscular Dystrophy: Exercise Programming

Modes	Goals	Intensity/Frequency/Duration	Time to Goal
Aerobic • Cycling • Walking/treadmill • Elliptical trainer • Rowing • Arm ergometry	• Maintain/increase aerobic capacity • Decrease cardiac risk factors	• 4-6 days/wk • 50-80% HR reserve • Until fatigue (goal: ≥ 20 min)	
Strength • Stretching	• Increase ROM • Prevent contractures	• Daily • Hold for 20 s/stretch	• 4-12 wk
Functional • Activity-specific task (i.e., wheelchair propulsion)	• Maintain and enhance proficiency in ADLs	• Daily as tolerated	

Special Considerations

- In some cases, performance may increase with the program; however, an attenuation of disease progression is usually seen (but is harder to quantify).
- It is very important to adapt the program to individual likes/dislikes (e.g., some may love walking).
- It is important for clients to "listen" to their bodies and stop if pain occurs or if function declines (medical assessment should be sought).

loss of isometric and isokinetic strength parallels the loss of functional capacities. In clients without a structural cardiomyopathy, there is usually a normal heart rate, ventilation, and rating of perceived exertion at a given relative exercise intensity of cycling; however, the loss of strength renders the absolute values higher than age-matched controls. Alterations in gait pattern (e.g., waddling, high stepping, excessive lordosis) can lead to an abnormally high oxygen cost per unit of work (speed) on a treadmill. For this reason, a cycle ergometer, and in severe cases a reclining ergometer, is most helpful in assessment

and in exercise prescription. The use of orthotics can reduce the oxygen cost of ambulation and it may be helpful to have the client tested with and without an orthosis.

Effects of Exercise Training

Several prospective studies have examined the effect of resistance exercise on muscle strength in clients with dystrophinopathies. In general, from the results of five studies on more than 100 DMD clients, it can be stated that there is no evidence that exercise induces a more rapid decline in strength (i.e., overuse). Overall, about half of the participants experienced mild improvements in strength and activities of daily living with moderate resistance exercise and stretching (usually 3 times/wk). In the more slowly progressive dystrophies (e.g., LGMD, FSHD, myotonic), several studies have used more traditional weight training programs ($\leq$ 80% of 1RM) and found increases in strength and functional capacity. In general, muscles with mild to moderate weakness are those that are most likely to show improvements. These muscles are weaker than antigravity strength and likely to show improvement with exercise. A more complete critical review of the literature can be found in the *ACSM's Resources for Clinical Exercise Physiology* (Tarnopolsky and Doherty, 2002).

Management and Medications

In spite of substantial advances in the understanding of the molecular bases for the dystrophies, there is currently no cure. As a result, management is focused upon the maintenance of function through exercise, orthoses, medication, and in some cases surgery. Therapeutic exercise is focused on the prevention of contractures (stretching), attenuating (and in some cases maintaining or even temporarily increasing) strength (strength training), and maintaining cardiovascular health (aerobic exercise). Aerobic exercise is important in preventing body fat accumulation and, because it reduces cardiovascular risk factors, in dystrophies where survival into adulthood is possible. Because most of the dystrophies primarily affect the proximal muscles, the main orthotic device that has been used is the knee-ankle-foot orthosis, which may prolong independent ambulation. In myotonic MD, where the weakness is distal, an ankle-foot orthosis is particularly helpful.

The main surgeries considered in clients with dystrophies are for release of contractures (e.g., ankles, adductors) and scoliosis correction. It is very important for therapeutic exercise to be continued as much as possible during the perioperative period to prevent deconditioning. A traumatic fracture can be the precipitating factor halting independent ambulation in clients who are "on the verge."

The only medications consistently shown to attenuate strength loss in clients with dystrophinopathies are corticosteroids. Overall, these result in about a 4 to 6% increase in strength that can delay degeneration beyond critical levels of function. Corticosteroids are associated with a loss of bone mass, attenuation in linear growth, increased body fat, insulin resistance, cataracts, and increased blood pressure. Given that children with DMD have low bone mass even prior to starting corticosteroids, it is important to measure bone mass prior to starting corticosteroids and to provide prophylaxis (calcium and vitamin D; if severe, bisphosphonates). Several trials of anabolic steroids and creatine monohydrate are scheduled to finish this year and preliminary results are somewhat encouraging.

Recommendations for Exercise Testing

Important qualitative information is obtained when exercise testing a person with MD. The following recommendations should be considered when completing these evaluations (see the Muscular Dystrophy: Exercise Testing table on page 255). The primary focus of exercise programming is on gaining muscle strength and muscular endurance. Therefore, testing is designed to guide such programming. Muscular power and peak aerobic power are of secondary importance, especially from a day-to-day clinical perspective.

- Manual muscle testing (i.e., 5-point Medical Research Counsel scale) is often used in a clinical setting; however, a very large decline in strength can go undetected before the grade changes.

- Objective testing in the clinic should include handgrip dynamometry and a handheld dynamometer at a minimum.

- Ideally, an isokinetic dynamometer (0°/s is isometric) should be used to follow clients at least every 12 months (or more frequently for more rapidly progressive dystrophies).

- Objective testing should be used before any therapeutic trial (e.g., drugs, surgery).

- Pulmonary function testing should be a part of the battery of standard tests available to the clinician (minimum of FVC and FEV_1).

- When using symptom-limited maximal graded exercise testing, heart rate, blood pressure, ECG, and rating of perceived exertion should be recorded.

- It is important to modify the testing and adapt the device to the individual.

- Body composition should be measured and followed using bioelectric impedance, DEXA scan, or air displacement. These data can be used to provide dietary advice to maintain an acceptable percentage of body fat and to follow lean mass. It is important that the same method be used longitudinally for each person because inter-test variance is high. Ideally, the same person should perform each test to minimize inter-tester variability.

Recommendations for Exercise Programming

The following are recommendations that need to be considered when developing an exercise program for the person with MD (see the Muscular Dystrophy: Exercise Programming table). Again, the focus is on gaining muscle strength and endurance.

• Provide manageable short-term goals to each individual and follow up closely in the initial stages of the program to ensure safety and encourage compliance.

• With weight training: start at a low percentage (~25%) of individual 1RM and with more than 10 repetitions. Gradually increase the percentage of 1RM as tolerated over a period of weeks to months. (This is a function of individual preference; however, some clients can eventually tolerate up to 75% of 1RM, 3 sets of 10 reps.) It is important to tell the client to "listen to your body" and to decrease the intensity if mild myalgias do not disappear after 24 hours or if the muscles cramp during activity. These symptoms should be reported to the attending clinician and the client should be evaluated.

• When muscles are weaker than anti-gravity strength, formal weights are essentially useless and the goal now becomes to exercise through the available range of motion and then to regain full range against gravity and to prevent contractures.

• For children, it is important to make the activities as game-like as possible.

• Stretching, to prevent contractures and to maintain overall flexibility, should be performed daily.

• Any client with dystrophy should exercise with a partner, drink plenty of fluids, and avoid strenuous exercise in high heat and humidity conditions.

Special Considerations

It is very important to know the characteristics of the dystrophy in order to adapt the exercise testing and prescription to the individual. Cardiac involvement is the most significant ancillary factor to consider in exercise prescription. Cardiomyopathy can be seen in DMD, BMD, and some forms of LGMD. This can limit exercise capacity by a central pumping limitation (decreased oxygen delivery). Cardiac conduction defects can be seen with EDMD and myotonic MD. This may also limit oxygen delivery by incomplete filling of the atria or dropped contractions. An ECG and an echocardiogram should be performed on all DMD, BMD, and LGMD clients with a cardiology consult before exercise prescription or testing.

Contractures are another important factor to consider in exercise prescription, for these may severely limit the ability to use certain testing or training devices. Exercise and range of motion are the mainstays of therapy in contracture treatment. Lack of motivation to exercise is a significant issue particularly in clients with myotonic MD and some more severely affected children with DMD.

Safety issues are important—for example, clients with myotonic MD often find that they have more myotonia in the cold; hence, they should avoid swimming in cold water. Myotonia can also be a significant disability in sports that require a rapid relaxation of the hand (e.g., throwing sports). Recent evidence has shown that clients with DMD (and likely many other types of dystrophy) have low bone mineral content. Thus, DEXA scanning on any client with MD who wishes to participate in contact sports may be a consideration. If the BMC is low, interventions can range from bisphosphonates and avoidance of all contact sports (severe) to recommending calcium supplements and follow-up (mild). Cataracts can limit the ability of clients with myotonic dystrophy to perform sports that require hand-eye coordination. A stationary cycle and cataract removal are possible suggestions for such a client.

Prednisone and Deflazacort (corticosteroids) are often used in children with DMD and in some with BMD. These drugs cause an increase in fat mass and reduce bone mineral content. With obesity, it may be appropriate to initiate exercise using weight-supported activities. Any child on prednisone should be followed yearly with a DEXA scan and all should be taking supplemental calcium and vitamin D. Exercise is the most potent modality to attenuate the negative effects of corticosteroids on muscle and bone and should be encouraged for all clients on these drugs. Finally, there has been the suggestion that clients with dystrophies are more likely to have malignant hyperthermia, a condition where the body's temperature and heat production increase massively and death can ensue. Although true malignant hyperthermia (autosomal dominant genetic channelopathy) is not likely to be more prevalent in the dystrophy population per se, the underlying muscle destruction could lead to an abnormally high release of myoglobin into the urine with resultant renal failure.

It is important to consider several issues when working with a client with dystrophy. Included in these are issues of safety, exercise intensity, mode of exercise, and psychological aspects.

Safety

Some dystrophies are associated with cardiomyopathy (e.g., dystrophinopathies, some types of LGMD) and others with conduction block (e.g., EDMD, myotonic

MD). An exercise stress test with a 12-lead ECG **must be** performed before embarking on an exercise program. Some clients may require an echocardiograph and a cardiology consult.

Even in the face of conduction block and cardiomyopathy, it is possible to design an exercise program using well-established guidelines for clients with primary cardiac problems. It is well known that plasma CK activity can fluctuate even without an antecedent trigger, so there is no good point in following CK activity, but do establish a baseline value. This may take several determinations until a mean value can be established and will also provide day-to-day variance in the measure. If a client loses strength more rapidly than expected, check the plasma CK, and if it is more than 2 standard deviations (SDs) above the individual's mean, decrease the exercise intensity and review for other factors that may have contributed to this rise. Clients with dark (tea-colored or foamy, indicative of myoglobinuria) urine should notify their physician and cease physical activity until evaluated. Finally, bone mass may already be low in someone with dystrophy and the mode of activity should be modified if bone mass is critically low.

Ergometry

Ergometers should be adaptable for arm cranking as well as cycling. The ergometer should be capable of functioning at very low work rates (≤ 5 watts). In addition, the work rate increments should be capable of increasing in 1- to 2-watt increments. A reclining cycle ergometer is sometimes required for those persons with poor balance or weakness to the degree that upright cycle ergometry would be dangerous.

Psychological Aspects

Participation in physical activity is important for every client with MD, for it is one of the few areas in which an afflicted person can feel a sense of control and self-direction. This allows a sense of self-determination and control over a disorder that often takes away their independence. Daytime somnolence is a particular factor in myotonic MD that may be correlated with a motivational personality. It is important to provide follow-up and support, particularly in the initial stages of the program, to enhance compliance and success.

CASE STUDY Limb Girdle Muscular Dystrophy

A 45-year-old male was diagnosed with autosomal dominant LGMD 10 years ago, after he had noted difficulty running around the bases in a baseball league. He stopped all activities because he was told that exercise would make his disease worse. Since then, he had gained 25 pounds and developed increasing difficulty climbing up the 10 steps to his bedroom (initially he was fatigued, then his legs became heavy). He required the use of his arms to pull himself up the stairs. He also had osteoarthritis in the knees, but was otherwise healthy and did not smoke.

S: "I'm afraid I'll have to sell my house and move to a single-floor dwelling."

O: Vitals: Height: 5'7" (1.7 m)   Weight: 198 lb (89.9 kg)   BMI: 31.1 kg/m²

Normal mental status, cranial nerves, reflex and sensory exam

Motor exam: Shoulder abductors 4/5; hip flexors 3/5; neck extension 4/5

More distal muscles graded at >4+/5

Routine blood tests (CBC, electrolytes, creatinine, BUN, and liver function): Normal

Serum CK: 430 U/l (normal: < 230 U/l).

Spirometry: Normal

Grip strength: Right 35 kg (77 lb); left 32 kg (70.5 lb) (normal)

Isometric knee extension: Right 5 kg (11 lb); left 4 kg (8.8 lb) (>2 SD below lower limit of normal)

A: 1. LGMD limiting ADLs (stair climbing)

2. Obesity

3. Osteoarthritis (knees)

P: 1. Increase strength in the limb and knee extensors.

2. Prescribe dietary counseling for weight loss.

(continued)

CASE STUDY **Limb Girdle Muscular Dystrophy** (continued)

Exercise Program

Goals:

1. Ability to ascend stairs
2. Increased knee extensor strength
3. Weight loss

Mode	Frequency	Duration	Intensity	Progression
Aerobic (cycling)	3 days/wk	8 min/session	THR (>120 contrac-tions/min)	Increase to 15-20 min @ HR > 140 contrac-tions/min, as tolerated
Strength (isometric knee extensions)	3 days/wk	1 set of 12 reps	40% of 1RM	Increase to 3 sets, 12 reps @ 70% of 1RM
Flexibility (all major muscle groups)	Daily	20-60 s/stretch	Maintain stretch below discomfort point	
Neuromuscular				
Functional				
Warm-up/Cool-down	Before and after each session	10-15 min	RPE <10/20	

Follow-Up

He developed some knee pain when he first increased to 70% of 1RM; however, this resolved with 1 week of decreasing to 60% and an occasional acetaminophen. After 12 weeks, he could climb stairs without using his arms. His isometric knee extension strength improved to (right) 8 kg (17.6 lb) and (left) 7 kg (15.4 lb) by dynamometry. Grip strength and weight were unchanged, but he decreased to 25% body fat.

Suggested Readings

Aitkens, S.G., M.A. McCrory, D.D. Kilmer, and E.M. Bernauer. 1993. Moderate resistance exercise program: Its effect in slowly progressive neuromuscular disease. *Archives of Physical Medicine and Rehabilitation* 74: 711-15.

Bar-Or, O. 1983. *Pediatric sports medicine for the practitioner.* New York: Springer-Verlag.

Bar-Or, O., and S.L. Reed. 1987. Rating of perceived exertion in adolescents with neuromuscular disease. In *Perception of exertion in physical work,* edited by G. Borg, 137-48. Stockholm: Wenner-Gre.

Brooke, M.H. 1986. *A clinician's view of neuromuscular diseases.* 2nd ed. Baltimore: Williams & Wilkins.

DeLateur, B.J., and R.M. Giaconi. 1979. Effect on maximal strength of submaximal exercise in Duchenne muscular dystrophy. *American Journal of Physical Medicine* 58: 26-36.

Florence, J.M., and J.M. Hagberg. 1984. Effect of training on the exercise responses of neuromuscular disease patients. *Medicine and Science in Sports and Exercise* 16: 460-65.

Fowler, W.M., Jr. 1988. Management of musculoskeletal complications in neuromuscular disease: Weakness and the role of exercise. *Archives of Physical Medicine and Rehabilitation* 2: 489-507.

Gozal, D., and P. Thiriet. 1999. Respiratory muscle training in neuromuscular disease: Long-term effects on strength and load perception. *Medicine and Science in Sports and Exercise* 31: 1522-27.

Mendell, J.R., R.T. Moxley, R.C. Griggs, M.H. Brooke, G.M. Fenichel, J.P. Miller, W. King, L. Signore, S. Pandya, J. Florence et al. 1989. Randomized, double-blind six-month trial of prednisone in Duchenne's muscular dystrophy. *New England Journal of Medicine* 320: 1592-97.

Milner-Brown, H.S., and R.G. Miller. 1988. Muscle strengthening through high-resistance with training in patients with neuromuscular disorders. *Archives of Physical Medicine and Rehabilitation* 69: 14-19.

Scott, O.M., S.A. Hyde, C. Goddard, R. Jones, and V. Dubowitz. 1981. Effect of exercise in Duchenne muscular dystrophy. *Physiotherapy* 67: 174-76.

Tarnopolsky, M., and T.J. Doherty. 2002. Muscular dystrophy and other myopathies. In *ACSM's resources for clinical exercise physiology: Musculoskeletal, neuromuscular, neo-*

plastic, immunologic, and hematologic conditions. Edited by J.N. Myers, W.G. Herbert, and R. Humphrey, 78-88. Philadelphia: Lippincott Williams & Wilkins.

Tarnopolsky, M., and J. Martin. 1999. Creatine monohydrate increases strength in patients with neuromuscular disease. *Neurology* 52: 854-57.

Tirosh, E., O. Bar-Or, and P. Rosenbaum. 1990. New muscle power test in neuromuscular disease: Feasibility and reliability. *American Journal of Diseases of Children* 144: 1083-87.

Tollback, A., S. Eriksson, A. Wredenberg, G. Jenner, R. Vargas, K. Borg, and T. Ansved. 1999. Effects of high resistance training in patients with myotonic dystrophy. *Scandinavian Journal of Rehabilitation Medicine* 31: 9-16.

Walter, M.C., H. Lochmuller, P. Reilich, T. Klopstock, R. Huber, M. Hartard, M. Hennig, D. Pongratz, and W. Muller-Felber. 2000. Creatine monohydrate in muscular dystrophies: A double-blind, placebo-controlled clinical study. *Neurology* 54 (9):1848-50.

CHAPTER 39

Epilepsy

Lorraine E. Colson Bloomquist, EdD, FACSM
University of Rhode Island

Overview of the Pathophysiology

Epilepsy, or convulsive or seizure disorder, is a chronic, neurological condition characterized by temporary changes in the electrical function of the brain. Transmission of information between nerve cells occurs by electrochemical process, so these abnormal electrical patterns in the brain activity result in seizures. During a seizure, several aspects of mental function can be affected, including awareness, movement, sensation, or a combination of these three. Epilepsy is feared by many people and can be inappropriately associated with negative connotations. This is unfortunate because the average person with epilepsy is of normal intelligence.

The National Institute of Neurological Disorders and Stroke (NINDS) estimates that:

- seizure disorders affect about 1% of the U.S. population (about 2.5 million people);
- approximately 10% of the population will have a seizure in their lifetime; and
- 3% will develop epilepsy.

The cause of epilepsy is unknown in about 80% of cases. Nonetheless, common causes for the other 20% include head trauma, tumors, infections, strokes, anoxia, and lead poisoning. Epilepsy is not inherited but may be a genetic predisposition and occurs in all ages and races. People with mental retardation or cerebral palsy may be prone to seizures.

Symptoms of epilepsy (in addition to seizures) include headache, changes in mood or energy, dizziness, fainting, confusion, memory loss, and babbling. An aura (e.g., a few seconds' warning) may signal seizure activity. Auras may include dizziness, tingling, peculiar smell or taste, a feeling of euphoria, auditory hallucination, and/or painful sensations.

Accurate diagnosis of epilepsy by a neurologist is critical to achieving successful treatment. Diagnostic methods may include blood tests and procedures such as CT scan, EEG, magnetic resonance imaging (MRI), and lumbar puncture (spinal tap). A physical examination and tests should be done to rule out other temporary and reversible causes of seizures. For example, both extremely low blood pressure and low blood sugar can cause seizures, but neither is considered a seizure disorder because treating the main problem (e.g., hypotension or diabetes) will prevent future seizures. To be diagnosed with epilepsy, a person must have had at least two documented seizures initiated by neurological causes.

Types of Seizures or Convulsions

There are more than 20 identified types of seizures, but the most common are generalized tonic clonic, absence, and complex partial, described in the following list. Other less common forms of seizures include simple partial, partial seizures with secondary generalization, tonic, atonic, myoclonic, and unclassified forms.

- Generalized tonic clonic (grand mal): Average duration is 70 ± 20 s, with loss of consciousness, sudden cry, fall, rigidity (tonic), erratic muscle contractions or jerks (clonic), possible incontinence, rapid heart rate, and cyanotic with blue lips or fingernails. The person may sleep or be difficult to arouse after the seizure, known as the postictal period.

- Absence (petit mal): Average duration is 3 to 10 s, and may include a blank stare, grimace, chewing, rapid eye blinks, or lack of awareness of surroundings. The person with absence seizures quickly becomes alert once the seizure stops but may have successive episodes.

- Complex partial (psychomotor or temporal lobe): Average duration is 1 to 5 min, and may include an aura, blank stare, chewing, lack of awareness of surroundings, wandering, acting dazed, mumbling, picking at clothing, trying to remove clothes, or being afraid and struggling. Postictal confusion can last a while and persons may not remember what they were doing.

Seizure Treatment

Medications, a ketogenic diet, vagus nerve stimulation, and surgery are various forms of treatment. See Management and Medications for immediate first aid (or for more information, go to the Epilepsy Foundation of America Web site: **www.efa.org**).

Effects on the Exercise Response

Exercise professionals should know that, with common sense and some restrictions, persons with seizures can participate in almost all sports and physical activities. The critical factor is that seizures be kept under control. The main worry is that persons would be doing something that could risk bodily harm if they had a seizure (e.g., racing cars, skydiving).

Activities not recommended are boxing, swimming under water, and soccer (because of heading). Those activities requiring special monitoring include swimming and anything from heights (e.g., rock climbing, rope climbing, spring board diving, balance beam, uneven bars, high bar, horseback riding).

Seizures rarely occur during exercise or activity itself, but rather after its completion or during rest. Regular exercise often inhibits seizure activity. Theories for this

phenomenon are that lowered blood pH (alkalosis), beta-endorphin release, and increased mental alertness and attention suppress the electrical activity. In addition, regular mental activity tends to decrease seizure frequency.

Precipitating factors to a seizure can include great excitement, frustration, anger or fear, strobe lights, hypoglycemia, hypoxia, changes in woman's menstrual cycle, hyperthermia, extreme fatigue, hyperventilation prior to breath holding (especially prior to swimming under water), breath holding during weightlifting, excessive alcohol intake, and a high blood pH (alkalosis).

Effects of Exercise Training

Because people with convulsive disorders are often overprotected, usually living a sedentary lifestyle and not being allowed to do "normal" activities, they tend to be physically unfit and avoid sports participation. Poor cardiorespiratory development from inactivity appears to be related to the frequency of seizures. The physiologic response and fitness improvements to exercise training should be the same as those of any other person at similar fitness levels.

Epilepsy: Exercise Testing

Methods	Measures	Endpoints*	Comments
Aerobic Cycle (ramp protocol 17 watts/min; staged protocol 25 watts/3 min stage) Treadmill (1-2 METs/stage)	• 12-lead ECG, HR • BP • RPE (6-20)	• Serious dysrhythmias • >2 mm ST-segment depression or elevation • Ischemia • T-wave inversion with significant ST change • SBP > 250 mmHg or DBP > 115 mmHg • Volitional fatigue	• Testing and screening may be warranted if risk factors/symptoms of CAD are present (see chapter 4 exercise testing table).
Muscular endurance and power 6- and 12-min walks	• Distance	• Time	• Useful for measurement of improvement throughout conditioning program.
Strength Free weights, machines	• 1RM or maximal voluntary contraction		

*Measurements of particular significance; do not always indicate test termination.

Medications	Special Considerations
• Phenobarbital, Dilantin, Depakote: Possible side effects include lethargy, incoordination, tremors, weight changes, liver damage, inattention, and rash.	• Know seizure first aid, learn medications used and time to be taken, know testing or exercise following a seizure, monitor after exercise for possible seizure.

Management and Medications

The best management is prevention. Discuss and plan the procedure preferred by an adult client. For example, if a person experiences an aura prior to a seizure, provide a mat or a place to go lie down and rest. Sufficient sleep and good nutrition are necessary. It is important that the person has his or her medicine available and that it is taken on time. Medic alert identification is also recommended. Assuring clients that they are safe and being monitored by caring, knowledgeable professionals is important to success.

Basic first aid for seizures is important in professional exercise training. General and immediate first-aid procedures for tonic clonic and absence seizures are provided here.

Tonic clonic

- Keep calm, and *do not* attempt resuscitation until the seizure is over.
- Try to break a fall to prevent the head from being struck.
- Place the person on his or her back, protecting under the head with a towel or jacket.
- Clear the area.
- Loosen the person's tie, belt, and collar.
- Place the person's head to the side or roll the person on his or her side to drain saliva.

- Keep your hands away from the person's teeth.
- *Do not* administer liquids.
- If the seizure lasts longer than three min, call an ambulance.
- If a second seizure begins soon after the first has ceased, call an ambulance.
- If the seizure occurs in water, call an ambulance (there is a danger of water aspiration).
- Look for medical identification (e.g., medic alert ID).
- Observe that the person is breathing.

Absence

- Do not touch, but observe the person's movement.
- Keep the person away from the pool side, the top of stairs, or anywhere he or she could fall.
- Remove harmful objects in the area.
- Speak quietly and in a friendly manner.
- Stay with the person until full consciousness returns.

After a seizure, arrange for safe transportation and follow-up evaluation by medical staff.

The National Epilepsy Foundation lists 26 anticonvulsant medications (or anti-epileptic drugs [AEDs]) used for people with epilepsy. Some persons require more than one drug to control their seizures. Commonly used medications include:

- Dilantin (phenytoin);
- Tegretol (carbamazepine);

Epilepsy: Exercise Programming

Modes	Goals	Intensity/ Frequency/Duration	Time to Goal
Aerobic • Large muscle activities (walking, biking, rowing, swimming, jogging— whatever the client enjoys most)	• Increase $\dot{V}O_2$peak, work rate, and endurance	• 60-90% peak work rate • 3-5 days/wk • 20-40 min/session • Progressively increase intensity and duration	• 4-6 mo
Strength • Isotonic/Isokinetic exercises	• Improve general fitness • Prevent muscle atrophy	• Low resistance, high reps to start	

Medications	Special Considerations
• See exercise testing table.	• Avoid boxing, underwater swimming, and soccer (heading). • Monitor swimming, all aquatic activities, and activities performed at heights (e.g., rope climbing, gymnastics, diving, horseback riding). • Normalize program as much as possible.

- Depakene / Depakote (valproic acid);
- Luminol (phenobarbital);
- Zarontin (ethosuximide);
- Klonopin (clonazepam);
- Neurotin (gabapentin); and
- Mysoline (primidone).

Side effects are related to medication used and dosage. Effects are usually seen early when used, or after changes in dosage. Some possible side effects are tremor, dizziness, nausea, vomiting, rash, fatigue, lethargy, increased or decreased appetite, elevated liver enzymes, ataxia, concentration/coordination difficulty, and menstrual changes. Dosage (blood levels) and side effects need to be monitored. Most side effects seen early subside, and many persons experience no side effects.

Recommendations for Exercise Testing

When seizure activity is controlled, any exercise test used with the regular population may be used with epileptics.

Clients should be monitored, especially after testing, for possible seizure activity, but a normal environment is important. Exercise has not been shown to precipitate seizures, but the tester should be alert, especially during maximal testing. Knowledge of medication being taken, the time it is taken, and possible side effects is helpful. Anticipate that the average client is below average fitness level. The client should *not* be tested immediately after a seizure (postictal state) (see the Epilepsy: Exercise Testing table on page 262).

Recommendations for Exercise Programming

If seizures are controlled, the American Medical Association is in favor of allowing epileptics to participate in collision and contact sports. Exceptions and precautions such as monitoring swimming and activities from heights are discussed in Effects on the Exercise Response. Working to help the client feel normal is important for reinforcing a positive self-image. The safest activities for epileptics tend to be individual sports (see the Epilepsy: Exercise Programming table on page 263).

CASE STUDY Epilepsy

A 60-year-old man was a successful teacher when he developed epilepsy. He had several episodes that occurred while operating a vehicle, including driving over a curb and stopping just before hitting a building, driving through an intersection to hit a turning car, and being unaware he had driven off the side of the road. Sometimes he felt tingling on the side of his face and would rub it. Occasionally, he would babble incoherently for several seconds. He had no recall of a 3-month trip to Europe. He had no prior history of seizures, but he had been unconscious as a child after a sledding accident and had played college football with no known head injury. An EEG clearly showed excessive activity on both sides of his brain, the left being more active than the right. An MRI showed no evidence of brain damage. Dilantin and Tegretol both caused him to have a red, itchy rash, but Depakote controlled his seizure activity. He wanted an exercise program to help control his weight and improve his fitness.

S: "I want to get in better shape."

O: Vitals: BP: 130/80 mmHg   HR: 80 contractions/min   Respirations: 14 breaths/min

Elderly male in no distress

Neurological: Cranial nerves intact; slight tremor, mild ataxia, normal sensory/proprioception motor and reflex exam

Lungs: Clear

Heart sounds: Normal without rubs, gallops, or murmurs

Normal peripheral pulses, no edema

Labs:
  ECG: Normal

Graded exercise test (Bruce protocol):
  Exercise tolerance: 5 METs
  Peak HR: 150 contractions/min
  No significant ST changes or dysrhythmias

(continued)

CASE STUDY Epilepsy *(continued)*

Medications: Valproic acid

A: 1. Absence seizures, etiology unknown

2. Deconditioning

P: 1. Monitor blood levels, liver function tests, and side effects.

2. Initiate a walking program.

Exercise Program

Goals:

1. Increase functional capacity

2. Reinforce lifestyle changes/medical management

Mode	Frequency	Duration	Intensity	Progression
Aerobic	3 days/wk	20 min/session	THR (55-70% HRmax) RPE 11-14/20	Increase to 40 min @ 60-70% THR after 12 wk
Strength (all major muscle groups)	3 days/wk	1 set of ≤ 10 reps	50-70% of 1RM	Increase to 2 sets of 10-12 reps after 12 wk
Flexibility (all major muscle groups)	3 days/wk	20 s/stretch	Maintain stretch below discomfort point	Discomfort point should occur at higher ROM
Neuromuscular				
Functional				
Warm-up/Cool-down	Before and after each sesson	10-15 min	RPE <10/20	Maintain

Suggested Readings

Cantu, R. 1998. Epilepsy and athletics. *Clinics in Sports Medicine* 17 (1): 61-69.

Cordova, F. 1993. Epilepsy and sport. *Australian Family Physician* 22: 558-62.

Dunn, J. 1997. Other conditions requiring special consideration in physical education. In *Special physical education,* edited by T. Grutz, 305-308. 7th ed. Madison, WI: Brown & Benchmark.

Ellerstein, B., H.R. Eriksen, R. Hege, D.I. Mostofsky, and H. Ursin. 1993. Exercise and epilepsy. In *The neurobehavioral treatment of epilepsy,* edited by D.I. Mostofsky and Y. Loyning, 107-22. Hillsdale, NJ: Erlbaum.

Epilepsy Foundation of America. Web site: **www.efa.org**.

Epilepsy Foundation of Northeast Ohio. Web site: **www.efneo.org**.

Gates, J. 1993. Epilepsy and sports participation. *Physician Sportsmedicine* 19: 98-104.

Gates, J., and R. Spiegel. 1993. Epilepsy, sports and exercise. *Sports Medicine* 15 (1): 1-5.

Roth, D.L, K.T. Goode, V.L. Williams, and E. Faught. 1994. Physical exercise, stressful life experience, and depression in adults with epilepsy. *Epilepsia* 35: 1248-55.

Schmitt, B., L. Thun-Hohenstein, H. Vontobel, and E. Boltshauser. 1994. Seizures induced by physical exercise: Report of two cases. *Neuropediatrics* 25: 51-53.

Sherrill, C. 1998. Cerebral palsy, stroke, traumatic brain injury. In *Adapted physical activity, recreation and sport,* edited by T. Grutz, 495-499. 5th ed. Madison, WI: Brown & Benchmark.

University of Maryland Medicine: Web site. **www.marylandepilepsy.com**.

van Linschoten, R., F.J. Backx, O.G. Mulder, and H. Meinardi. 1990. Epilepsy and sports. *Sports Medicine* 10: 9-19.

CHAPTER 40

Multiple Sclerosis

Janet A. Mulcare, PhD, FACSM
Andrews University

Overview of the Pathophysiology

Multiple sclerosis (MS) is a demyelinating disease affecting the central nervous system (CNS). The pathological definition of MS includes the demonstration of areas of specific demyelination that are disseminated in both time and space in the white matter of the CNS. The loss of myelin, the fatty material that insulates nerves, adversely affects rapid, smooth conduction along the neural pathways in the CNS. This loss of myelin reduces the speed of conduction, subsequently interfering with smooth, rapid, coordinated movement. As a result, MS-associated problems range from minimal effects to severe disability.

Effects on the Exercise Response

Depending on the level and nature of impairment associated with the disease, individuals may experience a variety of symptoms that may directly affect their responses to a single exercise session. These symptoms may include:

- spasticity;
- incoordination;
- impaired balance;
- fatigue;
- muscle weakness, paresis (partial paralysis), and paralysis;
- sensory loss and numbness;
- cardiovascular dysautonomia (dysfunction of the autonomic nervous system causing possible problem with cardioacceleration and reduction in blood pressure response);
- tremor; and
- heat sensitivity.

Effects of Exercise Training

Exercise training has no effect on the prognosis or progression of MS. However, exercise may improve short-term physical fitness and functional performance (e.g., strength, endurance, aerobic fitness).

- Fatigue can reduce exercise tolerance.
- Impaired balance may affect the choice of exercise mode.
- Heat intolerance may affect intensity, duration, mode, and environmental demands.
- Spasticity may require special foot strapping and may cause hip adduction and abduction.
- Sensory loss may preclude upright activities such as walking or running.
- Muscle paresis can reduce exercise intensity and duration.

Management and Medications

Several new medications are now commonly prescribed to persons immediately following diagnosis of the disease. These drugs include interferon beta-1a, interferon beta-1b, and glatiramer acetate. Clinical trials have shown a reduction in both the number and severity of exacerbations with these drugs. Often, individuals with MS are prescribed various medications simply to manage the symptoms associated with the disease (see the Multiple Sclerosis: Exercise Testing table or a summary of the drugs used with this disease).

Recommendations for Exercise Testing

Common symptoms that affect ambulation (e.g., lower extremity sensory decrement/loss, foot drop, balance difficulty, muscle spasticity, tremor) often make treadmill testing impractical for this population. Therefore, the preferred mode of clinical exercise testing is either upright or recumbent leg cycle ergometry (see the Multiple

Sclerosis: Exercise Testing table). If a combination arm/leg ergometer is available, the increase in activated muscle mass may improve test results by eliciting greater cardiopulmonary stress. In both types of ergometry, toe clips and heel straps are recommended to ensure foot stability and counteract spasticity, tremor, and weakness in the lower extremities. However, it is recommended that arm and leg movements be mechanically linked to reduce the need for motor coordination. Individuals who are more severely impaired with significant lower extremity paresis or paralysis may use arm cranking as a viable alternative to leg cycling. However, the primary problem associated with arm cranking is that arm muscle fatigue occurs before a true cardiopulmonary maximum is elicited.

Other recommendations for performing exercise testing with this population follow.

- Use a continuous or discontinuous protocol of 3- to 5-minute stages.
- Begin with a warm-up of unloaded pedaling or cranking.

- Increase the work rate for each stage by approximately 12 to 25 watts and 8 to 12 watts for legs and arms, respectively.
- Monitor heart rate and blood pressure.
- Typical test termination criteria are volitional fatigue, achievement of maximal heart rate, or decrease/plateau in oxygen consumption ($\dot{V}O_2$) with increasing work rate.

Research has shown that $\dot{V}O_2$peak varies greatly among individuals with MS and is to some extent related to the individual's lower extremity impairment. Because very little data are available that can be reported by gender, age, and impairment level, it is difficult to provide standard values as guidelines. In the absence of cardiovascular dysautonomia or severe muscle paresis, research has shown that most individuals are able to reach 85 to 90% of their age-predicted maximal heart rate. Therefore, this may be a viable means for gauging maximal exercise capacity in the absence of supportive metabolic data.

Multiple Sclerosis: Exercise Testing

Methods	Measures	Endpoints*	Comments
Aerobic Schwinn AirDyne™ Recumbent or semi-recumbent cycle (17 watts/min) Ramp protocol (12-25 watts/3-min stage) Discontinuous protocol (3-5 min/stage)	• Expired gas analysis • HR, rate pressure product • RPE (6-20) • BP	• $\dot{V}O_2$peak, METs • Peak HR • Volitional fatigue • SBP > 250 mmHg or DBP > 115 mmHg • Hypotensive response	• $\dot{V}O_2$peak, METs, and RPE are the best predictors for developing an exercise program because of possible abnormal cardioacceleration responses. • Attenuated BP response may occur.
Endurance Air-Dyne™ or cycle ergometer 6- and 12-min walk tests	• Distance	• Note time, distance, symptoms at rest stops	• Also a good indicator for developing an exercise program.
Strength Isokinetic	• Peak power output and peak torque of major muscle groups		• Has been shown to have moderate correlation with aerobic power.
Flexibility Goniometry	• Angles at full extension/flexion		• Helpful in explaining gait abnormalities.
Neuromuscular Gait analysis Balance (Berg balance scale) Functional reach			• Used to determine and quantify asymmetry, muscle weakness or paresis, and functional changes.

*Measurements of particular significance; do not always indicate test termination.

Medications	Special Considerations
The following drugs are prescribed for relapsing-remitting MS. All reduce the severity and number of exacerbations. • Amantadine: May temporarily reduce fatigue. • Baclofen: High dosage may cause muscle weakness and fatigue. • Amitriptyline, fluoxetine, hyoscyamine sulfate: May cause muscle weakness. • Prednisone: May cause muscle weakness, reduced sweating, hypertension, diabetes, and/or osteoporosis. • Interferon beta-1a (Avonex): May produce flu-like symptoms. • Interferon beta-1b (Betaseron): May produce flu-like symptoms. • Glateramer acetate (Copaxone).	• Prediction of $\dot{V}O_2$peak from submaximal performance has been shown to result in > 15% error in this population. • Patients may experience foot drop, affecting exercise capacity. • Reduced sensation is variable over the extremities; may be symmetrical or asymmetrical. Sensations of numbness and tingling are also common. • Paresis and paralysis are more prevalent in lower extremities and antigravity muscles. • Muscle imbalance may exist between agonist and antagonist muscles. • Some clients may have significant cognitive deficit. This may require careful instructions and cueing during testing. RPE scale may be difficult for them to understand. • Because of difficulty to adjust to temperature change, the testing room should be kept cool or therm neutral. • Incontinence is common. Opportunities for voiding before and during testing should be planned. • Morning is usually the optimal time to test. • If possible, recumbent cycling is desirable over upright cycling because of balance problems. Toe clips or heel straps are needed because of ankle/foot clonus or leg spasticity. • There are no studies examining the effects of these drugs on the exercise response. Flu-like symptoms may reduce exercise tolerance. • Consider controlling resistance in arms and legs separately to minimize premature fatigue.

Recommendations for Exercise Programming

Exercise prescription for individuals with MS should focus on maintenance and, when possible, improvement of their current level of joint flexibility, muscular strength and endurance, and cardiopulmonary endurance. Because fatigue is a common complaint, any intervention that can increase energy by improving efficiency should be incorporated into a well-balanced exercise program. This might include activities related to the areas already mentioned as well as activities that focus on weight control or reduction (see the Multiple Sclerosis: Exercise Programming table).

Special Considerations

When working with a person who has MS, exercise personnel need to keep in mind possible psychological dimensions as well as the variability of progression of the disease itself. There are also considerations relating to safety and the exercise environment. Many individuals with MS have some level of cognitive deficit that will affect their understanding of testing and training instructions. They may also have memory loss sufficient to require written instructions to supplement verbal cues. These individuals may require additional time for information processing as well as multiple forms of information presentation to ensure understanding.

It is common for the symptoms of MS to recur, resulting in progressive impairment. In some individuals, this progression is slow and may take years, while in others the disease may progress significantly within weeks or months. Therefore, the manner in which an exercise program progresses will vary among individuals. During a period of complete remission, persons with MS should be encouraged to follow the guidelines outlined in the exercise programming table. With use of a given target heart rate as a means for tracking physiological responses, work rate can be increased to match training adaptations.

Exercise professionals should be aware of the various symptoms experienced by persons with this disease and

Multiple Sclerosis: Exercise Programming

Modes	Goals	Intensity/ Frequency/Duration	Time to Goal
Aerobic • Cycling • Walking • Swimming	• Increase or maintain cardio-vascular function	• 60-85% peak HR • 50-70% $\dot{V}O_2$peak • 3 days/wk • 30 min/session	• 4-6 mo
Strength • Weight machines • Free weights • Isokinetic machines	• Increase functional capacity	• Do not perform on endurance training days	
Flexibility • Stretching	• Increase or maintain ROM	• Perform before strength or endurance training • 5-7 days/wk	

Medications	Special Considerations
• See exercising testing table. • There are no studies examining the effects of these drugs on exercise response. • Flu-like symptoms may reduce exercise tolerance.	• Incontinence is common. Opportunities for voiding before and during testing should be planned. • Morning is usually the optimal time to test. • If possible, recumbent cycling is preferred over upright cycling because of balance problems. Toe clips or heel straps are needed because of ankle/foot clonus or leg spasticity. • May experience attenuated HR or BP response during exercise. May have attenuated or absent sudomotor response. • Maintaining hydration is critical. • Secondary medical problems are common, with hypertension and obesity being common CAD risk factors. • Much of the disability incurred is also related to secondary deterioration from sedentary lifestyle. • Non-weight-bearing activities should be relegated to clients having balance problems, orthopedic complications, or sensory loss to the lower extremities. • Muscle weakness in the lower extremities often causes premature fatigue. Symptoms may change over the course of the exercise program and may require adjustments of intensity and duration. • Depression may affect adherence, so constant reinforcement and counseling are necessary for some clients.

should recognize the effects such symptoms may have on exercise performance. The exercise professional should also be sensitive to daily variation in symptoms that can be influenced by changes in medications, sleep disorders, and increases in environmental or circadian temperature. Daily training expectations should be flexible to accommodate these factors. Personnel should be knowledgeable regarding transfers, lifting, and assistance techniques for individuals with physical disabilities.

If individuals experience an exacerbation, they should not be encouraged to exercise until the disease status returns to full remission, meaning that the symptoms manifested during the exacerbation have diminished or disappeared. When possible, this should be confirmed by the client's neurologist or primary care physician. Once it is determined that the person is in remission, a new baseline of exercise performance should be established and goals should be adjusted. For the client whose disease is progressing slowly, increased impairment may be very subtle and distinct improvement may not be as obvious. In cases of the progressive non-remitting type of MS, the goal of the exercise program may be simply to slow any further physical deterioration and optimize remaining function.

Some persons with MS have either attenuated or absent sudomotor (sweating) responses. This impairment can further compound the already heightened sensitivity to increases in internal and external temperature that appear to adversely affect many individuals with MS. Therefore, even for moderate-intensity aerobic exercise, room temperature should be kept neutral (72 to 76° F [~20 to 22° C]). Fans should be provided upon request. Persons with MS should be encouraged to drink water before, during, and after each exercise session. For moderate-intensity aquatic exercise, water temperature between 89 and 91° F (~28 and 29° C) is sufficiently comfortable and offers significant heat-dissipating potential. There is some evidence that precooling prior to aerobic exercise may

have a beneficial effect on performance. In contrast, surface cooling during submaximal exercise does not appear to increase exercise time.

The general lack of uniformity among research protocols in this area and the variability in aerobic exercise capacity among persons with MS make it difficult to develop absolute standards for comparison. Therefore, expected outcomes from training are often less evident. Preliminary data show that after a six-mo program of moderate aerobic exercise, individuals with MS may show an average aerobic fitness gain of 30%; however, the variability among individuals is extremely high (i.e., 2 to 54%). Evidence shows that as impairment increases, the magnitude of improvement in training response will be less and the length of time needed to observe improvements will be longer.

CASE STUDY   Multiple Sclerosis

A 42-year-old male with a 13-year history of MS had difficulty walking and had pain caused by spasticity. He had difficulty with most functional activities but required minimal assistance to stand and transfer from his bed to an electric wheelchair. He was concerned about some recent weight gain, and primarily wanted to walk short distances with a cane and control his weight. He had no history of heart disease.

S: "I want to be able to walk by myself."

O: Vitals: HR: 74 contractions/min   BP: 130/82 mmHg

Reduced flexibility of the hamstrings and gastrocnemius and soleus muscle groups

Hip flexion contractures bilaterally

Limited abduction of arms; retraction of shoulders (tight anterior chest muscles)

Strength:
   5/5 upper extremity strength
   3-4/5 strength in both lower extremities (hip flexors, hamstrings and ankle dorsiflexors)
   Marked lower trunk weakness

Motor control:
   Moderate-severe bilateral lower extremity spasticity
   Antigravity muscle dysfunction during reciprocal flexion and extension

Functional activities:
   Ambulated 250 ft (76.2 m) using a walker
   Dragged toes during leg swing

Medications: Baclofen, Betaseron

A: 1. MS with moderate-severe motor dysfunction in lower extremities; weakness and spasticity

2. Deconditioning from chronic inactivity

3. Decreased ROM, global

P: 1. Prescribe a comprehensive exercise program, including stretching, strength training, and aerobic exercise.

Exercise Program
Goal:
   Independent ambulation (as far as possible)

(continued)

CASE STUDY Multiple Sclerosis *(continued)*

Mode	Frequency	Duration	Intensity	Progression
Aerobic (recumbent cycling, treadmill [harness], Schwinn Air-Dyne™)	Daily	20-30 min/session	THR (60-85% of maximal HR)	As tolerated to 30-40 min
Strength (leg press, partial squats, arm/leg raises [on hands and knees, hook lying])	2-3 days/wk	1-2 sets of 10-12 reps	To fatigue	Increase to 2-3 sets as tolerated
Flexibility (positional stretching)	Daily	1 min for normal muscles; 20 min for contracted muscles		
Neuromuscular				
Functional				
Warm-up/Cool-down	Before and after each session	5-10 min		

Special Considerations

- Toe clips are needed during pedaling.
- Positional stretches of ≥ 20 min are required for plastic deformation of muscle contractures muscles.
- Harness/partial body weight support facilitates longer exercise duration and reduces fear while walking.
- Reverse pedaling with resistance improves hip and ankle flexor strength for walking.

Suggested Readings

Mulcare, J.A., and J.H. Petajan. 2002. Multiple Sclerosis. In *ACSM's resources for clinical exercise physiology: Musculoskeletal, neuromuscular, neoplastic, immunologic, and hematologic conditions.* Edited by J.N. Myers, W.G. Herbert, and R. Humphrey. 29-37. Philadelphia: Lippincott Williams & Wilkins.

Petajan, J.H. 2000. Weakness. In *Multiple sclerosis: Diagnosis, medical management, and rehabilitation*, edited by J.S. Burke and K.P. Johnson. New York: Demos.

Petajan, J.H., E. Gappmaier, A.T. White, J.K. Spencer, L. Mino, and R.W. Hicks. 1996. Impact of aerobic training on fitness and quality of life in MS. *Annals of Neurology* 34: 432-41.

Ponichtera-Mulcare, J.A. 1993. Exercise and multiple sclerosis. *Medicine and Science in Sports and Exercise* 25: 451-65.

Ponichtera-Mulcare, J.A., T. Mathews, P.J. Barrett, and R.M. Glaser. 1997. Change in aerobic fitness of patients with multiple sclerosis during a 6-month training program. *Sports Medicine Training and Rehabilitation* 7: 265-72.

Ponichtera-Mulcare, J.A., T. Mathews, R.M. Glaser, and S.C. Gupta. 1995. Maximal aerobic exercise of individuals with multiple sclerosis using three modes of ergometry. *Clinical Kinesiology* 49 (1): 4-12.

Schapiro, R.T. 1987. *Symptom management in multiple sclerosis.* New York: Demos.

CHAPTER 41

Polio and Post-Polio Syndrome

Thomas J. Birk, PhD, MPT, FACSM
Wayne State University

Overview of the Pathophysiology

Poliomyelitis is an acute viral disease that attacks the anterior horn cells of lower motor neurons. This results in a flaccid paresis/paralysis and atrophy in affected muscle groups. Recovery from the self-terminating disease is generally good, and most individuals with polio lead active and productive lives. However, up to 40 years after contracting acute poliomyelitis during peak epidemic periods, at least one-fourth of the affected population have developed symptoms similar to those of the initial onset of the disease. Common symptoms include fatigue, weakness, and muscle and joint pain. Other symptoms include sleep disorders and intolerance of cold. The collection of these symptoms has been termed post-polio syndrome (PPS). Paramount to the diagnosis is new and increasing pain and weakness. New pain and weakness coupled with positive EMG and nerve conductin velocity findings facilitate greater diagnostic accuracy.

Apparently, the muscle weakness is secondary to chronic overload and eventual loss of motor units through the aging process. When a critical level of less than 50% of the original total number of motor units is reached, symptoms of fatigue, weakness, and pain become apparent. Other factors contributing to weakness, fatigue, and pain include excessive body fat (overloading already weakened leg muscles) and repetitive physical tasks (overloading a smaller muscle mass).

Effects on the Exercise Response

The majority of persons with PPS whose lower extremities have been affected will have altered acute responses to exercise. They can be expected to exhibit significantly diminished leg strength and aerobic capacity when compared with asymptomatic post-polio individuals of similar age. This appears secondary to a loss of motor units whereby fewer motor units can be activated to generate muscle tension, resulting in diminished strength and endurance. Thus, an additional burden is placed on the remaining motor units, and this can hasten onset of fatigue. Aerobic power is diminished in many persons with PPS and appears to be related to muscle weakness and deconditioning. A lack of lower extremity muscle strength also limits walking speed.

Labile exercise blood pressures are potential risks that should be initially monitored. Secondary to premature peripheral fatigue, maximal heart rates are usually 20 to 30 contractions/min less than what would be expected for asymptomatic post-polio persons of similar age. Concomitantly, maximal oxygen consumption ($\dot{V}O_2$max) is typically up to 20% lower than what would be seen for similarly aged counterparts.

Effects of Exercise Training

Although there are few well-controlled prospective studies, the literature suggests that lower extremity strength and aerobic capacity can be significantly increased in persons with PPS. The relative improvements in aerobic capacity have equaled those for asymptomatic post-polio persons of similar age. However, complications of prolonged high-intensity exercise were joint edema, possible deformity, and general muscle discomfort. Consequently, the best results were achieved at moderate intensities. Documented beneficial changes in stable PPS include:

- increases of 15 to 20% in aerobic capacity with moderate-intensity exercise after at least eight weeks of training; and
- increases in quadriceps and hamstring muscle strength after at least six weeks of moderate to hard resistive training.

Management and Medications

Primary means of managing and treating PPS have included energy conservation, bracing/splinting, and medication. Strength and moderate-intensity aerobic exercise training have been used as adjunctive therapy. For conservation of energy, it is advisable to perform exercise testing and training in the morning of relatively nonstressful days to avoid physical overstressing and effort overextending. To avoid excessive fatigue, encourage the use of a wheelchair or scooter if long periods of standing and/or walking are anticipated or planned.

Some guidelines for bracing and splinting follow.

• Support the joint around which muscles have significantly weakened and when abnormal structural problems indicate excessive "wear and tear."

• Fitting and braces/splints should allow for sufficient range of motion during exercise.

• Braces and splints increase muscular efficiency during activities of daily living, not during exercise.

• Fasten one or more limbs to ergometer pedals or cranks when necessary.

Medications are prescribed by a physician for pain, chronic fatigue, and sleep disorders. Nonsteroidal anti-inflammatory drugs and muscle relaxants have been used to reduce symptoms of peripheral pain. Antidepressants (e.g., Elavil, Pamelor, Sinequan, Prozac, Zoloft) inhibit neurotransmitters (norepinephrine, serotonin), decreasing fatigue and improving sleep. These medications, particularly the tricyclic antidepressants such as Elavil, may increase heart rate and decrease blood pressure during rest and exercise. Electrocardiogram abnormalities have included false positive and false negative exercise test results, as well as possible T-wave changes and dysrhythmias, especially in persons with a cardiac history. Exercise may help to alleviate some of the prevalent anticholinergic side effects such as constipation and lethargy. The therapeutic effect of these medications may be delayed from 2 to 4 weeks after the beginning of therapy.

Bromocriptine mesylate, a postsynaptic dopamine receptor agonist, has inhibited early-morning fatigue in one report but has not been used with exercise. Pyridostigmine, an anticholinesterase drug, has been purported to diminish fatigue but significant results are as yet lacking.

Recommendations for Exercise Testing

Exercise testing of persons with PPS should incorporate the following principles:

• optimally utilize available muscle mass;

• avoid use of a painful and/or recently weakened limb during an exercise test;

• use equipment that does not require complex motor coordination; and

• use submaximal exercise tests.

Four-limb ergometry is preferred, but for persons with severe lower limb involvement, an arm crank ergometer is recommended (see the Polio and Post-Polio Syndrome: Exercise Testing table on page 274). Four-limb ergometry activates the greatest possible muscle mass, and if necessary the use of a painful and/or recently weakened limb or muscle group can be minimized while the other limbs are still allowed to exercise. Because it increases the active muscle mass, use of a four-limb ergometer presents a greater challenge for the cardiopulmonary system. The four-limb ergometer should include a cycling mechanism for the legs and either a cycling or push/pull mechanism for the arms. Work rate should be measurable, accurate, and repeatable.

Although the treadmill is most commonly used by those without PPS, it is less preferred as a means of graded exercise testing for people with PPS, even though the majority are ambulatory. Typically, a symptomatic and weakened lower extremity will fatigue locally before cardiopulmonary systems are challenged.

The testing protocol should deviate from standard procedures by using a submaximal intensity over an increased period of time. Although some persons with PPS can be maximally tested, excessive residual fatigue and possible further reduction of motor units could result from excessive maximal testing.

A submaximal intensity eliciting at least a "somewhat hard" rating of perceived exertion, performed continuously for at least six minutes, facilitates an accurate estimation of aerobic fitness while minimizing possible motor unit damage. Terminating the test at a "hard" rating of perceived exertion (15/20) should enable the tester to challenge the cardiopulmonary system to reach 85% of age-predicted maximum heart rate. If 85% is not reached and coronary artery disease is not suspected, an additional stage of higher intensity can be used and should not unduly debilitate the subject unless new and increasing peripheral pain and weakness were present prior to testing.

Exercise MET values may range from 2 to 9 METs, depending on the limitation of skeletal muscle. Heart rate responses to acute maximal exercise may range from 120 contractions/min (for elderly persons using only the arms) to 175 to 180 contractions/min (for middle-aged persons using all four limbs). Both exercise systolic and diastolic blood pressures are generally similar to those observed for post-polio persons without PPS. Blood lactate concentration responses may range from 2 to 8 mmol/l during exercise testing. Ventilatory responses during exercise are approximately 10 to 20% lower than those observed in asymptomatic post-polio persons of similar age. Ratings of perceived exertion tend to focus on the peripheral component reflecting peripheral muscular fatigue. Consequently, the most limiting factors appear to be peripheral fatigue and pain, as opposed to central cues such as dyspnea. Premature muscle fatigue and low $\dot{V}O_2$max explain the lower maximal ventilation. Peak external power outputs during four-limb ergometry range from 15 to 200 watts.

Exercise testing considerations may include utilization of stirrups and/or straps for pedals and straps/gloves for hands on the handlebars or arm crank handles. These adaptations will secure weakened limbs to equipment, thus providing more efficient application of force and protection of impaired limbs. Discontinuous protocols are advised for individuals with chronically weakened muscles because this facilitates higher central physiological responses while delaying fatigue of exercising muscles.

Polio and Post-Polio Syndrome: Exercise Testing

Methods	Measures	Endpoints*	Comments
Aerobic Schwinn Air-Dyne™ (or any upper/lower limb ergometer) Arm ergometer	• $\dot{V}O_2$ peak, physical work capacity • 12-lead ECG, HR • BP • RPE (6-20) • METs	• Serious dysrhythmias • >2 mm ST-segment depression or elevation • Ischemic threshold • T-wave inversion with significant ST change • SBP > 250 mmHg or DBP > 115 mmHg • Volitional fatigue	• Use only if diagnosed CAD or related symptoms are present. • Calculate efficiency index. • Estimates functional capacity and predicts type or amount of ADLs and occupational tasks possible.
Endurance 6- and 12-min walk 1-mi (1.6K) walk	• Distance • Time	• Note time, distance, symptoms at rest stops	• Can be adopted as a fitness indicator. • 1-mi (1.6K) walk may be too long in some cases.
Strength Weight machines Dynamometers	• Submaximal endurance of stable and unstable limbs • Maximal voluntary contraction	• Fatigue	• Dynamometer: hip and knee flexion/extension and ankle dorsi- and plantar flexion should be measured; no more than a 6-s effort at 45° angle. • Monitor and document changes caused by intervention or neuromuscular changes.
Flexibility Sit and reach Goniometry	• Distance • Angle at full flexion/extension	• Full ROM • Full ROM	• Sit-and-reach measures middle and lower back flexibility, which is important for static and dynamic balance. • Goniometry measures specific joint active and passive ranges.

(continued)

Polio and Post-Polio Syndrome: Exercise Testing (continued)

Methods	Measures	Endpoints*	Comments
Neuromuscular Gait and balance analyses			• Gait and balance analyses are useful in determining static and dynamic balance and locomotion if ambulatory.
EMG/Nerve conduction studies	• Conduction velocities • Action potential wave forms		• Nerve conduction studies, along with EMG, are useful in diagnosis and prognosis of stable motor units and their available readiness.
Functional Sit to stand	• Balance and symmetry	• 10 reps completed; extensive use of arms; fatigue	• Use for ADLs and occupational tasks.
Lifting	• Balance, symmetry, and safety in techniques	• Potentially poor technique; fatigue	

*Measurement of particular significance; do not always indicate test termination.

Medications	Special Considerations
• Tricyclic antidepressants: Can affect motivation. • Antidepressants (e.g., Elavil, Pamelor, Sinequan, Prozac, Zoloft): Inhibit neurotransmitters (i.e., serotonin, norepinephrine).	• Weakness and pain may be present in the lower limbs of patients with braces or orthotic appliances. • Full or partial loss of sensation as well as fasciculations and paresthesia may be present in lower limbs. • A 4-limb ergometer (e.g., Schwinn Air-Dyne™) with foot straps and/or pegs to rest inactive or nonfunctional limbs should be used. • Consider use of discontinuous protocols in readily fatigued individuals.

Recommendations for Exercise Programming

The primary purpose of an exercise program for individuals with PPS is similar to that for their asymptomatic counterparts: to prevent premature onset of hypokinetic diseases and maintain adequate muscle strength and endurance for occupational and leisure pursuits. However, individuals without PPS can usually perform a wider range of intensities and durations without long-lasting residual complications, whereas the person with PPS usually has a narrower range of acceptable exercise intensities. If persons with PPS overestimate their maximum intensity, they may risk premature acceleration of motor unit loss. The following principles of aerobic exercise prescription are based on symptoms and history. Recent symptoms of pain and weakness warrant a preparticipation medical exam and neuromuscular evaluation (see the Polio and Post-Polio Syndrome: Exercise Programming table on page 276 for specific programming suggestions).

Exercise should involve as much stable musculature as possible. This should include four-limb ergometry, therapeutic aquatics, and other non-weight-bearing activities. Conventional weight-bearing activities such as walking and running may be appropriate for some individuals less involved and without a history of muscle atrophy.

An exercise intensity of 60 to 70% of peak oxygen consumption ($\dot{V}O_2$peak) or moderate-to-somewhat hard ratings of perceived exertion, is recommended if there is no new weakness or symptoms. An intensity of less than 50% of $\dot{V}O_2$peak is recommended if there is recent weakness and/or symptoms. Clients with severe atrophic polio and who have recent weakness should not exercise.

A frequency of 3 sessions/wk is recommended. An alternate-day basis would be optimal to attain beneficial physiological changes without overtaxing the reduced number of motor units.

Polio and Post-Polio Syndrome: Exercise Programming

Modes	Goals	Intensity/ Frequency/Duration	Time to Goal
Aerobic • Schwinn Air-Dyne™ (or any upper and lower limb ergometer) • Arm ergometer	• Increase cardiovascular condition • Increase endurance of stable and maintain unstable limbs • Increase efficiency of ADLs and ambulation	• 40-70% $\dot{V}O_2$peak or maximal HR reserve • 3 days/wk • 20-30 min/session (intervals initially for sedentary clients)	• Indeterminant • Increase, if tolerated, to 40 min continuous
Strength • Isotonic exercises (restrictive devices) • Isometric exercises	• Increase strength of stable and maintain unstable limbs • Increase efficiency of ADLs and ambulation	• 3 sets of 10-15 reps • 2-3 contractions at 67% of 1RM every 20° of ROM of stable musculature/ joints • 3 days/wk	
Flexibility • Stretching (passive)	• Increase ROM (if deficient) • Prevent contractures	• Perform with both stable (unless painful) and unstable (mild intensity) musculature/joints • 5-7 days/wk	

Medications	Special Considerations
• See exercise testing table.	• Spasms and fasciculations (involuntary twitching of muscle fibers) indicate a need to decrease work period and increase recovery period. • Progressive sudden fatigue indicates overly high intensity. • Clients may lack motivation and/or compliance secondary to clinical depression. • Rest periods during the day may be necessary during the initial stages of the exercise program. • Reevaluation recommended every 3-6 mo.

If the client is deconditioned or has been sedentary for more than 1 year and has not had new weakness or symptoms, an initial total exercise duration of up to 20 min/session in 2- to 4-min intervals is recommended. If the client is an irregular exerciser, use less than 25 min/session and divide the session into 5-min intervals or less. If the client is an active regular exerciser, use 30 to 40 min continuously. If weakness and symptoms are recent, 15 total min/session, divided into 3-min intervals, is recommended.

Routine exercise is appropriate in most cases of PPS. Furthermore, some individuals without recent weakness or symptoms but with a history of ventilator use or of four-limb involvement should have a thorough preparticipation medical examination and be supervised for two months to ensure safety. Any questions about exercise prescription should be directed to a physician and appropriately trained health professional. Increased fatigue, weakness, or pain in a particular area should alert the individual to decrease intensity or duration of exercise, or both. If symptoms continue for more than two weeks and are exacerbated by exercise, then exercise should be terminated and appropriate medical follow-up is suggested.

Special Considerations

Most sedentary individuals with PPS are encouraged to consult a physician or appropriately trained health professional before beginning an exercise program. These professionals can supervise and monitor responses to exercise over a two-month period. This will facilitate beneficial physical and psychological tolerance to exercise. Depression has a higher incidence in persons with PPS than in the asymptomatic post-polio population. Appropriate supervision should help the person with PPS not only with the physical but also with the mental obstacles of beginning and continuing an exercise program.

After the initial two-month period of supervision and perhaps follow-up with a health professional, persons with PPS should be able to self-monitor and adjust their exercise program. However, it is recommended that exercisers with PPS perform a submaximal evaluation every 3 to 6 months. This would allow a comparison of responses and help ensure fitness improvement and maintenance. If questions or concerns arise, an appropriately trained health professional should be consulted. The individual's own physician and an ACSM-certified rehabilitation therapist would be appropriate.

CASE STUDY Post-Polio Syndrome

A 47-year-old woman was diagnosed with paralytic polio at age 5. She did not use assistive devices until 2 years ago when balance and ambulation became more difficult. She used crutches for ambulation secondary to left lower extremity weakness, which rapidly and significantly worsened after 3 min of walking. She had gained 20 lb (9.1 kg) over the prior 9 months. She took over-the-counter nonsteroidal anti-inflammatory drugs for lower extremity pain and fatigue (6/10 worst, 3/10 best). She did not exercise regularly, and recently had difficulty with sleep patterns. She was unemployed, and lived with her adult daughter.

S: "My legs get weak after just a little bit of walking."

O: Vitals: Height: 5'2" (1.57 m)   Weight: 187 lb (84.8 kg)   BMI: 34.3 kg/m^2
              HR: 85 contractions/min   BP: 148/86 mmHg

Obese middle-aged female, flat affect but not depressed mood

Stands in lumbar hyperextension with anterior pelvic tilt, mild right lumbar scoliosis

Majority of weight on right side while standing with Lofstrand crutches

Left lower extremity:
  Knee hyperextended, moderate-severe atrophy mid-thigh to ankle, mostly flaccid
  Sensation diminished to light touch, vibration, sharp-dull, and temperature

Reflexes absent

EMG: Significant motor unit amplitude and duration with increased fasciculations (on left)

Passive flexibility: Grossly normal

Active flexibility:
  Hip flexion: 45°
  Hip extension: 20°
  Hip abduction: 20°
  Hip internal rotation: 15°
  Knee flexion: 45°

Balance (standing with crutches): Mild perturbation-step strategy

Sit and reach: 4 in (10.2 cm)

Sit to stand: 3 reps in 45 s before fatigue

Gait (with Lofstrand crutches):
  Ataxic with moderately excessive lumbar pelvic rotation
  Minimal hip extension/flexion
  Knee flexion/extension and heel plant/toe off
  Step and stride length reduced by 75%
  After 1 min, step and stride lengths decrease an additional 15%

Strength:
    Left lower extremity: Grossly 2-2+/5 (3 reps), all movements
    Left lower extremity knee (flexion/extension) and ankle (plantar flexion/ dorsiflexion): Grossly 3/5 (3 reps)
    Pain increased by 3rd rep (from 2/10 to 4/10)
    Right lower extremity: Grossly 4/5 (3 reps), all movements
Aerobic: Estimated max 4 METs

A:
1. PPS of left lower extremity
2. Scoliosis
3. Obesity
4. Exercise intolerance from PPS, obesity, deconditioning

P:
1. Fit for assistive devices:
knee-ankle-foot orthosis, and
electric scooter for ADLs or on feet > 10 min.
2. Prescribe an exercise/rehabilitation program.
3. Dietary counseling is needed for weight loss.

Exercise Program
Goals:

1. Perform ADLs with assistive devices
2. Increase leg strength
3. Decrease leg pain
4. Increase aerobic capacity
5. Weight loss

Mode	Frequency	Duration	Intensity	Progression
Aerobic (Schwinn Air-Dyne™)	3 days/wk	3-4 min/interval; 20 min/session	50-70% of HR reserve	Use lower extremity up to 60 s at a time
Strength (lower extemities, all muscle groups)	Daily	Left: 6 reps, 3 days/wk Right: 70% of 1RM	Left: 40% of 1RM Right: 70% of 1RM	Maintain
Flexibility				
Neuromuscular (rhythmic stabilization/ isometric contractions)	5 days/wk	60 s/stretch	Antigravity	Maintain
Functional				
Warm-up/Cool-down	Before and after each sesson	5-10 min	RPE <10/20	

Follow-Up
Her aerobic capacity increased 15% in 6 weeks without further exacerbation of left lower extremity symptoms. Her left lower extremity increased by 10% after 8 weeks without an increase in pain. Pain at rest decreased to 0-1/10, and after 8 weeks wasn't increased with activity until 15 min of walking. Static balance improved somewhat after 10 weeks.

Suggested Readings

Agre, J.C., and A.A. Rodriquez. 1990. Neuromuscular function: Comparison of symptomatic and asymptomatic polio patients to control subjects. *Archives of Physical Medicine and Rehabilitation* 71: 545-51.

Agre, J.C., A.A. Rodriquez, and T.M. Franke 1997. Strength, endurance, and work capacity after muscle strengthening exercise in postpolio subjects. *Archives of Physical Medicine and Rehabilitation* 78: 681-87.

Birk, T.J. and K.H. Pitetti. 2002. Postpolio and Guillain-Barré syndrome. In *ACSM's resources for clinical exercise physiology: Musculoskeletal, neuromuscular, neoplastic, immunologic, and hematologic conditions*. Edited by J.N. Myers, W.G. Herbert, and R. Humphrey. 68-77. Philadelphia: Lippincott Williams & Wilkins.

Birk, T.J. 1993. Poliomyelitis and the post-polio syndrome: Exercise capacities and adaptations. Current research, future directions, and widespread applicability. *Medicine and Science in Sports and Exercise* 25: 466-72.

Dalakas, M.C., H. Bartfield, and L.T. Kurland. 1995. The postpolio syndrome: Advances in the pathogenesis and treatment. *Annals of the New York Academy of Science* 753: 314-20.

Dean, E., and J. Ross. 1988. Modified aerobic walking program: Effect on patients with post-polio syndrome symptoms. *Archives of Physical Medicine and Rehabilitation* 69: 1033-38.

Einarsson, G. 1991. Muscle conditioning in late poliomyelitis. *Archives of Physical Medicine and Rehabilitation* 72: 11-13.

Grimby, G., G. Einarsson, M. Medberg, and A. Aniansson. 1989. Muscle adaptive changes in post-polio subjects. *Scandinavian Journal of Rehabilitative Medicine* 21: 19-26.

Jones, D.R., J. Speier, J. Canine, R. Owen, and G.A. Stull. 1989. Cardiorespiratory responses to aerobic training by patients with post-poliomyelitis sequelae. *Journal of the American Medical Association* 261: 3255-58.

Spector, S.A., P.L. Gordon, I.M. Feuerstein, K. Sivakumar, B.F. Hurley, and M.C. Dalakas. 1996. Strength gain without muscle injury after strength training in patients with postpolio muscular atrophy. *Muscle and Nerve* 19: 1282-90.

Willen, C., A. Cider, and K.S. Summerhagen. 1999. Physical performance in individuals with late effects of polio. *Scandinavian Journal of Rehabilitative Medicine* 31: 244-49.

CHAPTER 42

Amyotrophic Lateral Sclerosis

Karen Lo Nau White, PhD, PT, FACSM
Oregon State University

Overview of the Pathophysiology

Amyotrophic lateral sclerosis (ALS) is the most common form of motor neuron disease in adults. The primary feature of this progressive disease is degeneration of lower and upper motor neurons. Degeneration of the lower motor neurons results in progressive muscular atrophy and weakness, while degeneration of the upper motor neurons results in spasticity and hyperreflexia. The average age at diagnosis of ALS is 55 years. The mean survival time is 2.5 to 3 years after onset of symptoms, with a range of 6 months to 30 years. While 50% of persons with ALS live less than 3 years after diagnosis, 20% live more than 5 years, and 10% live longer than 10 years. Factors that signify a better prognosis include a younger age and a slower progression of symptoms prior to diagnosis.

The major factor contributing to disability is the muscular weakness consequent to lower motor neuron degeneration. Weakness can occur in any of the skeletal muscles, although the ocular and sphincter muscles are generally spared. Initial signs and symptoms of weakness are typically asymmetric and localized, and typically occur in the muscles of the distal upper or lower extremities, trunk, or bulbar musculature. If weakness is present in one extremity, generally the contralateral side will become affected next. Individuals who present with initial symptoms in the bulbar region (e.g., difficulty enunciating words, chewing, and swallowing) may not have significant extremity weakness until fairly late in their disease progression. Others have significant extremity weakness but never develop bulbar weakness. Problems that occur secondary to the weakness include decreased coordination, endurance, functional ability, and breathing capacity.

Amyotrophic lateral sclerosis is a progressive disease occurring at a steady rate without periods of remission. While an individual's rate of muscular weakness remains fairly constant over time, that rate of decline is highly variable among individuals, with some people losing strength very quickly and others changing so slowly that they remain at a high functional capacity for many years. In addition to differences in the rate of muscle weakness, there is a high degree of variability among individuals with respect to which muscles become affected and in what order they become affected.

Spasticity is a second ALS-related factor that can lead to disability. The increased tone can interfere with coordinated movements and range of motion. It may also lead to increased energy expenditure during activity. A third factor affecting functional ability is diminished pulmonary function secondary to weakness of the diaphragm and trunk musculature. Among individuals with ALS, pulmonary function is one of the best indicators of prognosis and survival time because death typically occurs secondary to a complication of respiratory failure.

During the early phases of ALS, it has been shown that denervated muscle fibers can become reinnervated by neighboring motor units. This process is important in maintaining muscular function for prolonged periods of time and may be a key element in the preservation of function among individuals with slow disease progression. However, one characteristic of the immature neuromuscular junction of the newly reinnervated muscle fiber is that it can experience transmission failure, a problem that does not occur in healthy neuromuscular junctions. This failure causes individuals with ALS to fatigue more quickly than persons without ALS. This is a transient process that repairs itself after a short rest period and results in no permanent damage to the motor neuron. In contrast, there is anecdotal evidence of permanent motor neuron death in severely overexercised muscle groups. This is an extreme and rare phenomenon that may occur because the surviving lower motor neurons become metabolically overtaxed from the severe overuse, causing premature death. For these reasons, individuals with ALS are encouraged to keep active but to rest frequently and avoid extreme overexertion.

Amyotrophic Lateral Sclerosis: Exercise Testing

Methods	Measures	Endpoints	Comments
Aerobic Recumbent cycle ergometer All-extremity ergometer	• HR • RPE (6-20) • BP • METs • $\dot{V}_E$		• Maximal testing is not appropriate for most individuals; submaximal or functional tests are sufficient. • HR and RPE are useful in determining exercise prescription. • BP measurement is useful to screen for hypertension. • METs can be used to estimate functional capacity and to predict the type and amount of ADLs possible. • $\dot{V}_E$ is useful in indicating whether dyspnea will be a limiting factor. • Choose a mode that involves all extremities or the extremities with the greatest function. • Provide trunk support to maximize safety.
Endurance 6-min walk	• Distance	• Note time, distance, symptoms at rest stops	• Use to determine safety and whether assistive devices are necessary.
Strength Weight machines Active ROM with light resistance	• Number of reps • Maximal voluntary contraction		• Expect strength to decrease as the disease progresses. • Test both upper and lower limbs. • Spasticity may influence results.
Flexibility Goniometer	• ROM of major joints		• Especially useful for persons with spasticity to indicate which joints need stretching.
Neuromuscular Gait analysis			• Use to determine safety and whether assistive devices are necessary.
Functional Sit to stand ADLs	• Time • Level of assistance needed	• 10 reps if possible	• Use to determine whether assistive devices are necessary. • Use to determine functional capacity, especially dressing and personal hygiene.

Medications	Special Considerations
•Pyridostigmine (Mestinon): Blocks acetylcholinesterase; may improve endurance. •Baclofen, diazepam, and dantrolene: Reduce spasticity; clients may feel weaker, sedated, or dizzy. •Amitriptyline, doxepin, and imipramine: For emotional stability; can cause sleepiness and decrease motivation. •Riluzole: May prolong survival.	•Orthopedic: Risk of injury due to flaccid limbs (e.g., caught, bumped) with joint discomfort (especially in shoulders), laxity, or stiffness. Constant vigilance is necessary during exercise testing because of muscle weakness and poor balance. •Pulmonary: Decreased pulmonary function (restrictive in nature) secondary to respiratory muscle weakness; decreased vital capacity, inspiratory and expiratory pressures, and reserve volumes. Some positions can limit function. Some clients become very dependent. •Psychological: Clients may be emotionally labile, frustrated, and/or depressed. Decreased motivation may result from lack of improvement despite effort. •Gastrointestinal: Clients may have difficulty chewing and swallowing if bulbar area is affected. Presence of a feeding tube may affect exercise capacity immediately after insertion. •Urologic: Expect occasional urinary urgency.

Effects on the Exercise Response

When an individual with ALS exercises, typically the limiting factor will be that person's muscular strength and endurance. Muscular fatigue will occur before the cardiovascular system reaches its maximal capacity. Persons early in the disease process may still be functioning at near-normal levels and may be able to reach their maximal aerobic capacity, but these individuals are the rare exception. People who have pulmonary deficits may find breathing to be their limiting factor, and symptoms of dyspnea should be monitored closely. Persons with spasticity are limited by their decreased coordination; they may not be able to exercise at speeds fast enough to elicit a cardiovascular response or fatigue their muscles. Decreased coordination and balance secondary to muscular weakness also make many modes of exercise testing unsafe or impractical.

Effects of Exercise Training

There is no evidence that exercise reverses or even slows the progressive denervation caused by ALS. However, anecdotal evidence suggests that a portion of the weakness and atrophy associated with ALS results from disuse, and that this weakness (in innervated muscle fibers) can be minimized. Although the disease process cannot be reversed and the individual with ALS will lose function despite his or her efforts, exercise will strengthen the healthy muscle fibers. This may temporarily lead to a stronger muscle and may permit an individual to maintain

strength and a higher functional level for a longer time. Strengthening the muscles of respiration should likewise optimize the functional ability of the intact fibers and prolong the time before pulmonary impairments become restrictive. Improving or maintaining aerobic endurance may also have a positive impact on functional ability by maximizing the efficiency of the innervated muscle fibers. Maintaining full range of motion in joints that are too weak to be moved actively, or in joints affected by spastic muscles, will minimize pain associated with joint stiffness (e.g., a frozen shoulder) and make it easier for someone else to provide care (e.g., dressing, positioning, transfers) for individuals who can no longer take care of themselves.

Management and Medications

At this time, only one medication, riluzole, has been approved by the FDA for the treatment of ALS. Riluzole has been shown to prolong survival by a few months, a clinically small but statistically significant amount. Several other medications are currently being evaluated in clinical trials. Additional medical management revolves around controlling secondary symptoms. Medications are available to decrease muscle spasticity (e.g., baclofen, diazepam, dantrolene), decrease excessive saliva production (e.g., atropine, scopolamine, diphenhydramine), minimize emotional swings (e.g., amitriptyline, doxepin, imipramine, fluoxetine), suppress fasciculations (e.g., lorazepam), and control the discomfort of joint stiffness (e.g., carbamazepine, phenytoin, amitriptyline,

Amyotrophic Lateral Sclerosis: Exercise Programming

Modes	Goals	Intensity/ Frequency/Duration	Time to Goal
Aerobic •Recumbent cycling and walking	•Maintain work capacity and endurance	•30-50% of peak work rate •Daily •As long as possible without excessive fatigue	•Very short term due to rapid deterioration
Strength •Weight machines •Active ROM exercises	•Maintain strength of arms, legs, and trunk	•1 set of 8-12 reps •Light weights or no resistance •3-5 days/wk •Reduce resistance and reps as weakness progresses	
Flexibility •Stretching •Active and passive ROM exercises	•Increase or maintain ROM	•1-2 sessions/day	
Functional •ADLs	•Maintain capacity to perform as many activities as possible	•ADLs as much as possible when "traditional" exercise program is no longer possible	

Medications	Special Considerations
•See exercise testing table.	•Eventually all goals will have to be decreased as functional ability declines. •Modify goals frequently. •Try to avoid overeating. •Stress that, by doing their own daily living activities, clients are exercising. •Perform all exercise modes as long as possible without causing excessive fatigue. •Frequent rest periods may be necessary throughout the exercise program. •Individuals may be emotionally labile, frustrated, depressed, or discouraged, with little motivation to exercise because of the progressive nature of the disease. •Adapted or support equipment may be needed because of muscle weakness and reduced balance. •Ideally, exercise programs should be managed in conjunction with a trained medical professional, such as a physical or occupational therapist, who is familiar with the unique and progressive nature of ALS.

nortriptyline). Be aware that medications to reduce spasticity can increase weakness, sedation, and dizziness while antidepressant agents can cause hypotension and sedation. Other therapeutic interventions may include

- recommendations for adaptive equipment and assistive devices;

- nutritional supplementation and the placement of a feeding tube for those with bulbar involvement;

- a ventilator for those with severe respiratory muscle weakness;

- emotional support and counseling for the individual and the family;

- arrangements for home health personnel to assist with care giving; and
- discussion of issues related to dying (e.g., hospice, use of a ventilator, taking a patient off a ventilator, the use of lifesaving techniques).

Recommendations for Exercise Testing

Participant safety is one of the key elements to consider when exercise testing individuals with ALS. If the person has diminished balance or coordination, an exercise mode that will maximize safety and functional ability should be used (see the Amyotrophic Lateral Sclerosis: Exercise Testing table on page 281). Equipment may have to be modified to increase support. For more involved individuals, assessing their ability to complete functional tasks may be the most useful method of exercise testing. As a matter of fact, functional assessment is one of the primary tools for monitoring ALS progression. Results from exercise testing will be highly variable, depending on the phase of disease progression, from near normal to severely compromised. Before beginning a test, ask the individual about his or her daily activities to develop an estimation of functional capacity. This will help determine an appropriate exercise test protocol.

Recommendations for Exercise Programming

The purpose of an exercise program for people with ALS is to maximize the functional capacity of the innervated muscle fibers, to prevent limitations in range of motion, and to maximize aerobic capacity, endurance, and functional level for as long as possible. Modest improvements may occur in these parameters at the onset of an exercise program, but it is more realistic to expect all parameters to decline in spite of the exercise program. Because disease progression cannot be stopped and functional capacity will decline, the overall goal of an exercise program is to maintain a higher functional level than the person would have otherwise. Specific goals must be constantly modified to adapt to the progressive nature of the disease.

Individuals with ALS will become weaker and more limited despite any type of exercise program. This must be understood and accepted by both the health professional and the individual with ALS. Exercise is only beneficial when it does not cause excessive fatigue in the participant. Once exercise becomes so tiring or so difficult that it prevents someone from completing activities of daily living, it is no longer appropriate. Excessive fatigue may be detrimental to individuals with ALS; therefore, they need to be active enough to minimize disuse atrophy but cautious enough to avoid overexertion (see the Amyotrophic Lateral Sclerosis: Exercise Programming table on page 283).

Special Considerations

Little research is available on the effects of regular exercise on individuals with ALS. Therefore, specific exercise recommendations are not possible; however, common sense and moderation will be key elements of any exercise program. Goals should be practical, intensity and duration should be moderate, rest periods should be frequent, and expectations should be kept realistic. Disease progression cannot be stopped or even slowed down; exercise will affect only innervated muscle fibers.

Exercise is not appropriate for all people with ALS, and eventually all with the disease will come to the point where they should stop exercising. The people who will benefit the most from an exercise program are those in the early phases of the disease and those with a slow rate of disease progression. Ideally, exercise programs should be managed in conjunction with a trained medical professional, such as a physical or occupational therapist, who is familiar with the unique and progressive nature of ALS.

CASE STUDY Amyotrophic Lateral Sclerosis

A 34-year-old man developed upper extremity pain and weakness that progressed over 6 months to the point where he required help with eating, dressing, and grooming. He was diagnosed with ALS. The weakness progressed from shoulder to hand, affecting the left more than the right. At the time of presentation, he denied weakness in the lower extremities and wanted to preserve his strength as long as possible. He was advised that because he was already experiencing significant weakness in his arms, he should not engage in any type of arm resistance exercises. Two months later, he had to stop working when he developed weakness in his legs and physically could no longer do his job. He was advised to discontinue using the ankle weight exercises and was referred for a research study.

(continued)

CASE STUDY Amyotrophic Lateral Sclerosis (continued)

S: "My arms have been weak for a while, but now my legs are getting weak, too. It's happening so fast."

O: Vitals: Weight: 197.5 lb (89.6 kg)   Lean mass: 138.0 lb (62.6 kg)

Visible muscle wasting in all extremities and trunk

Fasciculations in all extremities and in tongue

Maximal isometric strength:
  Knee extension: Right 135.0 lb (61.2 kg); left 146.0 lb (66.2 kg)
  Ankle dorsiflexion: Right 7.5 lb (3.4 kg); left 13.5 lb (6.1 kg)
  Elbow flexion: Right 3.5 lb (1.6 kg); left 7.0 lb (3.2 kg)
  Grip strength: Right 2.5 lb (1.1 kg); left 0 lb (0 kg)

Recumbent cycle (discontinuous protocol, feet strapped to pedals):
  Peak output: 40 watts
  $\dot{V}O_2$peak: 22.5 ml $\cdot$ kg^{-1} $\cdot$ min^{-1}
  Peak HR: 123 contractions/min @ RPE 18/20

A:
1. ALS progressing rapidly
2. Nonambulatory, will soon be wheelchair dependent
3. Resistance training not appropriate
4. Walking and assisted ADLs will not risk excessive fatigue

P:
1. Formulate a low-level activity program to maintain function.
2. ROM exercises will maintain flexibility.

Exercise Program
Goals:

1. Maintain endurance and functional leg strength
2. Maintain trunk strength
3. Maintain passive ROM

Mode	Frequency	Duration	Intensity	Progression
Aerobic				
Strength				
Flexibility (passive: arms; active: legs)	Daily	60 s/stretch	Maintain stretch below discomfort point	Convert to passive stretching when necessary
Neuromuscular				
Functional				
Warm-up/Cool-down				

Follow-Up

In 6 months, he became unable to walk and required moderate assistance for transfers. He developed spasticity in his lower extremities and became completely dependent in all aspects of care. His speech was affected and communication was difficult. His exercise program was limited to passive ROM exercises done daily. Hospice care was recommended.

Suggested Readings

Amyotrophic Lateral Sclerosis Association. 1997. *Living with amyotrophic lateral sclerosis manual series*. Vols. 1-6. Woodland Hills, CA: Amyotrophic Lateral Sclerosis Association. Web site: **www.alsa.org**.

Bohannon, R.W. 1983. Results of resistance exercise on a patient with amyotrophic lateral sclerosis. *Physical Therapy* 63: 965-68.

Dal Bello-Hass, V., A.D. Kloos, and H. Mitsumoto. 1998. Physical therapy for a patient through six stages of amyotrophic lateral sclerosis. *Physical Therapy* 78: 1312-24.

Francis, K., J.R. Bach, and J.A. DeLisa. 1999. Evaluation and rehabilitation of patients with adult motor neuron disease. *Archives of Physical Medicine and Rehabilitation* 80: 951-63.

Jette, D.U., M.D. Slavin, P.L. Andres, and T.L. Munsat. 1999. The relationship of lower-limb muscle force to walking ability in patients with amyotrophic lateral sclerosis. *Physical Therapy* 79: 672-81.

Kent-Braun, J.A., and R.G. Miller. 2000. Central fatigue during isometric exercise in amyotrophic lateral sclerosis. *Muscle Nerve* 23: 909-14.

Pinto, A.C., M. Alves, A. Nogueira, T. Evangelista, J. Carvalho, A. Coelho, M. de Carvalho, and M.L. Saler-Luis. 1999. Can amyotrophic lateral sclerosis patients with respiratory insufficiency exercise? *Journal of Neurological Science* 169: 69-75.

Schiffman, P.L., and J.M. Belsh. 1993. Pulmonary function at diagnosis of amyotrophic lateral sclerosis. *Chest* 103: 508-13.

Simmons, Z., B.A. Bremer, R.A. Robbins, S.M. Walsh, and S. Fischer. 2000. Quality of life in ALS depends on factors other than strength and physical function. *Neurology* 55: 388-92.

CHAPTER 43

Cerebral Palsy

James J. Laskin, PhD, PT
University of Montana

Overview of the Pathophysiology

Cerebral palsy (CP) is a nonprogressive lesion of the brain occurring before, at, or soon after birth that interferes with the normal development of the brain. Cerebral palsy is characterized by limited ability to move and maintain balance and posture because of the damage to areas of the brain that control muscle tone and spinal reflexes. The resulting changes in muscle tone and spinal reflex sequelae depend on the location and extent of the injury within the brain. The medical classification of CP depends on the type of muscle tone and the injury site (see table 43.1).

In the United States, CP is one of the most common physical disabilities, occurring in (depending on the source) 1.5 to 5 of 1,000 live births. This brain injury has two common etiologies:

1. Failure of brain to develop properly:
   • Occurring within the first and/or second trimesters of embryonic development
   • Disruption of normal developmental process, which may be caused by genetic disorder, chromosomal abnormality, or faulty blood supply
2. Neurological disorder:
   • Injury to brain before, during, or after birth

• Lack of oxygen, bleeding in brain, toxic injury or poisoning, head trauma, metabolic disorder, or infection of nervous system

The Cerebral Palsy-International Sport and Recreation Association (CP-ISRA) has developed a classification system based on an individual's "function." This system includes not only those typically medically diagnosed with CP but also people with other conditions characterized by nonprogressive brain lesions (e.g., stroke, traumatic brain injury, tumor). Many Paralympic sports (e.g., swimming and track and field) have moved to a truly functional classification system that deals with sport-specific abilities and is able to classify athletes across disabilities. When discussing CP and exercise, however, the CP-ISRA system allows for the grouping of individuals of similar "abilities" including the following groups:

• **CP1:** Severe spastic or athetoid tetraplegia. The person is unable to propel a manual wheelchair independently and has nonfunctional lower extremities, very poor to no trunk stability, and severely decreased function in the upper extremity.

• **CP2:** Moderate to severe spastic or athetoid tetraplegia. The person is able to propel a manual wheelchair slowly and inefficiently and has differential function abilities between upper and lower extremities, and fair static trunk stability.

• **CP3:** Moderate spastic tetraplegia or severe spastic hemiplegia. The person is able to propel a manual wheelchair independently; may be able to ambulate with assistance; and has moderate spasticity on the lower

Table 43.1 Medical Classification of Cerebral Palsy

Category	Site of injury	Presentation
Pyramidal	Cortical system	Spastic, hyperreflexia, "clasp knife" hypertonia, prone to contractures
Extrapyramidal	Basal ganglia and cerebellum	Athetosis, ataxia, "lead pipe" rigidity, chorea
Mixed	Combination of above	Combination of above

From DeLuca, P.A. 1996. The musculoskeletal management of children with cerebral palsy. *Pediatric Clinics of North America* 43 (5): 1135-50.

extremities, fair dynamic trunk stability, and moderate limitations to function in the dominant arm.

- **CP4:** Moderate to severe spastic diplegia. The person ambulates with aids over short distances and has moderate to severe involvement of the lower extremities, good dynamic trunk stability, and minimal to near-normal function of the upper extremities at rest.

- **CP5:** Moderate spastic diplegia. The person ambulates well with assistive devices, has minimal to moderate spasticity in one or both lower extremities, and is able to run.

- **CP6:** Moderate athetosis or ataxia. The person ambulates without assistive devices and has poor static and good dynamic trunk stability, good upper-extremity range and strength, and poor throwing and grasp and release; lower-extremity function improves from walking to running or cycling.

- **CP7:** True ambulatory hemiplegia. The person has mild to moderately affected upper extremity, and minimal to mildly affected lower extremity.

- **CP8:** Minimally affected diplegia, hemiplegia, athetosis, or monoplegia.

Effects on the Exercise Response

Specific research examining the exercise responses in the individual with CP is quite limited. Historically, the person with CP has not participated in any form of physical fitness program, structured or unstructured. When tested, however, because of the spasticity/athetosis and the inefficient nature of their mobility, these individuals often present with higher than expected exercise response values. In general, the studies that have examined heart rate, blood pressure, expired air, and blood lactate have found that individuals with CP present with higher heart rates, blood pressure, and lactate concentrations for a given submaximal work rate than their able-bodied peers.

Individuals with CP are found to have slightly lower peak physiological responses (10-20%) than able-bodied controls. Reduced mechanical efficiency has also been reported in individuals with CP. This was attributed to the extra amount of energy required to overcome muscle tonus in spastic CP. Physical work capacity has been reported to be as much as 50% lower than that of able-bodied subjects. This appearance of low fitness may be the result of poor exercise habits, difficulty performing skilled movements, contralateral and ipsilateral muscle imbalances, and often poor functional strength. Fatigue and stress are two other factors that have a negative impact on the client's performance. It is not uncommon for a client to report a transient increase in spasticity and incoordination after a strenuous exercise session.

Effects of Exercise Training

Given the nature of this physical disability, there is no reason to expect that persons with CP cannot benefit from a regular program focusing on muscular strength, flexibility, and/or aerobic endurance. With the understanding that the risk for cardiovascular disease and stroke is greater in the sedentary physically disabled individual than in able-bodied counterparts, it is in fact imperative to counsel this population into some form of regular physical activity.

A small but growing body of literature shows that trainability of persons with CP can be achieved. The literature also documents anecdotal evidence of improved sense of wellness, body image, and capacity to perform activities of daily living, as well as the apparent lessening of severity of symptoms such as spasticity and athetosis. Reports from athletes with CP and their coaches consistently demonstrate improved peak oxygen uptake, higher ventilatory threshold, increased work rate at given submaximal heart rates, increased range of motion, improved coordination/skill of movements, and increased strength and muscular endurance, including skeletal muscle hypertrophy. However, many individuals will report an overall attenuation in spasticity with participation in a long-term exercise program. Not only will this decrease in muscle tone allow for improved function, but often the individual will relate a decreased use of their antispasmodic medications. These anecdotal reports are supported by the performances of the athletes at national and international competitions.

Management and Medications

As for any client, appropriate physical screening should be performed to rule out any contraindications or precautions with respect to exercise. These factors should be evaluated on typical health-screening forms and through a basic physical examination. Before the test battery is selected or the exercise prescription is developed, the client's specific needs, goals, and limitations must be addressed. By using the CP-ISRA classification system, the tester/programmer will gain insight into the type and mode of exercise that should be used as well as any special considerations that will help maximize the individual's performance. It is critical for the tester/programmer to consider that the symptoms of spasticity and athetosis increase with stress and fatigue.

Medications may be a confounding factor for exercise testing or development of the exercise prescription. The tester/programmer must be aware of the medication the client is currently using. Seizure or seizure tendencies are present in 60% or more of persons with CP. Anti-seizure medications are commonly prescribed for individuals with CP. Three commonly used drugs to control seizures are phenobarbital, phenytoin, and carbamazepine. Some anti-seizure medications have a depressant effect on the central nervous system, thus blunting the physiologic responses to exercise. The use of carbamazepine is recommended because it has the fewest side effects, which may include mental confusion or irritability, dizziness, nausea, weight loss, and sensitivity to sunburn. It is

Cerebral Palsy: Exercise Testing

Methods	Measures	Endpoints*	Comments

Aerobic
Ambulatory:
  Treadmill
  Cycle ergometer
  Schwinn Air-Dyne™
  Nu-Step™**
Wheelchair user:
  Wheelchair ergometer
  Arm crank ergometer
  Nu-Step™**
  Recumbent bike
	• ECG, HR
	
	• BP
	
	• RPE (6-20)
	• $\dot{V}O_2$max; METs
	• 12-lead ECG
		• Serious dysrhythmia
		• > 2mm ST-segment depression/elevation
		• Ischemic threshold
		• T-wave inversion with significant ST change
		• SBP > 250 mmHg or DBP > 115 mmHg
		
		• Volitional fatigue
			• Use exercise methods that are reciprocal in nature and cadences that are relatively slow if spasticity is a concern.
			• Record current medications/dosages; any change in medication usage may confound test-retest data.

Endurance
Using the methods listed above:
  6- and 12-min walk/push
  1-mi (1.6K) walk/push
  Multistage submaximal protocols
	• Distance
	• HR
	• RPE (6-20)
		• Note vitals, time, distance, symptoms at rest stops	• Same concerns as listed for Aerobic.
			• The specific measure and/or endpoint may have to be individualized.

Strength Free weights Weight machines Hydraulic resistance	• 8RM • 25RM • Number of reps in 1 min	• Volitional fatigue • Increased spasticity • Inability to maintain prescribed pace • Inability to continue to move through full ROM	• Same concerns as listed for Aerobic. • Ensure the client moves through the entire available ROM. • To minimize the effects of spasticity, use a slow cadence; a metronome may help keep the client at the right prescribed pace.
Flexibility Goniometry	• Joint angles at full flexion/extension	• Pain • Increased spasticity	• ROM may be limited due to spasticity, athetosis, and/or contractures.
Neuromuscular Gait Balance	***	***	• These are useful measurements because CP may affect motor regions or pathways in the CNS, which could influence the exercise prescription.

*Measurements of particular significance; do not always indicate test termination.

**Allows for combined upper and lower extremity activity.

***For details, see Umpred, D.A. 2001. *Neurological rehabilitation.* 4th ed. St. Louis: Mosby.

Medications	Special Considerations
• Anti-seizure medications (including phenobarbital, phenytoin, and carbamazepine) and antispasmodic medications: May decrease aerobic capacity and results from other tests because of a decrease in attention span and/or motivation.	• Because of spastic and/or athetoid complications, straps, wraps, or gloves may be required to keep the hands and/or feet secure; watch for pressure areas and/or skin breakdown. Also remember that the client may experience increased spasticity if straps, wraps, or gloves are causing pain or discomfort. • In case of a fall, provide a spotter during treadmill exercise.

Cerebral Palsy: Exercise Programming

Modes	Goals	Intensity/Frequency/Duration	Time to Goal
Aerobic • Ambulatory: Schwinn Air-Dyne™ Any upper and lower limb ergometer • Wheelchair: Arm ergometer	• Increase aerobic capacity and endurance	• 40-85% $\dot{V}O_2$peak or HR reserve • 3-5 days/wk • 20-40 min/session • Emphasize duration over intensity	• Variable
Endurance • Ambulatory: 6- to 15-min walks • Wheelchair: 6- to 15-min pushes	• Improve distance covered	• 1-2 sessions/wk	• Variable
Strength • Free weights or weight machines	• Improve muscle strength of involved and uninvolved muscle groups	• 3 sets of 8-12 reps • 2 days/wk • Resistance as tolerated	• Variable
Flexibility • Stretching (involved and uninvolved joints)	• Improve ROM directly related to capacity for ADLs	• Before and after aerobic and endurance exercise	• Variable

Medications	Special Considerations
• See exercise testing table.	• Duration is more important than intensity for all exercise modes listed. • See exercise testing table.

also important to note that, in some instances, the paradoxical effect of hyperactivity may be a result of these medications.

Antispasmodic and muscle relaxants are two other classes of medications frequently prescribed to individuals with CP. Often with a decrease in muscle tone, the individual is able to perform physical activities with greater ease. However, a serious side effect of these drugs is drowsiness and lethargy. These medications act sys-

temically; therefore, an already low-tone trunk may be compromised in its ability to act as a base of support, thus further limiting extremity function. Increasingly, these medications (specifically baclofen) are being delivered directly via an intrathecal pump. This pump is implanted subcutaneously and does not pose any concern for exercise or exercise testing. However, during the period of time that the dosage is being titrated to maximize the effectiveness of the intervention, the clinician may see marked decreases in muscle tone with corresponding decreased coordination and weakness.

Recommendations for Exercise Testing

There is limited research available to substantiate testing protocols, principles, and techniques for the CP population. The commonly used modalities to test individuals with CP include leg cycle ergometry, Schwinn Air-Dyne™ ergometry, wheelchair ergometry, and the treadmill. Wheelchair ergometry is the preferred mode of testing the cardiorespiratory fitness of nonambulatory individuals with CP. The treadmill will give the optimal response for ambulatory individuals with adequate balance and coordination (see the Cerebral Palsy: Exercise Testing table on page 289).

The selection of testing methods is dependent on the abilities of the client. The principle of specificity is essential to selection of the test method that best complements an individual's physical capacities and is easily tolerated. For the wheelchair user, wheelchair ergometry or arm crank ergometry will be the common choice for testing. The use of personal wheelchairs will increase comfort with and tolerance of testing during wheelchair ergometry. Practice time should be allowed with holding gloves and, in most cases, is necessary to ensure that termination of the exercise test results from cardiorespiratory and muscular limitations and not the condition itself.

Leg cycle ergometry, Schwinn Air-Dyne™ ergometry, or treadmill may be the elected testing method for ambulatory individuals with CP. Balance and coordination are also a concern with ambulatory CP and should be taken into consideration in the choice of the testing method. Clients may be unable to perform leg cycle ergometry because of inadequate hip flexion caused by excessive spasticity, fixed deformities, or both. Practice time should also be allowed when the feet are strapped to the pedals during leg cycle ergometry or Schwinn Air-Dyne™ ergometry.

Recommendations for Exercise Programming

The progressive goal of all exercise training is to improve health and increase daily functional activities. Traditional contraindications for exercise prescription will also apply to the individual with CP. As with exercise testing, research pertaining to exercise prescription for the individual with CP is limited. Because of the nature and variability in presentation of CP, the practitioner will be required to implement some very creative adaptations. The average individual with CP will benefit most from a balanced program of muscular strength, flexibility, and aerobic endurance. The practitioner must take into consideration the client's abilities, interests, and personal goals. Specific exercises should be designed such that the client can be independent. As always, progression should be gradual and should increase at the individual's own rate in accordance with the principle of specific adaptations to imposed demands (see the Cerebral Palsy: Exercise Programming table).

Special Considerations

It is imperative for the practitioner to understand that a large proportion of individuals with CP have concomitant cognitive, visual, hearing, speech/swallowing difficulties, or a combination of these. The practitioner must be very careful not to assume decreased cognitive ability on the basis of the presence of drooling or the quality of the verbal skills of a person with CP. It is important to assess each client as an individual with very specific needs and concerns.

Special considerations for exercise training include strapping the hands or feet to the pedals during arm and leg cycle ergometry, respectively. Also, the use of gloves for wheelchair exercise testing is recommended. Gradual progression is recommended during the initial stages of exercise. Supervising personnel should be present when the treadmill is being used because of balance problems associated with CP. The importance of spotting on treadmill exercises, because of potential loss of coordination and balance during testing, cannot be overemphasized. Anecdotal experience suggests that when one is collecting expired gases during performance testing utilizing a mouthpiece or mask, it is necessary to be vigilant about checking the quality of the seal. Some individuals with CP present with mouths that have developed in such a way that there is a very acute angle of the mandible, making satisfactory seal difficult.

CASE STUDY Cerebral Palsy

A 26-year-old man had previously participated in a variety of unsupervised exercise programs at the local rehabilitation center. He had problems with spastic diplegia, resulting from trauma at birth. As a child, he underwent rigorous physical therapy and was very fit in high school. His spasticity had gotten much worse since then and, over the last few years, he had less energy and found it more difficult to perform routine ADLs. Walking to catch the bus left him short of breath. He also felt that the increased spasticity was causing joint pain in his hips and knees. He reported having gained over 25 lb (11.3 kg) during the previous 2 years. He was a nonsmoker and did not drink alcohol. Currently he was on no medications. He had no chronic cardiovascular diseases such as hypertension or diabetes, but did have a very strong family history of them. He was unemployed and thinking about getting some training in computer programming.

S: "I think I'm getting worse."

O: Vitals: HR: 85 contractions/min   BP: 110/90 mmHg

Young male, moderately overweight

Knees and hips without inflammation or effusion

Ambulated with Lofstrand crutches in a swing through gait

Unable to stand unsupported

Mild ataxia in both upper extremities

Full active and passive ROM in upper extremities but must move very slowly to avoid spasticity

Significantly reduced passive and active ROM:
  Knee flexion contracture: Right 10°; left 13°
  Hip flexion contracture: Right: 12°; left 20°
  Dorsiflexion bilateral ankles: 0°

Upper extremity strength: Normal

Lower extremity strength: Limited from spasticity

Submaximal aerobic test (modified 3-stage Nu-Step Recumbent Stepper™):
  Work rate setting 1 (65 steps/min): 95 contractions/min
  Work rate setting 2 (65 steps/min): 116 contractions/min
  Work rate setting 3 (65 steps/min): 122 contractions/min

8RM strength test:
  Chest press: 65 lb (29.5 kg)
  Seated row: 55 lb (24.9 kg)
  Seated abdominal curl: 45 lb (20.4 kg)
  Lat. pull-down: 75 lb (34 kg)

Medications: Tylenol

A: 1. Cerebral palsy with spastic diplegia

2. Easy fatigability

P: 1. Prescribe a weight-loss diet.

2. Initiate an exercise program.

Exercise Program

Goals:

1. Improved aerobic capacity, overall strength, and flexibility

2. Weight loss

(continued)

CASE STUDY Cerebral Palsy *(continued)*

Mode	Frequency	Duration	Intensity	Progression
Aerobic (recumbent stepper, Schwinn Air-Dyne™)	3-5 days/wk	2-3 10-min sessions	Work rate #2-3 65 steps/min on stepper	Increase to 45 min over 4-8 wk
Strength (weight lifting; all major muscle groups)	3-5 days/wk	2 sets of 8-12 reps Resistance as tolerated	To fatigue	Progress as tolerated to total exercise time of 60-90 min
Flexibility (floor stretches and stationary cycle for lower extremity)	3-5 days/wk	60 s/stretch	Maintain stretch below discomfort point	Progress as tolerated up to 20 min for contracted muscles
Neuromuscular				
Functional				
Warm-up/Cool-down	Before and after each sesson	5-10 min		

Suggested Readings

Albright, A.L. 1996. Baclofen in the treatment of cerebral palsy. *Journal of Child Neurology* 11: 77-83.

Cerebral Palsy-International Sport and Recreation Association (CP-ISRA). 1991. *Classification and sports rules manual.* 5th ed. Nottingham, England: CP-ISRA.

Damiano, D.L., and M.F. Abel. 1998. Functional outcomes of strength training in spastic cerebral palsy. *Archives of Physical Medicine and Rehabilitation* 79: 119-25.

DeLuca, P.A. 1996. The musculoskeletal management of children with cerebral palsy. *Pediatric Clinics of North America* 43 (5): 1135-50.

Fernandez, J.E., K.H. Pitetti, and M.T. Betzen. 1990. Physiological capacities of individuals with cerebral palsy. *Human Factors* 32: 357-466.

Jones, J. 1988. *Training guide to cerebral palsy sports.* Champaign, IL: Human Kinetics.

Laskin, J.J. and M.A. Anderson. 2002. Cerebral Palsy. In *ACSM's resources for clinical exercise physiology: Muscu-

loskeletal, neuromuscular, neoplastic, immunologic, and hematologic conditions.* Edited by J.N. Myers, W.G. Herbert, and R. Humphrey. 125-38. Philadelphia: Lippincott Williams & Wilkins.

Lockette, K., and A. Keys. 1995. *Conditioning with physical disabilities.* Champaign, IL: Human Kinetics.

Massin, M., and N. Allington. 1999. Role of exercise testing in the functional assessment of cerebral palsy children after botulinum A toxin injection. *Journal of Pediatric Orthopedics* 19: 362-65.

Miller, P.D., ed. 1995. *Fitness programming and physical disability.* Champaign, IL: Human Kinetics.

Morton, R. 1999. New surgical interventions for cerebral palsy and the place of gait analysis. *Developmental Medicine and Child Neurology* 41: 424-28.

Paciorek, M., and J. Jones. 1994. *Sports and recreation for the disabled.* Carmel, IN: Cooper Publishing.

Pitetti, K.H., J.E. Fernandez, and M.C. Lanciault. 1991. Feasibility of an exercise program for adults with cerebral palsy: A pilot study. *Adapted Physical Activity Quarterly* 8: 333-41.

CHAPTER 44

Parkinson's Disease

Elizabeth J. Protas, PhD, PT, FACSM
Texas Women's University

Rhonda K. Stanley, PhD, PT
University of Maryland

Overview of the Pathophysiology

Parkinson's disease is a progressive neurologic disorder involving the extrapyramidal system. The disease is associated with a reduction in the neurotransmitter dopamine, primarily in the substantia nigra, a component of the basal ganglia. The dopamine reduction results from the death of dopaminergic cells within the basal ganglia. The loss of dopamine results in the symptoms of resting tremor, bradykinesia (slow movements), rigidity, and gait and postural abnormalities. Symptoms do not occur until there is greater than 80% loss of the dopaminergic cells.

The most common form of Parkinson's disease is an idiopathic neurodegenerative disorder that usually occurs in individuals over the age of 50. It is found slightly more frequently in men than in women and may be less prevalent in African blacks and Asians. There is no known cause of Parkinson's disease; however, both genetics and environment (e.g., exposure to toxins) are thought to be factors in the disease. Other factors that may be contributing mechanisms are aging, autoimmune responses, and mitochondrial dysfunction. Parkinson's disease may be classified in a number of ways:

- age at onset (< 40 [juvenile]; between 40 and 70; > 70);
- clinical symptom (tremor predominant, akinetic-rigidity predominant, postural instability–gait difficulty predominant);
- mental status (dementia present/absent);
- clinical course (benign, progressive, malignant); and
- disability (Hoehn and Yahr stage 1.0-5.0).

These classifications are useful for gross categorization of an individual with Parkinson's disease, and some have prognostic implications. For example, a malignant clinical course is the situation in which symptoms have been evident for less than one year but disability has progressed rapidly. The prognosis is poor in this instance.

The motor symptoms that occur with Parkinson's disease affect many aspects of movement. Tremors can be evident both at rest and with action. Rigidity often begins in the neck and shoulders and spreads to the trunk and extremities, making movement difficult. The ability to move fingers, hands, arms, or legs rapidly is drastically reduced (bradykinesia), and motor control to rise from a chair is lessened. Standing posture is characterized by increased kyphosis and flexed knees and elbows, as well as adducted shoulders. Gait is described as slow and shuffling, with shortened festinating steps (involuntary hurrying), decreased arm swing, and difficulty initiating a step (start hesitation). Postural righting reflexes are compromised and lost (an individual with a Hoehn and Yahr disability level stage of 3.0 is unable to recover balance on a pull test). Falls can become a recurring problem. Episodes of decreased movement or freezing become more frequent during walking. Passage through doorways or narrowed spaces becomes more difficult. Activities of daily living can be affected by minute, illegible handwriting (micrographia), the inability to cut food or handle utensils, difficulty swallowing food, difficulty turning in and rising from bed, and needing assistance with dressing and bathing. Individuals with Parkinson's disease have problems with both the volume and the understandability of their speech. Communication disorders are exacerbated by a loss of facial expression (hypomimia). The motor symptoms contribute to the impairment displayed by individuals with Parkinson's disease.

Effects on the Exercise Response

The effect of Parkinson's disease on exercise is not well characterized. Considerable intra- and inter-person variability exists, increasing the difficulty of generalizing about exercise responses in this population. Symptoms may fluctuate from hour to hour, day to day, and week to week, regardless of the exercise intervention strategy precision.

Autonomic nervous system dysfunction is commonly found in Parkinson's disease. This can cause problems with thermal regulation during exercise, as well as altered heart rate and blood pressure responses with position changes and during exercise. Sweating patterns, heart rates, and blood pressure should be observed during exercise.

Movement disorders and muscular rigidity decrease the exercise efficiency of individuals with Parkinson's disease. Reduced efficiency results in higher heart rates

Parkinson's Disease: Exercise Testing

Methods	Measures	Endpoints*	Comments
Aerobic Leg or arm ergometer	• 12-lead ECG, HR	• Serious dysrhythmias • >2mm ST-segment depression or elevation • Ischemic threshold • T-wave inversion with significant ST change	• Prevalence of dysrhythmias is high. • Use HR response to determine impact of medications. • Autonomic dysfunction is common.
	• BP	• SBP > 250 mmHg or DBP > 115 mmHg • Hypotensive response	
	• $\dot{V}O_2$max, METs		• $\dot{V}O_2$max and METs useful in prescribing exercise.
	• RPE (6-20)	• Volitional fatigue	
Endurance 6- and 12-min walk	• Distance	• Note vitals, symptoms, time, distance at rest stops	• Aerobic training may improve walking velocity.
Strength Weight machines	• Maximal voluntary contraction		• Use with electromyography to determine strength deficits.
Flexibility Goniometry	• Joint angles at full extension/flexion		• Especially important to measure ROM of neck, trunk, shoulders, hip, and knees.
Neuromuscular Gait and balance analyses Reaction time Balance Gait	• Pull test, 360° turn, functional turn • Timed walk, velocity, cadence, step length	• Level of difficulty	• Use gait analysis if functional gait training and/or motor control intervention is necessary. • Classify disability level and define existing balance deficits. • Reaction time is important to determine whether driving competence is questionable.
Functional Sit and stand Bed mobility	• Time		• Multiple attempts in the sit and stand may suggest quadriceps weakness and/or poor motor control. Weight training should specifically target quadriceps.

*Measurements of particular significance; do not always indicate test termination.

Medications	Special Considerations
• Levodopa/carbidopa: Can produce exercise bradycardia and transient peak-dose tachycardia and dyskinesia. • Pramipexole, ropinirole, and pergolide: May lower BP and exacerbate dyskinesia. • Selegiline: Associated with dyskinesia; produces mood elevation.	• Orthopedic: Joint dysfunction is common in individuals after age 50 and may interfere with exercise training. Caution against overuse syndromes with exercise training. • Cardiac: High-risk age group; medications can produce dysrhythmia, tachycardia, and bradycardia. • Neurologic: Orthostatic hypotension. • Muscular: Painful dystonia, particularly at night. • Metabolic: Higher resting metabolic rate. • Psychological: Depression is very common. Hallucinations, delusions, and vivid dreaming can occur. Clients report a sense of invincibility when on and vulnerability when off medications. • Thermoregulatory: Decreased or absent sweating. • GI discomfort is a common side effect of medications. • Environmental: It is critical that testing occur at peak dose of medications, which is usually 45-60 min after the first dose. • Equipment adaptation: A mask rather than a mouthpiece is recommended for expired air collection. • Use safety harness for persons who freeze or have poor balance.

and oxygen consumption responses during submaximal exercise. Walking may be severely impaired, but other exercise responses such as stair climbing are easily accomplished. Freezing and start hesitation may make certain activities more difficult than others. During single sessions of exercise, significant loss of upright posture (increasing kyphosis) can occur.

Effects of Exercise Training

Little is known about aerobic exercise training in individuals with Parkinson's disease. Aerobic training can improve function, can fail to impact function, or can reduce function in individuals with Parkinson's disease. It cannot be assumed that aerobic training will be beneficial in this population because of the complexity of the problem, the progressive nature of the disease, and the impact of medications on the condition.

Management and Medications

Drugs have been the most successful way to treat many of the symptoms of Parkinson's disease. Drug management is aimed at correcting or preventing neurochemical imbalances in relation to dopamine deficiency, decreased epinephrine and norepinephrine, and relative increase in the amount of acetylcholine. The most common antiparkinsonian medications are:

- dopaminergics (e.g., levodopa, levodopa/carbidopa, amantadine, pergolide, bromocriptine, pramipexole, ropininrole);
- anticholinergics (e.g., benztropine, trihexyphenidyl); and
- monoamine oxidase type B (MAO-B) inhibitors (e.g., deprenyl, selegiline).

Most of the medications have both peripheral and central side effects. The most common side effects are gastrointestinal upset, confusion, delusional states, hallucination, insomnia, and changes in mental activity. Long-term use of drug therapies, particularly dopaminergics and MAO-B inhibitors, can result in movement disorders (e.g., dyskinesias), dystonias, and clinical fluctuations of motor disability. More than 50% of all persons with Parkinson's disease treated for more than five years with drug therapies have reduced responses to the drugs and display clinical fluctuation of motor disability.

Most individuals with Parkinson's disease are taking multiple medications to alleviate their symptoms. Sometimes the attending neurologist proceeds by trial and error to determine which combination and dosage of drugs work best for an individual. A key drug for Parkinson's disease is levodopa, a metabolic precursor to dopamine that can pass through the blood–brain barrier. In the brain, levodopa is metabolized into dopamine and increases the amount of dopamine available in the basal ganglia. Levodopa is also metabolized in peripheral muscle; this can lessen the amount available to cross into the brain's circulation. Carbidopa is added to the levodopa in the drug Sinemet to reduce the peripheral metabolism of levodopa and increase the amount that passes through the blood–brain barrier. The impact of exercise conditioning on the peripheral metabolism of levodopa is not established.

The importance of drug therapy in the medical management of these individuals, the declining effectiveness

Parkinson's Disease: Exercise Programming

Modes	Goals	Intensity/ Frequency/Duration	Time to Goal
Aerobic • Leg and arm ergometry • Rowing	• Maintain or improve work capacity	• 60-80% peak HR • 3 days/wk • ≤ 60 min/session	• ~ 3 mo
Endurance • Short walking bouts (20-30 m; well supervised)	• Increase work capacity	• Speed dependent on individual • 4-6 sessions/day	
Strength • Weight machines	• Maintain strength of arms, shoulders, legs, and hips	• Use light weights • 1 set of 8-12 reps • 3 sessions/wk	
Flexibility • Stretching	• Increase or maintain ROM	• 1-3 sessions/wk	
Functional • ADLs • Postural changes	• Maintain capacity to perform as many ADLs as possible		

Medications	Special Considerations
• See exercise testing table.	• Walking is a problem for individuals with balance deficits; however, some may be able to jog without risk of falling. • HR responses to the same power levels may vary from day to day because of autonomic fluctuations. • Duration should be increased slowly (every 4-5 wk). • Duration and intensity should receive equal priority. • Orthopedic: Dyskinesia and dystonia can aggravate problems such as degenerative joint disease. There is some evidence that exercise may reduce joint pain. • Cardiac: Use caution with any medication change. • Muscular: Supervised training is recommended to minimize muscular problems. • Metabolic: Observe for changes in medication dosages after 4-5 wk of aerobic training. • Psychological: Mask-like face makes it difficult to interpret patient's reaction or RPE. • Thermoregulatory: Sweating begins to occur with exercise conditioning. • Environmental: Time of day for exercise and medication should be kept as constant as possible.

of the drugs over time, and the variability of individual responses to the drugs make understanding of the influences on drug absorption, metabolism, and effectiveness critical. Most of this has not been carefully studied; however, reduced absorption may be affected by strenuous exercise, concomitant use of anticholinergic drugs, autonomic dysfunction, recent food intake, amount of protein in the diet, iron supplementation, and level of aerobic fitness.

There are a number of implications for graded exercise testing within the context of the antiparkinsonian medications.

- Medication plasma level may influence exercise performance.

- Whenever possible, test at peak dose, usually 45 min to 1 hour after medication has been taken.

- Some individuals who fluctuate clinically may demonstrate a brief, intense peak-dose tachycardia.

- Some people may have intense and severe dyskinesias at peak dose.

- Some medications are associated with cardiac dysrhythmias.

- Caution should be used in testing an individual who has had a recent change in medications because the impact may be unpredictable.

- A single exercise session may increase, decrease, or not affect the time to peak dose-response.

- Individuals who fluctuate clinically should be tested both on and off medications to establish performance ranges.

A number of these concerns for exercise testing are equally applicable to exercise training; however, some additional considerations should be noted.

- Some people display an impaired chronotropic response to aerobic exercise, making it difficult to reach target heart rates.

- Heart rate responses to the same exercise activity may vary greatly from day to day, depending on the medication plasma level.

- Heart rates should be carefully observed during aerobic exercise for evidence of this variability.

- Exercise outcomes may be dependent upon *consistently* exercising at the same time after the last medication dose.

- Observe for changes in parkinsonian symptoms during exercise training that might be related to changes in drug absorption or metabolism (e.g., increases or decreases in dyskinesias, bradykinesia, dystonias, freezing, tremor).

- Noting the time to peak dose onset may be useful in following an individual's medication response to exercise training.

Recommendations for Exercise Testing

People with Parkinson's disease who have balance deficits or freezing episodes should not be tested on treadmills without the use of safety support harnesses. An appropriate cycle ergometer protocol may be selected if harness support is not available. Individuals with Parkinson's disease have difficulty maintaining a seal around a mouthpiece during the collection of expired air. A mask is preferable (see the Parkinson's Disease: Exercise Testing table on page 295).

There is some evidence that persons in stage 2.0 on the Hoehn and Yahr scale have aerobic capacities comparable to those of healthy individuals. This is probably a reasonable assumption for individuals in stage 1.0; however, greater variability and lower capacities may be anticipated for stages 3.0 and 4.0, when greater disability exists. Persons with Parkinson's disease are in an age group that is at high risk for latent cardiovascular disease.

Many of these individuals can ride a leg cycle ergometer or perform an arm crank protocol even if they are in an "off" period and unable to walk without assistance. Frequently non-routine motor behaviors are easily accomplished. Don't make assumptions about what an individual can do. Try the activity as long as the client is safe.

Recommendations for Exercise Programming

The approaches to exercise for Parkinson's disease fall into five categories: flexibility, aerobic training, functional training, strengthening, and neuromuscular. Any exercise prescription should keep the goals of the exercise clearly in mind (see the Parkinson's Disease: Exercise Programming table on page 297). Different interventions will have different outcomes and expectations.

Parkinson's disease is a complex problem that is often difficult to evaluate. There may be direct, indirect, and composite effects of Parkinson's disease. Direct effects are those that occur directly as a result of Parkinson's disease—for example, tremor and rigidity. Indirect effects, such as aerobic deconditioning or loss of range of motion from inactivity, occur along with the disease. Composite effects may be a combination of the direct central nervous system changes and compensatory musculoskeletal symptoms, such as changes in axial mobility and balance problems. Exercise interventions could have a minimal effect on the symptoms resulting directly from the disease process, but appropriately designed interventions may alter the indirect and/or composite effects of musculoskeletal and cardiopulmonary changes.

Parkinson's disease can interfere with motor planning and motor memory. Repeated demonstrations along with written and visual cues are needed to ensure adherence. In some instances, supervision may be necessary for participation in an exercise intervention.

CASE STUDY Parkinson's Disease

A 62-year-old woman had bilateral total knee replacements and was referred to physical therapy for knee rehabilitation after the surgery. The program included strengthening of the knee and hip muscles, gait training, ROM exercises, general exercise for endurance, and pain reduction. After completing the rehabilitation program, however, she still had difficulty walking. She showed shortened step lengths and was referred to a neurologist who made a diagnosis of idiopathic Parkinson's disease. Antiparkinsonian medications were prescribed, and she was referred to physical therapy. She had difficulty in performing activities of daily living (e.g., bathing, grooming, rising from a chair and bed, turning over in bed), and complained of getting tired easily. She also lacked confidence in making conversation and had a fear of choking.

S: "I'm afraid of freezing and falling."

O: Elderly woman in no distress; masked facies and neck flexed with stooped shoulders; cranial nerves intact; slurred speech; poor finger-to-nose and heel-to-shin coordination

Romberg's sign: Positive; slight flexion of knees while standing; reduced ROM in neck, shoulders, trunk, hips, knees, and ankles; normal strength; festinating gait with reduced arm swing

Gait study:
  Slow, shortened steps, narrowed base of support and instability (festinating gait)
  50-ft (15.2-m) walk time: 16 s
  Gait velocity: 0.73 m/s
  Step length: Left 36.6 cm (14.4 in); right 38.4 cm (15.1 in)

Pull test: Unable to recover balance (Hoehn and Yahr stage 3.0)

360° turn: 6.7 s

Functional reach: 8.5 in (21.6 cm)

A: 1. Status post-bilateral knee replacement surgery

2. Parkinson's disease
   Gait and balance impairment
   Difficulty in transfers (turning in bed, getting up)
   Decreased flexibility
   Decreased endurance
   Impaired orofacial functions

P: 1. Prescribe Sinemet/anticholinergic medication.

2. Initiate a physical rehabilitation program.

Exercise Program
Goals:

1. Be able to ambulate with confidence
2. Improved balance
3. Self-sufficiency with transfers
4. Improved endurance

Mode	Frequency	Duration	Intensity	Progression
Aerobic (walking, swimming[a])	3 days/wk	30 min	Self-selected	As tolerated
Strength (resistance[b])	2 days/wk	3 sets	Hold for 10 s each	As tolerated
Flexibility (stretching[c])	1 day/wk	20 s/stretch 30 min total	3 reps, hold for 10 s each	
Neuromuscular (gait and balance[d], orofacial[e])	1 day/wk 2 days/wk	15-20 min	3 reps, hold for 10 s each	
Functional (transfer exercises[f])	1 day/wk	15-20 min	3 reps, hold for 10 s each	
Warm-up/Cool-down				

a. Perform during peak drug response.

b. Resistance exercises include shoulder shrugs, shoulder squeezes, trunk twists, hip bridges, straight leg raises, leg kicks, toe/heel raises, standing against the wall, and wall push-ups.

c. Stretching exercises include head turns and tilts, chin tucks, arm stretches, wrist circles, finger/thumb circles, back extensions, hamstring stretches, bringing the knees to the chest, hip rolls, calf stretches, and ankle circles.

d. Gait training requires an attentional strategy—for example, reminding about larger steps, using visual or auditory cues to improve step length, and walking with alternate arm swing. Balance training includes tandem walking, sideways walking, backward walking, standing on one limb, alternate standing on toes and heels, and turning the head and looking over the shoulders while standing.

e. Orofacial exercises include chin tucks in and out, eyebrow lifts, deep breathing, sticking the tongue out and in, saying "u-k-r" loudly, lip presses, whistling, circling the tongue inside the lips, long blowing through the mouth, big smiles, face squeezes, and cheek stretches.

f. Transfer training includes bed turns (sequential trunk rolling and pushing up) and getting up (leaning forward, shifting weight, and standing up quickly).

Suggested Readings

Ahlskog, J.E. 2000. Initial symptomatic treatment of Parkinson's disease. In *Parkinson's disease and movement disorders*, edited by C.H. Adler and J.E. Ahlskog, 115-28. Totowa, NJ: Humana.

Burleigh-Jacobs, A., F.B. Horak, J.G. Nutt, and J.A. Obeso. 1997. Step initiation in Parkinson's disease: Influence of levodopa and external sensory triggers. *Movement Disorders* 2: 206-15.

Canning, C.G., J.A. Alison, N.E. Allen, and H. Groeller. 1997. Parkinson's disease: An investigation of exercise capacity, respiratory function, and gait. *Archives of Physical Medicine and Rehabilitation* 78: 199-207.

Formisano, R., L. Pratesi, F.T. Modarelli, V. Bonifati, and G. Meco. 1992. Rehabilitation and Parkinson's disease. *Scandinavian Journal of Rehabilitative Medicine* 24: 157-60.

Goetz, C.G., J.A. Thelan, C.M. Macleod, P.M. Carvery, E.A. Bartley, and G.T. Stebbins. 1993. Blood levodopa levels and the unified Parkinson's disease rating scale function: With and without exercise. *Neurology* 43: 1040-42.

Jankovic, J., and E. Tolosa, eds. 1998. *Parkinson's disease and movement disorders*, 3rd ed. Baltimore: Williams & Wilkins.

Morris, M.E. 2000. Movement disorders in people with Parkinson's disease: A model for physical therapy. *Physical Therapy* 80: 578-97.

Myai, I., Y. Fujimoto, Y. Ueda, H. Yamamoto, S. Nozaki, T. Saito, and J. Kang. 2000. Treadmill training with body weight support: Its effect on Parkinson's disease. *Archives of Physical Medicine and Rehabilitation* 81: 849-52.

Protas, E.J., R.K. Stanley, J. Jankovic, and B. MacNeill. 1996. Cardiovascular and metabolic responses to upper- and lower-extremity exercise in men with idiopathic Parkinson's disease. *Physical Therapy* 76: 34-40.

Reuter, I., M. Engelhardt, K. Stecker, and H. Bass. 1999. Therapeutic value of exercise training in Parkinson's disease. *Medicine and Science in Sports and Exercise* 31: 1544-49.

Roberts-Warrior, D., A. Overby, J. Jankovic, S. Olson, E.C. Lai, J.K. Krauss, and R. Grossman. 2000. Postural control in Parkinson's disease after unilateral posteroventral pallidotomy. *Brain* 123 (10): 2141-49.

Rogers, M.W. 1996. Disorders of posture, balance, and gait in Parkinson's disease. *Clinics in Geriatric Medicine* 12: 825-45.

Schenkman, M., T.M. Cutson, M. Kuchibhatla et al. 1998. Exercise to improve spinal flexibility and function for people with Parkinson's disease: A randomized, controlled trial. *Journal of the American Geriatric Society* 46: 1207-16.

Stanley, R., E.J. Protas, and J. Jankovic. 1999. Comparison of exercise responses in individuals with Parkinson's disease and healthy individuals. *Medicine and Science in Sports and Exercise* 31: 761-66.

Tintner, R., and J. Jankovic. 2001. Assessment and treatment of Parkinson's disease. *Clinical Geriatrics* 9: 62-74.

SECTION VIII

Cognitive, Psychological, and Sensory Disorders

Lorraine E. Colson Bloomquist
EdD, FACSM

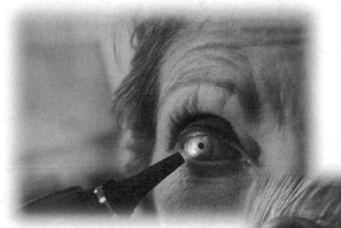

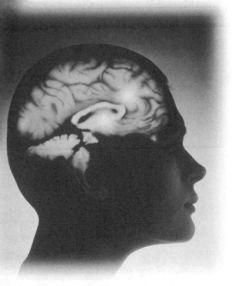

CHAPTER 45

Mental Retardation

Bo Fernhall, PhD, FACSM
Syracuse University

Overview of the Pathophysiology

According to the American Association on Mental Retardation, mental retardation is a significantly subaverage general intellectual function that exists concurrently with related limitations in two or more of the following adaptive skill areas: communication, self-care, home living, social skills, community use, self-direction, health and safety, functional academics, leisure, and work.

There are many potential causes of mental retardation, including genetic and maternal disorders, birth trauma, and infectious diseases. It is also believed that poverty, malnutrition, maternal drug use, and fetal alcohol syndrome, as well as severe stimulus deprivation, can contribute to mental retardation. With an estimated prevalence of 3%, mental retardation is the most common form of developmental disability in industrialized Western society.

The previously used process of classifying persons with mental retardation by IQ score has been replaced by simply determining the presence or absence of mental retardation on the basis of three criteria: age of onset, significantly subaverage general intellectual function, and limitations in two or more adaptive skill areas. The classification of mild, moderate, severe, and profound is still in wide use but is in the process of being replaced with a classification system based on the determination of level of support needed.

Levels of support are determined across four dimensions: (1) intellectual functioning and adaptive skills, (2) psychological and emotional considerations, (3) physical/health/etiology considerations, and (4) environmental considerations. Levels of support may be needed in any or all of the four divisions at the following levels:

- Intermittent: as needed, short-term support of a high or low intensity;
- Limited: a constant need for support of lesser intensity at extensive and pervasive levels;
- Extensive: a constant need for support on a daily basis in some environments; and

- Pervasive: a constant need for high-intensity support across environments.

However, all of the reported physical fitness research on persons with mental retardation refers to levels of mental retardation according to the old classifications (i.e., mild, moderate, severe, and profound). Therefore, the old classification will be used in this discussion.

Approximately 90% of all individuals classified with mental retardation fall into the category of mild mental retardation. Mild mental retardation can be characterized by:

- IQ scores between 52 and 70 on standardized scales (100 points is an average IQ);
- the ability to live independently, work, marry, and rear children; and
- often social isolation and living in or near poverty.

Individuals classified with moderate mental retardation constitute approximately 5% of this population and can be characterized by:

- IQ scores between 36 and 51 points;
- maladaptive behaviors, including problems with speech, social interaction, and a higher incidence of psychiatric disorders; and
- often the display of physical limitations, including gait problems.

Most individuals with Down syndrome (DS) fall into this category. Down syndrome is the most common chromosomal disorder leading to mental retardation. The presence of DS is often associated with several physical characteristics, such as small stature, short limbs and digits, digital malformations, small nasal and oral cavities (leading to mouth breathing and tongue protrusion), almond shaped and slanted eyes (often strabismic and myopic), joint laxity, and pulmonary hypoplasia. Temperamentally, people with DS tend to be friendly, cheerful, mannerly tactile, and occasionally stubborn.

Persons classified with severe mental retardation make up approximately 3.5% of this population and those of profound mental retardation comprise approximately 1.5%. These persons have the following characteristics:

- IQ scores of 20 to 35 (severe) or 19 or lower (profound);
- difficulty with activities of daily living and self-care;
- high incidence of physical and motor disabilities; and
- high incidence of institutionalization.

Effects on the Exercise Response

Exercising individuals with mental retardation can be challenging because of difficulties with task understanding, motivation, attention deficits, and motor disabilities. To help control for these factors, it is imperative that practice sessions be scheduled before the actual exercise test. The number of practice sessions needed depends on the individuals being tested. The practice session(s) will:

- familiarize the person with the test protocol, environment, and staff; and
- allow staff members to demonstrate, simplify instructions, and adjust the protocol to ensure validity of test results and safety of the person being tested.

For treadmill testing, walking protocols should be selected on the basis of the individual's ability. Selecting a walking speed that is too fast is likely to result in early test termination because of fear rather than fatigue. The practice sessions also help reveal whether a given individual is able to perform the intended protocol or exercise mode. Ambulatory limitations or poor coordination, or both, may prevent a person from performing on a treadmill; selecting an alternative exercise mode (e.g., cycle ergometer) may then become necessary.

People with mental retardation have maximal heart rates that are 8 to 20% lower than expected. On average, individuals with mental retardation without DS have maximal heart rates of 10 to 15 contractions/min below expected levels. Persons with DS have even lower maximal heart rates, on average approximately 30 to 35 contractions/min below expected levels. It is unknown whether mental retardation per se is the cause of the lower maximal heart rates or whether problems with motivation have produced poor effects. However, chronotropic incompetence has been identified as a physiologic condition existing in most individuals with DS. Furthermore, many individuals with DS exhibit the following characteristics, which could affect the exercise response.

- Up to 40% have congenital heart defects such as aortic arch defects, tetralogy of Fallot, septal defects, and valvular defects.

- Approximately 17% have atlantoaxial instability (lax ligaments/muscles surrounding the joint between vertebrae C1 and C2 that may slip out of alignment and cause spinal cord injury).
- Skeletal muscle hypotonia is present in the majority of individuals and is associated with poor muscle strength.
- Most individuals have poor pulmonary function, leading to reduced ventilatory ability during exercise.

If atlantoaxial instability exists, the following activities are contraindicated: exercises with strong neck flexion or extension, equestrian sports, gymnastics, diving, pentathlon, butterfly stroke, diving starts in swimming, high jump, alpine skiing, squat lifting, and team competition (soccer). Special Olympics requires X rays before sport participation in DS individuals from age 8 and older.

It is important to carefully screen all individuals with mental retardation before exercise testing to identify any conditions that may affect the exercise response or the safety of exercise. Pretest screening for signs and symptoms of premature coronary heart disease may also be indicated for individuals with mental retardation over the age of 30 years because of a high incidence of sedentary lifestyle, obesity, and very low exercise capacity.

For adult individuals with mental retardation between 20 and 30 years of age without the presence of apparent cardiovascular disease, maximal capacities as low as 4 METs have been reported, although the mean exercise capacity is usually between 6.5 and 8.5 METs in this population. Thus, it is not unusual to find very low functional capacity in individuals with mental retardation, although values as high as 18 METs have been reported. Muscle strength is associated with both aerobic capacity and endurance run performance in this population.

The information on exercise testing, as well as exercise training, applies only to individuals with mild to moderate mental retardation according to the old classification system. People with severe and profound mental retardation have not participated in studies utilizing conventional exercise testing and training, so it is unknown whether the protocols discussed in this chapter will apply to that subpopulation.

Effects of Exercise Training

Exercise training has been shown to be beneficial for most people with mental retardation. It is common to observe improvements in functional capacity after cardiorespiratory training and in strength after strength training. Strength training appears to yield expected improvements typically ranging from 20 to 50%. However, while endurance training will usually increase functional capacity, this may not be accompanied by an

Mental Retardation: Exercise Testing

Methods	Measures	Endpoints*	Comments
Aerobic Schwinn Air-Dyne™ or cycle ergometer (25 watts/2-min stage) Treadmill (Naughton, Balke protocols; speed 2-3.5 mph)	• HR • BP • $\dot{V}O_2$peak • METs	• SBP > 250 mmHg or DBP > 115 mmHg • Volitional fatigue	• Peak HR usually lower than age predicted. • $\dot{V}O_2$peak usually lower than age/gender predicted.

Strength
Adults:
  Rockport 1-mi (1.6K) walk
  1.5-mi (2.4K) run/walk
Children:
  20-m shuttle run
  600-yd (0.5K) walk/run
	• Time
	• Laps
	
	• Time
		• Distance
		• Inability to complete laps in required time
		• Distance
			• A pacer will be needed along the client's side.
			• Most clients will walk more than run.
			• Practice prior to testing is essential.

Strength Isokinetic Weight machines	• Peak torque • 1RM		• Speed of 60°/s should be used with isokinetic testing. • Constant supervision is of utmost importance.
Flexibility Sit and reach	• Distance		• Proceed with caution for persons with DS.

*Measurements of particular significance; do not always indicate test termination.

Medications	Special Considerations
• Clients may be taking antidepressants, anticonvulsants, hypnotics, beta blockers, and neuroleptics and thyroid replacement. • See appendix C.	• It is essential to familiarize individuals with protocol, staff, and environment. Simplify, demonstrate, and repeat. • Obesity and poor muscle strength and endurance, as well as poor cardiovascular capacities, are very common in this population. • Low peak HR is common, especially with Down syndrome. • Congenital heart defects may be found in persons with Down syndrome. • Motivation can be a problem in attaining maximal effort. Positively reinforce. • Seizures are prevalent, and many individuals are on anticonvulsive agents. • Poor kinesthetic sense could create problems with balance and gait. • Hyperflexion and hyperextension of the neck are contraindicated for persons with atlantoaxial instability. • Careful screening for cardiovascular disease in individuals over age 30 may be indicated.

increase in measured maximal oxygen consumption ($\dot{V}O_2$max), particularly in persons with DS. For persons without DS, standard improvements in $\dot{V}O_2$max (10-20%) should be expected.

Because motivation and task understanding are common problems, it is important to keep the exercise program simple and to demonstrate, repeat, and utilize motivational techniques. Token reward systems have been used with some success, and positive reinforcement and personal supervision are essential. Since obesity is prevalent in this population, weight reduction should be a primary goal in addition to exercise programs. However, exercise alone has not been effective for weight reduction in this population; thus, dietary intervention is necessary. For individuals with DS, exercise programs have not been as effective as for persons without DS, although a physiological reason for this difference has not been identified.

Management and Medications

Because of the very low levels of physical fitness and exercise participation of individuals with mental retardation, the goal is to improve the overall physical fitness profile. Although exercise training cannot have an impact on mental retardation per se, the condition and health profiles of persons with mental retardation can be significantly improved. This is important because individuals with mental retardation have higher rates of cardiovascular mortality at an earlier age than their peers without mental retardation. Furthermore, both cardiovascular fitness and strength are related to job performance in this population, and may be related to the ability to live independently. Considering that the rate of institutionalization is much higher in this population than in groups without mental retardation, improving functional capacity and strength may have an important economical and sociological impact.

Anticonvulsive and antidepressant medications are commonly used in this population. These medications have minimal impact on a single exercise session or chronic exercise adaptations, but may impact the level of concentration, motivation, and ability to understand instructions. The use of beta blockers is also not unusual; their effect combined with the inherently low maximal heart rate responses of persons with mental retardation may produce severely blunted exercise heart rates. Hypnotics are used to modify psychotic behavior while neuroleptics induce sleep or dull the senses. Hypothyroidism is common in persons with DS; thus, many of these individuals will be on thyroxine (T_4) replacement therapy. Because of the effect of thyroxine on cardiac contractility and heart rate, angina can be precipitated until a stable dose has been titrated. Exercise testing and training should be cautiously applied or avoided until euthyroid status has been reached.

Recommendations for Exercise Testing

Persons with mental retardation, particularly those with DS, should be evaluated for potential congenital cardiovascular problems prior to exercise testing. To help ensure valid testing, the following recommendations should be followed (see the Mental Retardation: Exercise Testing table).

- Provide ample time for laboratory familiarization and practice testing.
- Provide safety features to ensure that participants do not fall or fear falling.
- Tailor the protocol to the individual.
- Provide an environment in which the individual feels like a participating member.
- Demonstrate first and give simple, one-step instructions.
- Reinforce verbally and regularly.
- Ask individuals to repeat instructions to ensure they understand.

For treadmill testing:

- walking protocols should be used and the walking speed should be individualized;
- only grade should be increased throughout most of the test (speed can be increased at the end of the test to elicit a maximal response, provided grade is not increased at the same time); and
- work stages of 1 to 2 minutes should be used.

Because many individuals with mental retardation have ambulatory limitations or poor coordination leading to poor balance, treadmill protocols are not always appropriate. However, standard cycle ergometer protocols have not been shown to be valid for this population. Only the Schwinn Air-Dyne™ has been shown to be both valid and reliable. Exercise testing that uses the Schwinn Air-Dyne™ should start at 25 watts and increase 25 watts every 2 minutes. Field tests such as the Rockport 1-mi (1.6K) walk, or the 1.5-mi (2.4K) run/walk, can be used in adults with mental retardation. For children with mental retardation, the 600-yd (0.5K) run/walk or the 20-m shuttle run are recommended.

Strength testing can be performed on most equipment, including isokinetic machines. Standard protocols can be followed, with the low levels of strength of the population kept in mind. Because of safety concerns and problems with motivation, concentration, and task understanding, the use of free weights is not recommended.

Flexibility should be measured in most people with mental retardation, but caution should be applied for persons with DS because of joint laxity in these individuals. The most common test used is the sit and reach (although this is often considered a functional test). Coordination and functional testing can be useful, but none of these tests have been uniformly applied; nor have they been validated in this population.

Mental Retardation: Exercise Programming

Modes	Goals	Intensity/Frequency/Duration	Time to Goal
Aerobic • Walking, walking/jogging • Schwinn Air-Dyne™ • Swimming • Aerobics (or other exercise to music) • Cycling	• Weight control or loss • Improve cardiovascular fitness • Improve work capacity	• 60-80% peak HR • 3-7 days/wk • 20-60 min/session	• 4-6 mo
Strength • Weight machines	• Increase strength of large muscle groups	• 70-80% of 1RM • 3 sets of 8-12 reps • Monitor closely	• 10-12 wk

Medications	Special Considerations
• See exercise testing table and appendix C.	• Because of motivation problems, constant supervision and encouragement are necessary. • The following activities are contraindicated for persons with atlantoaxial instability: equestrian sports, gymnastics, diving, pentathlon, butterfly stroke, diving starts in swimming, high jump, alpine skiing, squat lift, football (soccer and American-style), and any other activity that may cause hyperflexion or hyperextension of the neck. • Aerobic endurance programs should focus on participation most days of the week. Intensity, as measured by HR, can be ignored during low-intensity sessions, which are recommended 2-3 days/wk. Standard exercise intensity sessions are used on the remaining days.

Recommendations for Exercise Programming

Exercise programming for individuals with mental retardation can be conducted in a manner similar to that used with other populations. They especially need a structured environment, a standard routine, repetition, consistency, demonstration (they learn best visually), a reward system, and regular positive reinforcement. Some important considerations are outlined here (see the Mental Retardation: Exercise Programming table).

• Exercise intensity should be between 60% and 80% of maximal functional capacity.

• Exercise should be supervised, since it is unlikely that most persons with mental retardation will exercise on their own.

• It may take longer than anticipated to produce a training effect (i.e., 16 to 35 wk may be needed to improve $\dot{V}O_2$max), whereas improvements in functional capacity have been demonstrated in programs of shorter duration.

• Motivational techniques, such as token rewards, may be necessary to maintain adherence to the program.

• Strength training appears to be essential because the majority of individuals with mental retardation exhibit poor muscle strength. Leg strength is related to both aerobic capacity and endurance run performance in this population. Furthermore, strength may have important ramifications for vocational productivity and independence.

Special Considerations

The focus of any program for individuals with mental retardation should be on participation and personal enjoyment. It is important to personalize the program as much as possible to keep the individual interested in exercise. Because motivation is a primary obstacle in this population, innovative ideas that increase the enjoyment of the activities for each person become important. Activities set to music appear to be effective and may increase adherence. Swimming has been a very successful activity because these individuals float well (as a result of being overweight), balance problems are not of concern, and it is a safe and individual activity. With close supervision, weight training has also been highly successful. Sport participation in such programs as the Special Olympics, while important for other reasons, has not been shown to produce any physiological training improvements. Large group programs have been equally ineffective. Therefore, the emphasis should be on individualized programs.

CASE STUDY Mental Retardation

A 24-year-old female with DS had experienced some weight gain and a resulting reduction in Special Olympics performances. She had a diagnosis of mild mental retardation, but an IQ score was not available. She had a history of inner ear problems that were surgically corrected and she used a hearing aid. She had no history of congenital heart disease but was diagnosed with a hypothyroid condition at age 15. She was a nonsmoker and trained periodically.

S: "I want to do better in the Special Olympics."

O: Vitals: Height: 5'8" (1.72 m)   Weight: 141 lb (63.9 kg)   BMI: 21.6 kg/m^2
            HR: 99 contractions/min   BP: 90/58 mmHg

Whole body plethysmography: 42% body fat

Resting metabolic rate: 1260 kcal/day

Graded exercise test:
   Stopped at 4.4 mph and a grade of 12.5% because of fatigue
   Peak HR: 165 contractions/min
   $\dot{V}O_2$peak: 18.5 ml · kg^{-1} · min^{-1}
   Peak ventilation: 60 l/min
   Respiratory exchange ratio: 1:14

Strength tests:
   Hand grip: 29.3 lb (13.3 kg)
   Peak knee extension: 105.8 lb (48 kg)

Medications: Synthroid, oral contraceptives

A: 1. DS, with minor behavioral and attention span problems
    2. Low aerobic capacity, peak HR
    3. Weak upper and lower extremities
    4. Moderate obesity, normal metabolic status

P: 1. Prescribe aerobic exercise, using several modalities without a focus on intensity.
    2. Improve muscle strength.
    3. Decrease body weight and relative body fat using exercise and diet.
    4. Prescribe dietary counseling.

Exercise Program
Goals:
    1. Increased physical activity
    2. Increased muscle strength
    3. Weight loss

(continued)

CASE STUDY Mental Retardation *(continued)*

Mode	Frequency	Duration	Intensity	Progression
Aerobic (walking, jogging, swimming, cycling, low-impact aerobics)	6-7 days/wk	20-30 min/ session		Increase to 45 min over 3-6 wk as tolerated
Strength (circuit weights)	2-3 days/wk	1 set of 8-12 reps	60% of 1RM	Increase gradually to 80% of 1RM after 2 wk Increase to 2-3 sets after 2-6 wk
Flexibility				
Neuromuscular				
Functional				
Warm-up/Cool-down	Before and after each session	10-15 min		

Suggested Readings

Fernhall, B. 1993. Physical fitness and exercise training of individuals with mental retardation. *Medicine and Science in Sports and Exercise* 25: 442-50.

Fernhall, B., L. Millar, G. Tymeson, and L. Burkett. 1990. Graded exercise testing of mentally retarded adults: Reliability study. *Archives of Physical Medicine and Rehabilitation* 71: 1065-68.

Fernhall, B., K.H. Pitetti, J.H. Rimmer, J.A. McCubbin, P. Rintala, A.L. Millar, J. Kittredge, and L.N. Burkett. 1996. Cardiorespiratory capacity of individuals with mental retardation including Down syndrome. *Medicine and Science in Sports and Exercise* 28: 366-71.

Fernhall, B., K.H. Pitetti, M.D. Vukovich, N. Stubbs, T. Hensen, J.P. Winnick, and F.X. Short. 1998. Validation of cardiovascular fitness field tests in children with mental retardation. *American Journal of Mental Retardation* 102: 602-12.

Fernhall, B., and G. Tymeson. 1987. Graded exercise testing of mentally retarded adults: A study of feasibility. *Archives of Physical Medicine and Rehabilitation* 68: 363-65.

Fernhall, B., G. Webster, and G. Tymeson. 1988. Cardiovascular fitness of mentally retarded individuals. *Adapted Physical Activity Quarterly* 5: 12-28.

Pitetti, K.H., and K.D. Campbell. 1991. Mentally retarded individuals: A population at risk? *Medicine and Science in Sports and Exercise* 23: 586-93.

Pitetti, K.H., J.H. Rimmer, and B. Fernhall. 1993. Physical fitness and adults with mental retardation: An overview of current research and future directions. *Sports Medicine* 16: 23-56.

Pitetti, K.H., and D.M. Tan. 1991. Effects of a minimally supervised exercise program for mentally retarded adults. *Medicine and Science in Sports and Exercise* 23: 594-601.

Rimmer, J.H., and L. Kelly. 1991. Effects of resistance training program on adults with mental retardation. *Adapted Physical Activity Quarterly* 8: 146-53.

Rintala, P., J.A. McCubbin, S.B. Downs, and S.D. Fox. 1998. Cross-validation of the 1-mile walking test for men with mental retardation. *Medicine and Science in Sports and Exercise* 29:133-37.

Sherrill, C. 1998. Mental retardation, Special Olympics, and the INSA-FMH. In *Adapted physical activity, recreation, and sport,* edited by T. Gurtz, 520-49. 5th ed. Madison, WI: Brown & Benchmark.

CHAPTER 46

Alzheimer's Disease

James H. Rimmer, PhD
University of Illinois at Chicago

Overview of the Pathophysiology

Alzheimer's disease is a chronic degenerative disorder that is the most common cause of dementia among older people. Knowledge on the pathophysiology of Alzheimer's disease has grown tremendously over the last five years. While there is still no known cure, researchers are getting close to developing medications that can slow the progression of the disease and possibly even prevent it in those at risk for acquiring the disease. The pathophysiology of Alzheimer's disease begins in the entorhinal cortex and proceeds to the hippocampus, an important structure in memory formation. As the hippocampal neurons degenerate, short-term memory falters. It then gradually spreads to other regions of the brain, particularly the cerebral cortex, which is involved in functions such as language and reason. In the regions attacked by Alzheimer's disease, nerve cells or neurons degenerate, losing their connections of synapses with other neurons. Some neurons die. Atrophy of the cerebral cortex results in intellectual impairment, which progresses from increasing loss of memory to total disability. This deterioration is manifested in the brains of individuals with Alzheimer's disease at autopsy (a definite diagnosis of Alzheimer's disease is still only possible when an autopsy reveals the hallmark features of the disease).

Overwhelming data now show that tangles occur in dying nerve cells following the accumulation of beta-amyloid proteins. These sticky tangles are the twisted, abnormal, pretzel-like filaments that form inside the nerve cells as they die. Beta-amyloids "gum up" the space between the nerve cells, are toxic to nerve cells, and interfere with the normal function of the brain. Formation of the tangles, however, is the result of neuronal breakdown and is the end-stage event resulting from the accumulation of the beta-amyloid fibrils over time. Some experts have noted that if you compare Alzheimer's to heart disease where cholesterol levels must be lowered, in Alzheimer's disease a similar situation is present: the cholesterol equivalent is beta-amyloid, which must be lowered to reduce the progression of neurofibrillary tangles that exacerbate the disease over time.

Alzheimer's disease affects approximately 4 million Americans. It is listed as the primary cause of dementia. The prevalence of Alzheimer's disease rises exponentially with age. After age 65, the percentage of affected people approximately doubles with every decade of life. The highest rate of Alzheimer's disease occurs in people age 85 and over. Alzheimer's disease is more common in women than in men.

Despite the great increase in research on Alzheimer's disease over the past decade, the diagnosis of this disease before death remains an enigma. At present, there is no universally accepted set of criteria for a pathologic diagnosis. The disease was first recognized in 1907 by the German psychiatrist Alois Alzheimer. From 1907 to 1983, the diagnosis of the disease was based solely on exclusion criteria. That is, other conditions such as brain tumors, strokes, infections, head trauma, and other potential etiologies had to be ruled out before a person was diagnosed as having Alzheimer's disease. Alzheimer's disease is also characterized by the presence of dementia of insidious onset and a progressive deteriorating course. In 1984, the National Institute for Neurological and Communicative Disorders and Stroke-Alzheimer's Disease and Related Disorders Association (NINCDS-ADRDA) task force formalized and structured the disease into three categories: definite, probable, and possible Alzheimer's disease.

In definite Alzheimer's disease, the clinical picture of probable Alzheimer's disease is confirmed at autopsy by histopathologic findings of neurofibrillary plaques and tangles. In probable Alzheimer's disease, dementia is established clinically and confirmed by neuropsychological tests (cognitive loss accompanied by memory loss.) In possible Alzheimer's disease, the major clinical sign is unusual losses of memory. Other symptoms include deterioration of language and perception, judgment problems that compromise the person's ability to carry out activities of daily living, and behavioral problems such as agitation and paranoia.

Alzheimer's disease is progressive and degenerative. Although the life expectancy among persons with the disease is diverse, early mortality is seen among persons who develop it early in life and in men. However, persons with Alzheimer's disease can often live for years with this condition, dying eventually from pneumonia or other diseases. The duration of Alzheimer's disease from time of diagnosis to death can be 20 years or more, with the average length 4 to 8 years. Former U.S. President Ronald Reagan has had Alzheimer's disease for over a decade and continues to live today. At the present time, there is no cure for this disease and, for the most part, treatment has been limited. Nonetheless, the future care of Alzheimer's disease appears promising, and investigators are getting closer to finding new medications that can slow the progression of the disease.

Effects on Exercise Response and Training

The exercise literature is devoid of data on the use of exercise testing and training in persons with Alzheimer's disease. The recommendations on testing and training that follow are, for the most part, based on clinical experiences and practicality.

Management and Medications

A litany of drugs to treat the psychiatric symptoms frequently associated with dementia have been used in the management of Alzheimer's disease. They fall under the headings of antidepressants, hypnotics, and neuroleptics (to modify psychotic behavior). These drugs are used to control depression, psychotic behavior, agitation, aggression, and sleep disturbances. Possible side effects of these drugs include orthostasis, poor balance, and dysrhythmias. As a result of their age, many clients are also on other medications to control hypertension, arthritis, heart disease, Parkinson's disease, and other conditions often found in elderly populations.

Recommendations for Exercise Testing

Because Alzheimer's disease affects mental capacity, laboratory tests may be difficult to obtain or may be unreliable, especially during the later stages of the disease. Many individuals with Alzheimer's disease have a high level of agitation and would probably not tolerate lengthy testing. Thus, exercise testing may be of dubious merit in all but early Alzheimer's. If a decision is made that testing can be conducted on a client with Alzheimer's, it is recommended that several practice sessions be conducted before the actual maximal test. If the client becomes agitated or confused, the test should be stopped and scheduled for another day. Additionally, any testing should be conducted in the morning because most persons with Alzheimer's disease function better during the early hours of the day.

Recommendations for Exercise Programming

Exercise training for individuals with Alzheimer's disease has three major challenges: (1) problems arising from the declining physical and mental health of the participant; (2) behavioral changes that may cause the client to become agitated with the exercise program or the exercise setting; and (3) care givers' willingness to continue bringing the person to the exercise program as the disease progresses. For this reason, a low-level program at the client's usual ADL levels is the basic recommended program. For this level of involvement, exercise testing is unnecessary.

During the early stages of Alzheimer's disease, most clients will be able to participate in some form of physical activity. The main problem will involve memory loss. The client may forget to come to the exercise session or may find that he or she has forgotten how to do certain activities. Depression is quite common during the early stage of the disease and may result in the client's withdrawal from the program. The cornerstone of an exercise program for this population is consistency, patience, and enjoyment of the exercise sessions. The exercise leader must constantly provide verbal encouragement and support to maintain the client's interest in the program. During this stage, simple exercises like walking and performing light calisthenics will be easier than more complex routines.

The middle stage of Alzheimer's disease presents a different set of challenges for the exercise leader. At this point, the program should get simpler, and the leader should consider what reasonable criteria should be used to terminate the program. The major problem during this stage involves behavior. Because one of the hallmark symptoms of the disease is extreme agitation, it is not unusual for a client to be totally resistant to an exercise program. A client who has been attending exercise classes during the early stage may suddenly drop out. Memory loss during this stage is more pronounced, and the client may need physical assistance in performing the exercise routine. Extreme outbursts of anger and physical aggression are common during this stage. The exercise leader must work through this agitation with the support of the care giver. Often this behavior will last for only a few minutes and the client will immediately forget that the incident occurred. The exercise leader must remember that this is a symptom of the disease and therefore should not take these outbursts personally.

Alzheimer's Disease: Exercise Testing and Programming

See chapter 24, including testing and programming tables. If the client has a specific medical problem, see the corresponding chapter in this book (e.g., if the patient has a history of MI, see chapter 4 and tables). Exercise testing is generally not necessary.

Modes	Goals	Intensity/Frequency/Duration	Time to Goal
Aerobic •Walking •Chair exercises	•Enjoyment •Enjoyment	•As tolerated •10-15 min, as tolerated	•As tolerated •As tolerated
Strength •Therabands™	•Enjoyment •Maintain function	•10-12 reps, as tolerated	
Flexibility	•Enjoyment •Maintain function		

Medications	Special Considerations
•A wide variety of medications are commonly found in clients with Alzheimer's. See relevant chapters and appendixes B and C.	•Emotional instability or outburst may affect exercise test or program. •Constant supervision is of utmost importance. •ROM and strength exercise should be main focus with the disease. •Goals and expected progress should be limited in almost all cases. •Participation is more important than adherence to all aspects.

During the advanced and final stage of the disease, the client will require constant supervision and physical assistance. Language skills will be greatly diminished and language comprehension extremely limited. The exercise program must be done on an individual basis. Incontinence and limited mobility are common. Range-of-motion and strength exercises will be the major focus during this stage of the disease.

Special Considerations

It should be remembered that it is common for persons with Alzheimer's disease to have a higher level of restlessness and agitation at the end of the day, which some investigators have labeled "sundowning." Therefore, the exercise program should be conducted during the early hours of the day, preferably in the morning, when the client's agitation level is usually at its lowest.

If the client is exercising at home with a family member, a daily walk may be the optimal manner of establishing a structured routine. However, if the client refuses to exercise at home, a day care program attended once or twice a week may be a better setting. The hallmark exercise program is one that keeps the client active at various times during the day (e.g., 10-min exercise routines), has a low risk of injury from falls, and has a strong behavioral component (e.g., effective reinforcement strategies).

CASE STUDY Alzheimer's Disease

An active, healthy-appearing 73-year-old woman learned that she may have Alzheimer's disease, which upset her. She had two years of unusual losses of memory, including not remembering the house where her son lived and forgetting to add eggs when making her favorite bread. These occurrences were becoming more frequent, her language and perception were deteriorating, and she was depressed and having loud outbursts. Tests ruled out the possibility of brain tumors, stroke, infection, or trauma. She tried taking a cholinesterase inhibitor to improve her memory and function but experienced the side effects of nausea, vomiting, and anorexia. Over the prior year, she lost 15 pounds, became considerably weaker, and had difficulty performing activities of daily living. She had started using a cane to prevent falls and was referred to an exercise program to increase strength and improve balance.

(continued)

CASE STUDY Alzheimer's Disease (continued)

S: "My doctor says I might have Alzheimer's and need exercise to help prevent falls."

O: Vitals: Height: 5'4" (1.63 m)   Weight: 122 lb (55.4 kg)   BMI: 20.8 kg/m²

Elderly woman, anxious and ambulating with quad cane

Musculoskeletal exam: Grossly normal but lean

6-min walk: Estimated VO_2max 22 ml $\cdot$ kg^{-1} $\cdot$ min^{-1} (poor)

Sit and reach: 11.5 in (29.2 cm) (poor)

Functional performance: Failed to lift 3 lb (1.4 kg) weight higher than shoulder

Timed stand: 1 leg, 18 s; 1 leg with cane, 60 s

A: 1. Possible Alzheimer's
2. Generalized weakness/sarcopenia
3. Recent falls; unclear if balance deficit or secondary to weakness
4. Cardiorespiratory deconditioning

P: 1. Initiate a daily exercise program.
2. Follow up with testing every 6 mo.
3. Prescribe dietary counseling.

Exercise Program

Goals:

1. Maintain independence
2. Enjoy participation

Mode	Frequency	Duration	Intensity	Progression
Aerobic (walking)	5 days/wk	10 min/session	Slow	Increase to 10-15 min/day, 5-7 days/wk
Strength Resistance (chest/shoulder press, triceps extension, biceps curls, wall squats, wall push-ups, chair push-ups)	3 days/wk	1 set of 10-12 reps	Theraband™ Complete all exercises in 10-15 min	Start seated; progress to standing as tolerated Increase to 3 sets of 12 reps over 3-6 wk
Flexibility (all major muscle groups)	5 days/wk	3-5 reps; hold for 10-30 s	Maintain below discomfort point	
Neuromuscular (walking, drills, without cane)	5 days/wk	Walk 5 paces, turn around, return	As tolerated	Increase 1 pace/wk until 20 paces/day
Functional				
Warm-up/Cool-down	Before and after each session	5-10 min		

Suggested Readings

American Psychiatric Association. 1980. *Diagnostic and statistical manual of mental disorders,* 3rd ed. Washington, DC: American Psychiatric Association.

Bowlby, C. 1993. *Therapeutic activities with persons disabled by Alzheimer's disease and related disorders.* Rockville, MD: Aspen.

Breteler, M.M.B., J.J. Claus, C.M. van Duijn, L.J. Launer, and A. Hofman. 1992. Epidemiology of Alzheimer's disease. *Epidemiologic Reviews* 14: 59-82.

Glickstein, J.K. 1988. *Therapeutic interventions in Alzheimer's disease.* Rockville, MD: Aspen.

McKhann, G.D., D. Drachman, M. Folstein, R. Katzman, D. Price, and E.M. Stedlan. 1984. Clinical diagnosis of Alzheimer's disease: Report of the NINCDS-ADRDA work group under the auspices of the Department of Health and Human Services Task Force on Alzheimer's Disease. *Neurology* 34: 939-43.

National Institute on Aging. 1995. *Alzheimer's disease: Unraveling the mystery.* [Online]. Available: **www.alzheimers.org/ unravel.html**.

Parks, R.W., R.F. Zec, and R.S. Wilson. 1993. *Neuro-psychology of Alzheimer's disease and other dementias.* New York: Oxford University.

Rimmer, J.H. 1994. *Fitness and rehabilitation programs for special populations.* Dubuque, IA: Brown & Benchmark.

Teri, L.T., S.M. McCurry, D.M. Buchner, R.G. Logsdon, A.Z. LaCroix, and W.A. Kukull. 1998. Exercise and activity level in Alzheimer's disease: A potential treatment focus. *Journal of Rehabilitation Research and Development* 35: 411-19.

Volicer, L., K.J. Fabiszewski, Y.L. Rheaume, and K.E. Lasch. 1988. *Clinical management of Alzheimer's disease.* Rockville, MD: Aspen.

Wolf-Klein, G.P. 1993. New Alzheimer's drug expands your options in symptom management. *Geriatrics* 48: 26-36.

CHAPTER 47

Mental Illness

Gary S. Skrinar, PhD, FACSM
Boston University

Overview of the Pathophysiology

As defined by the American Psychiatric Association and the Surgeon General's report, mental illness is conceptualized as a clinically significant behavioral or psychological syndrome or pattern that occurs in an individual and that is associated with present distress (e.g., a painful symptom) or disability (i.e., impairment in one or more important areas of functioning), with a significantly increased risk of suffering death, pain, or disability, or an important loss of freedom. Whatever its original cause, mental illness must be currently considered a manifestation of a psychological, biological, or behavioral dysfunction in a person.

It is estimated that 5.5 million people in the United States suffer from severe mental illness, the most common diagnoses being bipolar disorders, personality disorders, and schizophrenia. Of this group, it is estimated that 1.8 million have schizophrenia, a mental illness that has a devastating impact on people's lives. Historically, schizophrenia has been more resistant to treatment and rehabilitation efforts because of the lack of clear etiological understanding, residual symptoms, and debilitating side effects of psychotropic medications. In general, the causal factors responsible for psychiatric disabilities are unclear. Most experts attribute the most common diagnoses of mental illness to a variety of factors: genetic, biological (biochemical, neurophysiological, neuroanatomical), psychosocial, and sociocultural.

Effects on the Exercise Response

Specific diagnosis of mental illness per se (e.g., depression, schizophrenia, personality disorders) does not modulate the exercise response to a single exercise session (i.e., exercise testing) unless concurrent pharmacological therapy has a dual role (i.e., propranolol minimizes social phobia but also influences cardiovascular function). In addition, it is not uncommon for persons with psychiatric disabilities to be afflicted with a secondary medical condition. In this case, consideration must be given to the particular secondary problem and its effect on the response to a single session of exercise.

Effects of Exercise Training

Exercise programming has been safely and successfully conducted with diverse populations of persons, including individuals with psychiatric disabilities. Changes in fitness, performance time, and body composition are important and can be expected in this population if standard components of exercise prescription are followed. Programs that include supervision by both exercise and psychiatric rehabilitation personnel are preferred. Concomitant positive changes in the psychological profile may include the following:

• Improved mood;

• Improved self-concept;

• Improved work behavior; and

• Decreased depression and anxiety.

The majority of studies reviewed indicate that exercise provides an antidepressive effect and is recommended for inclusion in both inpatient and outpatient treatment programs. A number of studies have substantiated the benefits of exercise in the treatment of depression. From a rehabilitation and health care perspective, it is important to recognize that emotional and physical fitness are central to people's ability to control their lives and create options in living, learning, and working. Exercise is a key component of this process.

Management and Medications

Since people with severe psychiatric disabilities are almost always on some type of pharmacological therapy (e.g., antianxiety, antidepressant, anti-psychotic), a review of the client's current medications is of utmost importance. In situations in which maximal testing is

Mental Illness: Exercise Testing and Programming

For testing and programming methodologies, see guidelines for the general population in *ACSM's Guidelines for Exercise Testing and Prescription*, 6th edition. If the client has a specific medical problem, see the corresponding chapter in this book (e.g., if the patient has a history of MI, see chapter 4 and testing and programming tables).

Medications	Special Considerations
• Beta blockers: Will attenuate HR response. • Proxilin: May increase BP. • Nefazodone: Infrequent tachycardia, hypertension, ventricular extrasystoles, and angina pectoris. • Anti-psychotic medication: Possible gait disturbances in relation to tardive dyskinesia; frequently causes dehydration. • Antidepressants: Insomnia, weight gain, and dizziness. • Anti-anxiety medication: Drowsiness, potentiation of alcohol effects, and withdrawal.	• Allow time for the individual to practice the test or mode of exercise. • Familiarize the client with staff and surroundings. • Anxiety disorders, social phobias, and lack of motivation are commonly caused by emotional condition and/or medication. • Cycle testing is generally preferable in clients with drug-induced side effects. • Emphasize low to moderate intensity and enjoyment of participation.

being conducted, physician supervision is advisable. The following is a list of the most common drugs used in pharmacological therapy that usually do not preclude exercise testing:

- *Anti-psychotic:* clozapine, fluphenazine, olanzapine, risperidone

  Effects: sedation, nausea, vomiting, weight gain

- *Antidepressant:* fluoxetine, nefazodone, sertraline, venlafaxine

  Effects: insomnia, weight gain, dizziness

- *Antianxiety (anxiolytic):* alprazolam, buspirone, diazepam, lorazepam

  Effects: drowsiness, potentiation of alcohol effects, withdrawal

Some medications prescribed for certain diagnoses of mental illness have the same action as for other disabilities but are utilized for different purposes. For example, propranolol is a beta blocker employed for individuals with angina and hypertension. For these individuals, propranolol generally reduces the oxygen requirement of the heart at any given exercise intensity, thereby reducing angina. Propranolol is also used to decrease social phobias in individuals with anxiety disorders. In the latter situation, the beta blocker reduces the amount of nervous system stimulation and consequently the anxiety associated with social situations. However, propranolol will still have the same cardiovascular effect on the person with social phobias as it does for individuals with angina. Because many clients who take psychopharmacologic medications also take medications for medical conditions, and may also use alcohol and/or nicotine, the risk of adverse drug-drug interactions in these individuals should be assessed and addressed.

Recommendations for Exercise Testing

When exercise testing is being conducted, both field and laboratory evaluations should be preceded by extensive orientation sessions. The psychological/emotional status of people with psychiatric disabilities varies from day to day and is frequently influenced by the medications being taken. This psychological status may affect the motivation and ability to perform exercise protocols that depend on volitional maximal efforts. People with psychiatric disorders may be either uncomfortable or unaccustomed to treadmill testing, probably as a result of the effects of medication (e.g., fatigue, dehydration, depression), of gait disturbances associated with tardive dyskinesia (side effect of anti-psychotic medications), and of anxiety responses associated with certain diagnoses. Because of its stability, the bicycle ergometer offers a less intimidating and more dependable mode of testing for this population. It is recommended that this form of testing be considered whenever possible to reduce the anxiety associated with treadmill testing, which may increase a person's sense of vulnerability and lack of control. It is not necessary, particularly in light of anxiety usually present, to measure oxygen consumption via a metabolic cart (see the Mental Illness: Exercise Testing and Programming table).

Recommendations for Exercise Programming

Exercise prescription for people with mental illness should follow standard ACSM protocol for the general population. Because the achievement of maximal values is infrequent during initial testing, a more conservative approach may be necessary with regard to intensity (i.e., low to moderate) prescription. Because inactivity, high body fat, and low self-esteem are common in this popu-lation, it is recommended that a structured, supervised program be initially employed to reinforce the elements of exercise programming and exercise education.

CASE STUDY   Depression

A 50-year-old woman had a long history of affective and eating disorders, beginning at age 16, which probably stemmed from sexual abuse early in life. Despite these difficulties, she earned a bachelor's degree while in a state hospital and was working on a master's degree. She'd had many years of psychotherapy, but for the last 10 years was mainly managed with antidepressive medications. She had been heavy since youth and had made many attempts to lose weight through exercise programs. These attempts had been marginally successful at decreasing her weight but were associated with her fears about loss of control. She had a problem with bingeing, use of laxatives, and self-induced vomiting. She was referred for another exercise program to help control her weight and blood pressure, as adjunctive therapy for depression.

S: "I've been struggling with depression for eight years. I haven't worked for months. I lie in bed many hours a day."

O: Vitals: Height: 5'5" (1.65 m)   Weight: 180 lb (81.7 kg)   BMI: 30 kg/m²
                HR: 80 contractions/min   BP: 150/100 mmHg

Obese middle-aged woman, normal appearance

Chronic severe depression (Beck depression inventory)

Medications: Zoloft, Verapamil

A: 1. Major depression

2. Eating disorder: Bulimia with bingeing eating disorder

3. Obesity

4. Hypertension

P: 1. Continue psychotherapy and psychiatric treatment.

2. Initiate a comprehensive rehabilitation program stressing health and wellness.

Exercise Program

Goals:

1. Sustain a moderate exercise program

2. Improve self-esteem and reduce anxiety and depression

Mode	Frequency	Duration	Intensity	Progression
Aerobic	≥ 4 days/wk	20-30 min/ session	RPE 11-14/20	Limit to 30 min/session
Strength Resistance (all major muscle groups)	2 days/wk	1 set of 8-12 reps	50-70% of 1RM	Increase gradually to 2 sets
Flexibility (all major muscle groups)	5 days/wk	20-60 s/stretch	Maintain stretch below discomfort point	
Neuromuscular				
Functional				
Warm-up/Cool-down	Before and after each session	5-10 min		

Suggested Readings

American Psychiatric Association. 1994. *Diagnostic and statistical manual of mental disorders*. 4th ed. Washington, DC: American Psychiatric Association.

Center for Mental Health Services and National Institute of Mental Health. 1992. *Mental health, United States*, edited by R.W. Manderscheld and M.A. Sonnenschen. Department of Health and Human Services Publication No. (SMA) 92-1942. Washington, DC: Superintendent of Documents.

Greist, J.H., M.H. Klein, R.R. Eschens, J.W. Faris, A.S. Gurman, and W.P. Morgan. 1979. Running as treatment for depression. *Comprehensive Psychiatry* 20: 41-54.

Hutchinson, D.S., G.S. Skrinar, and C. Cross. 1999. The role of improved physical fitness in rehabilitation and recovery. *Psychiatric Rehabilitation Journal* 22 (4): 355-59.

Martinsen, E.W., A. Medhus, and L. Sandvik. 1985. Effects of aerobic exercise on depression: A controlled study. *British Medical Journal* 291: 109.

Nadel, G., and S. Horvath. 1967. Fitness evaluation of psychiatric patients. *International Neuropsychology* 3: 191.

Pelham, T.W., and P.D. Campagna. 1991. Benefits of exercise in psychiatric rehabilitation of persons with schizophrenia. *Canadian Journal of Rehabilitation* 5: 159-68.

Plante, T.G., and J. Rodin. 1990. Physical fitness and enhanced psychological health. *Current Psychology: Research and Reviews* 9: 1-22.

Skrinar, G.S., K.V. Unger, D.S. Hutchinson, and A.D. Faigenbaum. 1992. Effects of exercise training in young adults with psychiatric disabilities. *Canadian Journal of Rehabilitation* 4: 151-57.

U.S. Department of Health and Human Services. 1999. *Mental health: A report of the Surgeon General*, Rockville, MD: U.S. Department of Health and Human Services, Substance Abuse and Mental Health Services, National Institutes of Health, National Institute of Mental Health.

CHAPTER 48

Deaf and Hard-of-Hearing

Lorraine E. Colson Bloomquist, EdD, FACSM

University of Rhode Island

Overview of the Pathophysiology

Approximately 0.5% of the U.S. population has no useful hearing. They can participate in all types of physical activities but may require some minor adaptations. *Hearing loss* is a generic term that applies to people who are hard-of-hearing or deaf.

- Hard-of-hearing is a condition that makes understanding speech difficult through use of the ears alone, with or without a hearing aid.
- Deaf is a condition in which a person is unable to understand speech through use of the ears alone, with or without a hearing aid.

Three major types of hearing loss include conductive, sensorineural, and mixed. Conductive loss of hearing is a condition in which sound does not pass through the external and middle ear to reach the inner ear, resulting in the condition hard-of-hearing. Tympanic tubes for ventilation may be surgically inserted to relieve pressure, dry and ventilate the middle ear, and equalize the air pressure on the two sides of the eardrum. Conductive loss of hearing is caused:

- in the external ear by buildup of impacted wax, injury, or infection; and
- in the middle ear by otitis media produced by colds, sinus infections, allergies, or small or blocked Eustachian tubes.

Otosclerosis, progressive deafness of unknown etiology, is caused by formation of spongy bone, especially around the oval window, resulting in stiffening of stapes, preventing proper vibration.

In the more serious sensorineural loss, the inner ear hearing apparatus of the cochlea is affected. This is the site at which sensory receptors convert sound waves into neural impulses that are transmitted to the brain for translation. In sensorineural hearing loss, balance is sometimes affected (as in Ménière's disease) because the vestibular apparatus is also located in the inner ear. Most people who are born deaf have this type of loss. Causes are a result of the following:

- idiopathic (unknown) factors (50% of cases);
- hereditary factors (60 different types have been identified);
- meningitis;
- mumps;
- scarlet fever;
- encephalitis; and
- measles.

Illnesses of the mother during pregnancy (e.g., herpes viruses, measles, toxoplasmosis), as well as head trauma and premature birth, produce hearing defects. Aging and noise pollution are statistically the most important causes of hearing deterioration. City life, noisy work environments, machinery, rock concerts, and loud personal earphones all cause hearing damage.

Mixed type of hearing loss is a combination of the two conditions already identified and is common in senior citizens.

Effects on the Exercise Response

Hearing loss generally does not change the exercise response to a single exercise session. Individuals can participate at a high level in most sports with some special considerations. If profoundly deaf, they may not hear music but can still feel vibrations in the floor or through a handheld balloon. However, persons with a hearing loss may exhibit poor balance and have difficulty with spatial orientation and peripheral or depth perception. Also possible are lower than average physical fitness levels, lower self-image, and lack of self-confidence. Individuals may also appear restless and hyperactive from constantly tuning in visually and moving to touch everything around them. As a result of difficulty in language communication, they may have fewer social skills. Because of difficulty in reading, grades in school may be lower than average (if early onset exists).

Effects of Exercise Training

Regular exercise by people with hearing loss produces the same positive physiological, psychological, and skill benefits as for individuals with no hearing loss. Additional benefits may include:

- more opportunities to improve socialization skills in group activities;
- practice and improvement in balance;
- learning to work with and relate to a new leader in a group; and
- improved self-image, confidence, and spatial orientation.

The assistive device used primarily for conductive hearing loss is the hearing aid. Today's hearing aids are very sophisticated and tailored to a particular loss. Hearing aids have the same component parts as public address systems and amplify in the same way. They do not clarify or make speech sound clearer. A value of the aid is that it helps people to learn to recognize their own names and assist in their speech. Four basic types of hearing aids are available, according to the position worn:

- on the chest or body (young children and persons with multiple disabilities);
- behind the ear (mainly school-aged children);
- in the ear (mainly adults, about 80% of total); and
- on the eyeglasses (mainly adults).

There are more than 200 kinds of assistive listening devices that amplify sounds and convert them to light or vibration systems. In large halls or gyms, for example, AM and FM radio frequencies can transmit voice sounds when the speaker wears a special device. Great technological strides are being made in serving those who are hard-of-hearing.

A recent and exciting innovation is the use of cochlear implants, which bypass damaged hair cells in the inner ear cochlea and convert speech and sounds into electrical signals and then send these signals to the auditory nerve. They do not amplify. Approximately 1 in every 1,000 children has hearing loss severe enough to require a cochlear implant; and approximately 40,000 people worldwide have received cochlear implants. These are recommended for those in whom a hearing aid would not help. The younger the recipient, the greater the effect, but this relatively safe surgery can be done at any age.

Implants are surgically placed by an otolaryngologist in the inner ear and are activated by an external speech processor worn on a belt or in a pocket. A microphone is worn outside the body as a headpiece behind the ear. The speech processor translates sound into distinctive electrical signals that travel up a thin cable to the headpiece and are transmitted across the skin via radio waves to the implanted electrodes in the cochlea. Some newer models have no external wire. When the auditory nerve is stimulated, the information is sent to the brain where it is interpreted as meaningful sound. An expensive treatment costing approximately $30,000 (U.S.), cochlear implantation can greatly improve the lives of those with profound hearing loss.

In normal people with deafness or hearing loss, no medications are prescribed. However, if the person has other primary problems (e.g., coronary artery disease), then one should note and consider specific medications when testing and developing the exercise prescription. In some cases, children may have Ritalin prescribed for hyperactivity. Possible side effects of this medication need to be considered, including the following:

- loss of appetite;
- abdominal pain;
- weight loss;
- insomnia;
- tachycardia; and
- long-term effects that may have implications for the cardiovascular system and normal growth.

Recommendations for Exercise Testing

If the person with a hearing loss does not have any signs or symptoms of other primary conditions, exercise testing can follow standard protocols. When signs or symptoms of other primary disease are present, however, exercise testing should follow recommended procedures for that particular disorder (see the Deaf and Hard-of-Hearing: Exercise Testing and Programming table on page 322).

The primary objectives of exercise testing are to:

- uncover hidden risk of vascular disease; and
- determine an appropriate intensity range for exercise prescription.

Deaf and Hard-of-Hearing: Exercise Testing and Programming

For testing and programming methodologies, see guidelines for the general population in *ACSM's Guidelines for Exercise Testing and Prescription*, 6th edition. If the client has a specific medical problem, see the corresponding chapter in this book (e.g., if the patient has a history of MI, see chapter 4 and testing and programming tables).

Medications	Special Considerations
• Ritalin: Children taking this for hyperactivity may experience tachycardia, appetite loss, abdominal pain, weight loss, and/or insomnia.	• Be aware that clients may have lower than average fitness levels. • Show videotape of test before beginning. Show instructions in writing. • Establish signs to designate "ready," "start," "stop," "faster," or whatever is necessary for the activity. • Speak in a normal voice if the client wears a hearing aid. • Maintain eye contact so that clients may speech (lip) read. • Remove hearing aids for contact sports, gymnastics, self-defense, and aquatics. • Review the client's clearance for aquatics. If client has tympanic tubes, provide ear plugs and keep his/her head out of the water. • Maintain the same daily routine so the client can adjust quickly.

Additional considerations for a person with a hearing loss may include:

- having all instructions described in writing, pictorially, signed, or on a video;
- allowing the person to describe or demonstrate the test protocol before the test begins;
- giving visual or tactile reinforcement to motivate the individual; and
- taking necessary steps to prevent the individual from tripping or falling.

Recommendations for Exercise Programming

People with hearing loss generally can participate in all types of physical activity. Prescription procedures are the same as for other clients.

Special Considerations

Communication is the major special consideration with prelingually deaf individuals who have never "lost" hearing and have not acquired speech that is understandable to persons with normal hearing. Deaf people may use a variety of manual sign language systems, including American Sign Language (ASL), Conceptually Accurate Signed English (CASE), Signed Essential English (SEE), or gestures only. Use of interpreters may be necessary to facilitate communication and provide access to medical and exercise services and programs. Some interpreters work as oral interpreters—that is, they interpret the speech of the oral deaf person to the hearing person and mouth the words of the hearing person for the benefit of the oral deaf person. Other sign language interpreters specialize in the different sign language systems.

The best speech (lip) readers are able to read only approximately 30% of the words they see. If the deaf individual is having difficulty understanding speech, the speaker should rephrase the wording. If difficulty persists, use paper and pencil to write the message down. The goal is effective communication, no matter how it is achieved.

When communicating with deaf individuals, face them, maintain eye contact, and speak directly to them (not the interpreter). Literally show the deaf person what you want from start to finish. Use as many visual cues and concrete examples as possible.

Exercise professionals working with people who have a hearing loss may need to consider the following recommendations and guidelines.

- Show a video demonstrating the routine or activity.
- Use visual and tactile cues.
- Remove hearing aids for contact sports, gymnastics, self-defense activities, and aquatics.

- Remove external apparatus with cochlear implants to reduce the chance of electrostatic discharge (ESD). Clients with cochlear implants must also be kept away from plastic mats, plastic ball pits, or plastic equipment to prevent ESD, which may damage the "maps" in the client's implanted electrodes.
- Speak normally if the person uses a hearing aid.
- Keep near the person and maintain eye contact to enable speech (lip) reading.
- Gum chewing, wearing a mustache, and covering the mouth when speaking hinders speech (lip) reading.
- Use facial expressions, body language, gestures, and common signs such as thumbs up or down for OK or not OK.
- Orient the client to all aspects of the facility with special attention to exits, use of the pool, and fire evacuation procedures.
- If the person's speech is unclear, do not pretend that you understand.
- Be sure strobe (visual) fire alarms or other alerting devices are installed in the facility. Alerting devices include flashing lights, flags, very loud sounds, or vibrations.
- Swimmers may need to use individualized molded ear plugs if a conductive disorder exits.
- Loud, constant background noise or music may cause headaches, reduce hearing aid effectiveness, and prevent hearing aid users from attending to one speaker.
- When tympanic membrane tubes are used, care should be taken to keep water out of the ears, to have swimmers wear individualized ear plugs in water, and to swim under advice from a physician.
- Teach clients to be visually aware, especially when they are near moving vehicles as in road or cross-country racing, cycling, and jogging.
- Avoid extra physical or visual movements behind a person speaking (called "visual noise").
- If balance difficulty is evident, avoid activities involving precarious positions such as balance beam or springboard diving.
- Avoid head-impact sports (e.g., soccer).

CASE STUDY Hard-of-Hearing

A 15-year-old athlete attended a school for people who are deaf or hard-of-hearing. Her hearing loss was sensorineural, congenital, profound, and bilateral, so she could not hear a whistle or spoken word. Nonwritten communication was possible only by speech (lip) reading and signing. Because of her exceptional athletic skills, she participated in basketball and track, practicing for 1.5 hours in the afternoons. In addition, she participated in community recreational softball and soccer leagues. In regular physical education classes, she compared favorably with other high school girls on the President's Physical Fitness Test. She was chosen to be on her state team in the 1998 State Scholar Athlete Games and competed in the Mini Deaf Olympics for two summers. She reacted quickly to facial expressions and common gestures used in sports. Team sports developed her skills in teamwork, interdependence, and communication with classmates. Sports were her main recreational activity because she had a high level of skill and could compete with the regular population in all sports.

S: "I want to be a better basketball player."

O: Neural exam intact, except VIIIth cranial nerve, which shows extreme hearing loss.

A: Profound sensorineural hearing loss
Otherwise normal athlete

P: 1. Encourage participation in her sports of preference, including team sports.
2. Notify officials to use visual signals during competition.

Exercise Program
Goal:
Play basketball in Deaf Olympics

(continued)

CASE STUDY Hard-of-Hearing *(continued)*

Mode	Frequency	Duration	Intensity	Progression
Aerobic	3-7 days/wk			Per basketball coach
Strength (free weights and machines)	3 -7days/wk			Per basketball coach
Flexibility (all major muscle groups)	3-7 days/wk			Per basketball coach
Neuromuscular				
Functional				
Warm-up/Cool-down	Before and after each session			Per basketball coach

Suggested Readings

Butterfield, S. 1988. Deaf children in physical education. *Palaestra* 4 (3): 28-30, 52.

Craft, D.H., and L. Lieberman. 1995. Visual impairments and deafness. In *Adapted physical education and sport,* edited by J.P. Winnick, 143-66. 2nd ed. Champaign, IL: Human Kinetics.

Lieberman, L.L., and J.F. Cowart. 1996. *Games for people with sensory impairments.* Champaign IL: Human Kinetics.

Longmuir, P.E., and O. Bar-Or. 2000. Factors influencing the physical activity levels of youths with physical and sensory disabilities. *Adapted Physical Activity Quarterly* 17 (1) 40-53.

National Education Steering Committee. 1994. *Maximizing opportunities for students who are deaf or hard-of-hearing.* Gloucester, Ontario: Canadian Deaf Sports Association, and Ottawa, Ontario: Canadian Hard-of-hearing Association.

Padden, C., and T. Humphries. 1988. *Deaf in America: Voices from a culture.* Cambridge, MA: Harvard University.

Sherrill, C. 1998. Deaf and hard-of-hearing conditions. In *Adapted physical activity, recreation, and sport,* edited by T. Grutz, 652-68. 5th ed. Madison, WI: Brown and Benchmark.

Sternberg, M. 1987. *American sign language dictionary.* New York: Harper & Row.

Stewart, D. 1999. Contrasts: The 14th Deaf World Winter Games. *Palaestra* 15 (3): 38-43.

Stewart, D. 1991. *Deaf sport: Impact of sports within the deaf community.* Washington, DC: Gallaudet University.

Stewart, D., J. Robinson, and D. McCarthy. 1991. Participation in deaf sport: Characteristics of elite deaf athletes. *Adapted Physical Activity Quarterly* 8 (2): 136-45.

Tripp, A., and B. Turner. 1986. Hinsdale South High School: A view from the mainstream. *Perspectives for Teachers of the Hearing Impaired* 5: 6-10.

CHAPTER 49

Visual Impairment

Lorraine E. Colson Bloomquist, EdD, FACSM
University of Rhode Island

Overview of the Pathophysiology

Visual impairment is a generic term that includes a range of visual acuity from legal blindness with partial sight to total blindness. Legal blindness is vision of 20/200 or less with the best correction (while wearing glasses). It is the ability to see at 20 feet what the normal eye sees at 200 feet (i.e., ≤ 1/10 of normal vision), blind by acuity. Blind by visual field means having a visual field of less than 10° of central vision, or having tunnel vision (retinitis pigmentosa). Total blindness is lack of visual perception or the inability to recognize a strong light shown directly into the eye, sometimes called "no light perception."

In approximately 95% of the people who are considered blind, there is some residual vision that needs to be used to allow the person to participate as normally as possible. Uncommon in school-aged children, visual impairment is the second least frequently occurring disability in childhood (next to deaf-blind). It is a major problem of old age, however, with approximately 500,000 persons in the United States classified as legally blind.

In younger populations, causes are attributed to birth defects, including congenital cataracts and optic nerve disease. Another now uncommon cause in children is retinopathy of prematurity (excessive oxygen in incubators), although there are many individuals aged 18 and older with this condition. Tumors, injuries, and infectious diseases are possible but less common causes. In persons who are elderly, diabetes, macular degeneration, glaucoma, and cataracts are leading causes. Visual impairment may occur concomitantly in people with cerebral palsy and mental retardation.

Effects on the Exercise Response

Visual impairment generally does not alter the exercise response to a single exercise session. However, some persons may have poor balance, forward head, low cardiovascular fitness, obesity, lack of confidence, timidity, self-stimulatory behaviors such as rocking, and fewer social skills. Verbal cues are essential during testing. Loss of visual field—that is, peripheral vision—may affect mobility.

Effects of Exercise Training

People with a visual impairment can participate in many vigorous physical activities with some adaptations. In fact, regular exercise by people with visual impairment produces the same positive physiological and skills benefits as for individuals without a disability. Additional benefits include:

- more opportunities to improve socialization skills;
- practice and improvement in balance skills, which may be low;
- improvement in self-image, confidence, and spatial orientation;
- improvement in cardiovascular fitness; and
- decrease in obesity.

Depending on the degree of visual impairment, the primary treatment is the use of corrective lenses, or wearing eyeglasses (note: eyeglasses do not correct vision impairments). Often people who are visually impaired wear glasses because they are also nearsighted or farsighted, as in the general population, but glasses are not the norm. Glasses do not correct vision above the 20/200 level (i.e., some people wear glasses, but this does not correct vision to normal, especially sunglasses for light sensitivity when one is outside).

Management and Medications

In normal, healthy adults with visual impairments, no medications are prescribed. People with glaucoma may need to use eye drops. However, if the person has other primary problems (e.g., coronary artery disease or diabetes), then specific medications should be noted and considered in testing and development of the exercise prescription (see chapters 4, 5, 6, and 21).

Visual Impairment: Exercise Testing and Programming

For testing and programming methodologies, see guidelines for the general population in *ACSM's Guidelines for Exercise Testing and Prescription,* 6th edition. If the client has a specific medical problem, see the corresponding chapter in this book (e.g., if the patient has a history of MI, see chapter 4 and testing and programming tables).

Medications	Special Considerations
• Moistening eye drops: May be needed by clients with glaucoma.	• Be aware that clients may have lower than average fitness levels. • Balance may be poor, so the client may need to use handrails for occasional support. • Play an audio tape describing the test, activity, or sport. Ask the client to repeat the instructions verbally before beginning. • Manually and verbally orient the client to all testing/ training facilities and equipment. • Use verbal cues to reinforce the client. • Pair the client with a partner for running and other activities. • Avoid jumping or other high-impact activities if the client has had a detached retina, high myopia, or a cataract surgically removed (aphakia). • Keep the facility clear of clutter.

Recommendations for Exercise Testing

If the person with a visual impairment does not have any signs or symptoms of other primary conditions, standard exercise testing protocols can be used. When signs or symptoms of other primary diseases are present, exercise testing should follow recommended procedures for that particular disorder (see the Visual Impairment: Exercise Testing and Programming table).

The exercise professional may need to follow these additional guidelines for a person with a visual impairment:

- Have all instructions described verbally or on audio tape.
- Allow the person to describe or demonstrate the test protocol before the test begins.
- Give tactile and verbal reinforcement to motivate the participant.
- Allow the person to stand close to the tester to use residual vision, or to lightly touch handrails or tester when necessary.

Recommendations for Exercise Programming

People with visual impairment generally can participate in all types of physical activity, understanding that blind by loss of field leads to greater difficulty in mobility than blind by acuity. The prescription procedure is the same as for any client, but it may be advisable to take one or more of the following special steps:

- Manually or verbally orient the person to facilities.
- Keep instructions in large print or braille or use a strong magnifying glass.
- Play an audio tape describing the routine or activity.
- Ensure that eyeglasses are securely held to the face.
- Allow the person to run or exercise with a partner.
- Have the person run with a short tether to a partner or holding a partner's upper arm.
- Give regular tactile and verbal cues and feedback to prevent boredom.
- Avoid tracking activities such as handball, tennis, and so on.
- Consider offering goal ball, a specialized team sport in which all are blindfolded and a large bell ball is used.
- Most individual sports, such as swimming, weight training, dance, track and field, golf, and aerobics, are appropriate.
- Ensure that people with aphakia (absence of natural lens of eye that occurs when a cataract has been surgically removed), detached retina, or high myo-

pia do not engage in high-impact activities such as jumping.

- Orient the person to all aspects of the facility with special attention to exits, use of the pool, and fire evacuation procedures.
- Keep areas clear of clutter for safe movement.
- Keep doors either closed or wide open.
- Keep equipment in the same place so that individuals can memorize locations.

- Paint or tape (use white) floors or walls where changes occur (e.g., stairs, ramps, pool edge, lockers).
- Keep areas well lit, especially around stairs, pool, equipment, and so on.
- A handrail or grab bar can be installed for accessing equipment.
- Keep a sound source, radio, or tape recorder at one end of the room or at the shallow end of the pool for direction orientation.

CASE STUDY Visual Impairment

A 20-year-old student at a high school for the visually impaired wanted to be physically fit and enjoy a lifetime of sports and exercise. She had congenital cataracts, wore glasses, and could only see shadows and light. She could see a person's face at a 1-ft distance. She also had moderately severe to severe hearing impairment and could only hear a whistle or someone shouting to her when wearing hearing aids in both ears. She communicated by speech and sign language, and used a cane for independent walking except when in the gym or exercising. She participated in regular physical education and was a member of the track team. She ran alone on the track with guide wires along the straight-away and bars on the curves. Her weekly program consisted of two structured 30-min exercise classes and one unstructured 60-min open gym time of cardiovascular circuit training on equipment. She liked to use the treadmill, bike, rowing machine, free weights, and Cybex™ machine, and she liked step aerobics.

S: "I want to be active all my life."

O: Young woman, no distress

Detects light, can't count fingers

Hearing impaired

Visual acuity: Left, 1/160; right, 1/700

A: 1. Severe hearing and visual impairments
2. Average aerobic and strength fitness for age

P: 1. Assistance from exercise specialist in learning safe modes of exercise is advised, including the following:
Use hand over hand with a leader, allowing her to feel the movements of the weights, equipment, and so on.
Model by allowing her to see (at close range) the movements of the leader's arms, legs, and body positions when performing the exercises and using equipment.
Access braille fitness equipment.
Exercise in a small, supervised group, but encourage independence.
2. Initiate progressive aerobic and strength training programs.
3. Compete in track/other sports.

Exercise Program
Goals:
1. Increased strength and aerobic capacity for participation in track
2. Independent use of exercise equipment

(continued)

CASE STUDY Visual Impairment (continued)

Mode	Frequency	Duration	Intensity	Progression
Aerobic	3-7 days/wk			Per track coach
Strength (machines and free weights)	3-7 days/wk			Per track coach
Flexibility (all major muscle groups)	3-7 days/wk			Per track coach
Neuromuscular				
Functional				
Warm-up/Cool-down	Before and after each session			Per track coach

Suggested Readings

Buell, C. 1984. *Physical education for blind children.* 2nd ed. Springfield, IL: Charles C Thomas.

Buell, C. 1982. *Physical education and recreation for the visually handicapped.* Rev. ed. Reston, VA: American Alliance for Health, Physical Education, Recreation and Dance.

Craft, D.H., and L. Lieberman. 1995. Visual impairments and deafness. In *Adapted physical education and sport,* edited by J.P. Winnick, 143-66. 2nd ed. Champaign, IL: Human Kinetics.

Dunn, J.M. 1997. *Special physical education.* 7th ed. Madison, WI: Brown & Benchmark.

Lieberman, L.L., and J.F. Cowart. 1996. *Games for people with sensory impairments.* Champaign, IL: Human Kinetics.

Paciorek, M., and J. Jones. 1994. *Sports and recreation for the disabled.* 2nd ed. Carmel, IN: Cooper Publishing.

Richards, P. 1986. *Popular activities and games for blind, visually impaired and disabled people.* New York: American Foundation for the Blind Press.

Sherrill, C. 1998. Blindness and visual impairment. In *Adapted physical activity, recreation, and sport,* edited by T. Grutz, 652-69. 5th ed. Madison, WI: Brown and Benchmark.

Tapp, K., J.G. Wilhelm, and L.J. Loveless. 1991. *A guide to curriculum planning for visually impaired students.* Bulletin No. 91540. Madison, WI: Wisconsin State Department of Public Instruction.

Winnick, J. 1985. The performance of visually impaired youngsters in physical education activities: Implications for mainstreaming. *Adapted Physical Activity Quarterly* 2 (4): 292-99.

Generic and Brand Names of Commonly Used Drugs by Class

Generic name	Brand name
I. Cardiovascular Drugs	
Alpha₁-Adrenergic Blocking Agents	
Doxazosin	Cardura
Prazosin	Minipress
Terazosin	Hytrin
Beta-Adrenergic Blocking Agents	
Acebutolol	Sectral, Monitan
Atenolol	Tenormin
Betaxolol	Kerlone
Bisoprolol	Zebeta
Carteolol	Cartrol
Metoprolol	Lopressor, Toprol, Betaloc
Nadolol	Corgard
Penbutolol	Levatol
Pindolol	Visken
Propranolol	Inderal
Sotalol	Betapace
Timolol	Blocadren
Selective Alpha- and Beta-Adrenergic Blocking Agents	
Carvedilol	Coreg
Labetalol	Normodyne, Trandate
Nonselective Adrenergic Blocking Agents	
Clonidine	Catapres
Guanabenz	Wyntensin
Guanadrel	Hylorel
Guanethidine	Ismelin
Guanfacine	Tenex
Methyldopa	Aldomet
Phenoxybenzamine	Dibenzyline
Reserpine	Serpasil

(continued)

(continued)

Generic name	Brand name
Calcium-Channel Blockers	
Amlodipine	Norvasc
Bepridil	Vascor
Diltiazem	Cardizem, Dilacor, Tiazac, Tiamate
Felodipine	Plendil, Renedil
Isradipine	DynaCirc
Nicardipine	Cardene
Nifedipine	Adalat, Procardia
Nimodipine	Nimotop
Nisoldipine	Sular
Verapamil	Calan, Isoptin, Covera, Verelan, Chronovera
Angiotensin Converting Enzyme (ACE) Inhibitors	
Benazepril	Lotensin
Captopril	Capoten
Enalapril	Vasotec
Fosinopril	Monopril
Lisinopril	Zestril, Prinivil
Moexipril	Univasc
Perindopril	Aceon, Coversyl
Quinapril	Accupril
Ramipril	Altace
Trandolapril	Mavik
Angiotensin II Receptor Antagonists	
Candesartan	Atacand
Eprosartan	Teveten
Irbesartan	Avapro
Losartan	Cozaar
Telmisartan	Micardis
Valsartan	Diovan
Peripheral Arterial Vasodilators (Non-Adrenergic)	
Hydralazine	Apresoline
Minoxidil	Loniten
Isoxsuprine	Vasodilan
Papaverine	Pavabid
Nitrate Vasodilators	
Amyl nitrite	Amyl nitrite
Isosorbide mononitrate	Ismo, Monoket, Imdur
Isosorbide dinitrate	Isordil, Sorbitrate, Dilatrate
Nitroglycerin, sublingual	Nitrostat
Nitroglycerin, translingual	Nitrolingual, NitroQuick

Generic name	Brand name
Nitroglycerin, transmucosal	Nitroguard
Nitroglycerin, sustained release	Nitrong, Nitrocine, Nitroglyn, NitroBid
Nitroglycerin, transdermal	Minitran, Nitro-Dur, TransdermNitro, Nitrodisc, NitroDerm, Deponit, Trinipatch
Nitroglycerin, topical	Nitro-Bid, Nitrol

Diuretics

Thiazides

Chlorothiazide	Diuril
Chlorthalidone	Hygroton, Thalitone
Hydrochlorothiazide (HCTZ)	Esidrix, Hydrodiuril
Indapamide	Lozide
Metolazone	Zaroxolyn, Mykrox

Loop Diuretics

Bumetanide	Bumex, Burinex
Ethacrynic acid	Edecrin
Furosemide	Lasix
Torsemide	Demadex

Potassium-Sparing Diuretics

Amiloride	Midamor
Spironolactone	Aldactone
Triamterene	Dyrenium

Other Diuretics

Acetazolamide	Diamox

II. Combination Cardiovascular Drugs

Adrenergic Blocker + Diuretic

Methyldopa + chlorothiazide	Aldoclor, Supres
Methyldopa + HCTZ	Aldoril
Clonidine + chlorthalidone	Combipres
Prazosin + polythiazide	Minizide
Reserpine + methyclothiazide	Diutensin
Reserpine + polythiazide	Renese-R
Reserpine + hydroflumethiazide	Salutensin
Reserpine + hydrolazine	Ser-Ap-Es

Beta Blocker + Diuretic

Nadolol + bendroflumethiazide	Corzide
Propranolol + HCTZ	Inderide
Metoprolol + HCTZ	Lopressor
Atenolol + chlorthalidone	Tenoretic
Timolol + HCTZ	Timolide

(continued)

(continued)

Generic name	Brand name
Bisoprolol + HCTZ	Ziac

ACE Inhibitor + Diuretic

Generic name	Brand name
Captopril + HCTZ	Capozide
Benazepril + HCTZ	Lotensin
Lisinopril + HCTZ	Prinzide, Zestoretic
Moexipril + HCTZ	Uniretic
Enalapril + HCTZ	Vaseretic

ACE Inhibitor + Calcium-Channel Blocker

Generic name	Brand name
Enalopril + felodipine	Lexxel
Benazepril + amlodipine	Lotrel
Enalapril + diltiazem	Teczem
Trandolapril + verapamil	Tarka

Angiotensin II Inhibitor + Diuretic

Generic name	Brand name
Candesartan + HCTZ	Atacand
Irbesartan + HCTZ	Avalide
Losartan + HCTZ	Hyzaar
Telmesartan + HCTZ	Micardis
Valsartan + HCTZ	Diovan

Potassium-Sparing Diuretic + Thiazide Diuretic

Generic name	Brand name
Spironolactone + HCTZ	Aldactazide, Spirozide
Triamterene + HCTZ	Dyazide, Hyazide, Maxzide
Amiloride + HCTZ	Moduretic, Moduret

Vasodilator + Diuretic

Generic name	Brand name
Hydralazine + HCTZ	Apresazide

III. Cardiovascular Inotrope and Rhythm Drugs

Cardiac Glycosides

Generic name	Brand name
Digitoxin	Crystodigin
Digoxin	Lanoxin, Lanoxicaps, Digitek

Antiarrhythmic Agents
  Class IA

Generic name	Brand name
Disopyramide	Norpace, Rythmodan-LA
Moricizine	Ethmozine
Pocainamide	Pronestyl, Procan SR, Procanbid
Quinidine	Quinora, Quinidex, Quinaglute, Quinalan, Quinate, Cardioquin

  Class IB

Generic name	Brand name
Lidocaine	Xylocaine, Xylocard
Mexiletine	Mexitil

Generic name	Brand name
Tocainide	Tonocard
Class I	
Flecainide	Tambocor
Propafenone	Rythmol
Class II—Beta blockers (see above)	
Class III	
Amiodarone	Cordarone, Pacerone
Bretylium	Bretylol, Bretylate
Sotalol	Betapace, Rylosol, Sotacar
Class IV—Calcium-channel blockers (see above)	

IV. Cardiovascular Anti-Atherosclerosis Drugs

Antihyperlipidemia Drugs

Bile Acid Binding Resins

Cholestyramine	Questran, Cholybar, Prevalite, LoCHOLEST
Colestipol	Colestid
Colesevelam	Welchol

Fibric Acid Derivatives

Clofibrate	Atromid
Gemfibrozil	Lopid, Lipidil Micro
Fenofibrate	Tricor

HMG CoA Reductase Inhibitors

Atorvastatin	Lipitor
Cerivastatin	Baycol**
Fluvastatin	Lescol
Lovastatin	Mevacor
Pravastatin	Pravachol
Simvastatin	Zocor

Nicotinamides

Nicotinic acid (niacin)	Nicobid, Nicolar, Slo-Niacin, Niaspan, Niacor

**(no longer available in the U.S. and Canada)

V. Anti-Thrombosis Drugs

Platelet Aggregation Antagonists

Aspirin	ASA
Cilostazol	Pletal
Clopidogrel	Plavix
Dipyridamole	Persantine
Dipyridamole + ASA	Aggrenox

(continued)

(continued)

Generic name	Brand name
Ticlopidine	Ticlid

Antithrombotics/Anticoagulants

Dalteparin	Fragmin
Danaparoid	Orgaran
Enoxaparin	Lovenox
Heparin	Calciparine, Hepalean
Tinzaparin	Innohep
Warfarin	Coumadin

Viscosity-Reducing Drugs

Pentoxifylline	Trental

VI. Respiratory Drugs

Sympathomimetic Bronchodilators

Albuterol	Proventil, Ventolin, Volmax, Ventodisk, Alromir, Asmavent, Salbutamol
Bitolterol	Tornalate
Epinephrine	Bronkaid, Primatene, AsthmaNefrin, MicroNefrin
Formoterol	Foradil Aerosolizer
Isoetharine	Bronkosol, Bronkometer
Isoproterenol	Isuprel, Medihaler-Iso
Levalbuterol	Xonopex
Metaproterenol	Alupent, Metaprel, Pro-Meta
Perbuterol	Maxair
Salmeterol	Serevent
Terbutaline	Brethine, Bricanyl

Anticholinergic Bronchodilators

Ipratropium	Atrovent

Xanthine Bronchodilators

Aminophylline	Phyllocontin
Dyphylline	Dilor, Lufyllin
Oxtriphylline	Choledyl
Theophylline	Theobid, Slo-Phyllin, Theo-24, Theo-Dur, Theolair

Corticosteroid Anti-Inflammatory Anti-Asthmatics

Beclomethasone	Beclovent, Vanceril
Budesonide	Pulmicort
Dexamethasone	Decadron Respihaler
Flunisolide	AeroBid
Fluticasone	Flovent
Triamcinolone	Azmacort

Generic name	Brand name
Asthma Prophylactic Drugs	
Cromolyn	Intal, Nasalcrom, Gastrocrom, Nalcrom
Nedocromil	Tilade
Anti-Leukotriene Anti-Asthmatics	
Montelukasat	Singulair
Zafirlukast	Accolate
Zileuton	Zyflo
Mucolytics/Expectorants	
Acetylcysteine	Mucomyst, Mucosil, Parvolex
Guaifenesin	Fenesin, Humibid, Robitussin
Potassium Iodide	SSKI
Combination Anti-Asthmatics	
Albuterol + ipratropium	Combivent, DuoNeb
Fluticasone + salmeterol	Advair Diskus
Isoproterenol + phenylephrine	Duo-Medihaler

VII. Respiratory/Allergy Drugs

Generic name	Brand name
Antihistamines	
Sedatives	
Azatadine	Optimine
Brompheniramine	Dimetapp, Dimetane
Cetirizine	Zyrtec, Reactine
Chlorpheniramine	Chlor-Trimeton, Chlo-Amine, Aller-Chlor
Clemastine	Tavist
Cyproheptadine	Periactin
Dexchlorpheniramine	Polaramine
Dimenhydrinate	Dramamine, Gravol
Diphenhydramine	Benadryl, Unisom, Nytol, Sleep-eze, Allerdryl, Allernix
Doxylamine	Unisom-Nighttime
Hydroxyzine	Atarax, Vistaril
Phenindamine	Nolahist
Tripelennamine	PBZ
Nonsedating	
Fexofenadine	Allegra
Loratidine	Claritin

VIII. Diabetes Drugs

Generic name	Brand name
Sulfonylureas	
Acetohexaminde	Dymelor
Chlorpropamide	Diabinese

(continued)

(continued)

Generic name	Brand name
Glimepiride	Amaryl
Glipizide	Glucotrol, Glucotrol XL
Glyburide	DiaBeta, Glynase PresTab, Micronase, Euglucon
Tolazamide	Tolinase
Tolbutamide	Orinase, Tol-Tab

Biguanides/Combination Biguanides

Metformin	Glucophage
Metformin + glyburide	Glucovance

Alpha-Glucosidase Inhibitors

Acarbose	Precose, Prandose
Miglitol	Glyset

Thiazoladinediones

Pioglitazone	Actos
Rosiglitazone	Avandia

Meglitinides

Nateglinide	Starlix
Regaglinide	Prandin, Gluconorm

Insulin (all rapidity of onset types)

Human	Humulin, Novolin, Lispro, Glargine, Lantus
Porcine	Iletin

Glucagon

Glucagon	Glucagon, GlucaGen

IX. Weight-Loss Drugs

Orlistat	Xenical
Sibutramine	Meridia

X. Gastrointestinal Drugs

H-2 Receptor Blockers

Cimetidine	Tagamet
Famotidine	Pepcid
Lansoprazole	Prevacid
Nizatidine	Axid
Ranitidine	Zantac

Gastric Secretion Inhibitors/Mucosa Protectors

Esomeprazole	Nexium
Lausoprazole	Prevacid
Misoprostol	Cytotec
Omeprazole	Prilosec, Losec

Generic name	Brand name
Pantoprazole	Protonix, Pantaloc
Rabeprazole	Aciphex
Sucralfate	Carafate, Sulcrate

Gastrointestinal Motility Agents

Cisapride	Propulsid, Prepulsid
Metoclopramide	Reglan, Maxesan

Anti-Inflammatories

5-Aminosalicylate	Pentasa
Sulfasalazine	Azulfidine, Salazopyrin

Digestive Enzymes

Amylase-lipase-pancrease	Pancrease, Creon, Cotazym, Viokase, Ku-Zyme, Donnazyme, Entozyme

XI. Analgesic Drugs

Non-Narcotic Analgesics

Acetominophen	Tylenol, Tempra, Atasol
Tramadol	Ultram

Barbiturate Analgesics

Phenobarbital	Phenobarbital
Primidone	Mysoline

Narcotic Analgesics

Butalbibal	Oxybutamin
Codeine	Codeine
Hydromorphone	Dilaudid
Hydroxycodone	Vicodin
Fentanyl	Duragesic
Meperedine	Demerol
Morphine	MS Contin
Oxycodone	Percodan, Oxycontin, Roxicodone, Speudol, Endocodone
Pentazocine	Talwin
Propxyphene	Darvon

Narcotics + Acetaminophen

Codeine + acetaminophen	Tylenol 3, Tylenol with Codeine
Hydrocodone + acetaminophen	Anexsia, Lorcet, Lortab, Maxidone, Vicodin, Zydone
Pentazocine + acetaminophen	Talacen
Propoxyphene + acetaminophen	Darvocet, Wygesic
Oxycodone + acetaminophen	Percocet, Percodan

(continued)

(continued)

Generic name	Brand name
XII. Analgesic/Anti-Inflammatory Drugs	

Nonsteroidal Anti-Inflammatory Drugs (NSAIDs)
  Prostaglandin Inhibitor NSAIDs

Generic name	Brand name
Aspirin	ASA, Anacin, Bufferin
Diclofenac	Voltaren, Arthrotec
Etodolac	Lodine
Ibuprofen	Motrin, Advil, Nuprin, Rufen
Indomethacin	Indocin, Indocid, Indotec
Fenoprofen	Nalfon
Flurbiprofen	Ansaid, Froben
Ketoprofen	Orudis, Actron, Oruvail, Orafen
Ketorolac	Toradol
Meloxicam	Mobic
Nabumetone	Relafen
Naproxen	Aleve, Naprosyn
Oxaprozin	Daypro
Phenylbutazone	Butazolidin
Piroxicam	Feldene, Fexicam
Salsalate	Disalcid
Sulfasalazine	Azulfidine, Salazopyrin
Sulindac	Clinoril
Tenoxicam	Mobiflex
Tolmetin	Tolectin

Cyclooxygenase II Inhibitor (Cox II) NSAIDs

Generic name	Brand name
Celecoxib	Celebrex
Rofecoxib	Vioxx

XIII. Anti-Inflammatory/Immunosuppressant Drugs

Glucocorticoid Immunosuppressants

Generic name	Brand name
Betamethasone	Celestone, Beben
Dexamethasone	Dexasone, Decadron, Dexone, Hexadrol
Fludrocortisone	Florinef
Hydrocortisone	Cortef, Solu-Cortef
Methylprednisolone	Medrol, Depo-Medrol, Solu-Medrol
Prednisolone	Prelone, Pediapred, Orapred
Prednisone	Deltasone, Orasone, Prednisone, Meticarten, Pred-Pak, Winpred, Sterapred, Metreton
Triamcinolone	Aristospan, Aristocort, Kenalog

XIV. Immunosuppressant Drugs

Immune Modulator Drugs (see also Anticancer and Anticancer Adjunct Drugs)

Generic name	Brand name
Azathioprine	Imuran
Chlorambucil	Leukeran

Generic name	Brand name
Cyclophosphamide	Cytoxan, Neosar, Procytox
Cyclosporine	Neoral, Sandimmune, Gengraf
Mycophenolate	CellCept
Penicillamine	Cuprimine, Depen
Tacrolimus	Prograf

XV. Anti-Arthritis Drugs
Gouty Arthritis

Allopurinol	Zyloprim
Colchicine	Colchicine
Probenecid	Benemid, Probalan, Benuryl
Sulfinpyrazone	Anturane
Colchicine + probenecid	Colbenemid

Osteoarthritis

Hylauronic acid and derivatives	Hyalgan, Synvisc

Rheumatic Immunomodulating Drugs

Etanercept	Eubrel
Gold (intramuscular/oral)	Ridaura, Myochrysine
Hydroxychloroquine	Plaquenil
Infliximab	Remicade (also used for Crohn's disease)
Leflunomide	Arava
Methotrexate	Rheumatrex, Folex, Trexall

XVI. Osteoporosis Drugs
Bone Resorption Inhibitors (Bisphosphonates)

Alendronate	Fosamax
Etidronate	Didronel
Pamidronate	Aredia
Risedronate	Actonel
Tiludronate	Skelid

Parathyroid Hormone

Calcitonin (human recombinant)	Cibacalcin
Calcitonin (salmon)	Calcimar, Miacalcin, Caltine

Estrogen Antagonists

Clomiphene	Clomid, Milophene, Serophene
Raloxifene	Evista
Tamoxifen	Nolvaclex, Tamone

XVI. Miscellaneous Metabolic Disease Drugs
Renal Failure Adjunctive Drugs

Calcium (phosphate binders)	PhosLo, OsCal, Tums, Caltrate

(continued)

(continued)

Generic name	Brand name
Iron	InFeD, Fergon, Palafer, Fer-In-Sol, Slow-Fe, FeoSol, Dexiron, Venofer

Mydriatic Drugs

Generic name	Brand name
Atropine	Atropine
Cyclopentolate	AK-Pentolate, Cyclogyl, Pentolait
Phenylephrine	Neo-Synephrine, Mydefrin, Relief
Scopolamine	Transderm Scop, Transderm-V
Tropicamide	Mydriacyl

Anti-Glaucoma Drugs
Cholinergic

Generic name	Brand name
Demecarium	Humorsol
Echothiophate	Phospholine

Beta-Adrenergic Blockers

Generic name	Brand name
Betaxolol	Betoptic
Carteolol	Ocupress
Levobunolol	Betagan
Levobetaxolol	Betaxon
Timolol	Timoptic

Sympathomimetics

Generic name	Brand name
Apraclonidine	Iopidine
Brimonidine	Alphagon
Dipivefrin	Propine

XVII. Sex Hormones

Androgens

Generic name	Brand name
Danazol	Cyclomen
Fluoxymesterone	Halotestin
Methyltestosterone	Metandren, Android, Methitest, Testred, Virilon
Nandrolone	Deca-Durabolin, Hybolin Decanoate
Testosterone	Androderm, Andriol, Depo-Testosterone, Androgel, Testoderm, Depotest, Testro-LA, Dalatestryl, Everone, Testro AQ, Virilon IM

Estrogens and Progesterones

Generic name	Brand name
Conjugated estrogen	Premarin, CES, Congest
Diethylstilbestrol	Stilbestrol, Honvol, Stilphostrol
Esterified estrogen	Estratab, Menest, Neo-Estrone
Estradiol	Alora, Climara, Estrace, Estraderm, Delestrogen, Menaval, Valergen, Vivelle, Esclim, Gynogen, Estinyl
Estrone	Aquest, Estragyn, Kestrone, Wehgen, Estragyn
Estropipate	Ogen, Ortho-Est

Generic name	Brand name
Oral Contraceptives	
Ethinyl estradiol + Norgestrel	Ovral
Ethinyl estradiol + Desogestrel	Ortho-Cept
Ethinyl estradiol + Ethyndiol	Demulen
Ethinyl estradiol + Levonorgestrel	Alesse
Ethinyl estradiol + Norethindrone	Loestrin, Minestrin
Ethinyl estradiol + Norgestimate	Cyclen
Levonorgestrel	Norplant, Plan B
Medroxyprogesterone	Depo-Provera
Medroxyprogesterone + estradiol	Lunelle
Mestranol + Norethindrone	Ortho-Novum
Norethindrone	Micronor, Nor-QD, Ovret
Norgestrel	Ovrette
Progestins for Non-Contraceptive Use	
Hydroxyprogresterone	Gesterol, Hylutin, Prodrox, Pro-Span
Medrogestone	Colprone
Medroxyprogesterone	Amen, Curretab, Cycrin, Depo-Provera, Provera, Alti-MPA
Megestrol	Megace
Norethindrone	Aygestin, Norlutate
Progesterone	Prometrium, Gesterol, Crinone

XVIII. Other Hormones

Generic name	Brand name
Human Growth Hormone	
Somatrem	Protropin
Somatropin (recombinant hGH)	Genotropin, Humatrope, Norditropin, Nutropin, Serostim
Hematopoietic Colony-Stimulating Factors (CSF)	
Erythropoietin (r-HuEPO)	Epogen, Procrit, Eprex
Filgastrim (G-CSF)	Neupogen
Sargramostim (GM-CSF)	Leukine
Opreluekin	Neumega
Hypophyseal Hormone Agonists/Antagonists	
Desmopressin (arginine vasopressin)	DDAVP, Stimate, Octustim
Somatostatin Analogs	
Octreotide	Sandostatin
Thyroid	
Levothyroxine	Synthroid, Levoxyl, Levothroid, L-thyroine, Levotec, Eltroxin, Levo-T
Liothyronine	Cytomel

(continued)

(continued)

Generic name   **Brand name**

XIX. Anticancer Drugs

Anticancer drugs come in several classes, with some drugs belonging to more than one class. This list is not comprehensive.

Alkalating Agents

Generic name	Brand name
Busulfan	Myleran, Busulfex
Carboplatin	Paraplatin
Carmustine	BiCNU
Cisplatin	Platinol
Chlorambucil	Leukeran
Cyclophosphamide	Cytoxan, Neosar, Procytox
Dacarbazine	DTIC
Ifosfamide	IFEX
Lomustine	CeeNU, CCNU
Melphalan	Alkeran
Procarbazine	Matulane, Natulan
Thiotepa	Thiotepa

Anthracycline Antibiotics

Generic name	Brand name
Doxorubicin	Doxil, Caelyx
Daunorubicin	Cerubidine, DaunoXome
Idarubicin	Idamycin
Epirubicin	Ellence
Valrubicin	Valstar

Anti-Microtubule Vinca Alkaloids

Generic name	Brand name
Etoposide (VP-16)	VePesid, Etophos
Vincristine	Oncovin, Vincasar, Vincrex
Vinblastine	Velban
Vindesine (vinblastine)	Eldisine
Vinorelbine	Navelbine

Antimetabolites

Generic name	Brand name
Capecitabine	Xeloda
Cladribine (2-CdA)	Leustatin
Cytarabine (ara-C)	Cytosar
Flourouracil (5-FU)	Adrucil, Efudex, Flouroplex
Floxuridine	FUDR
Fludarabine	Fludara
Gemcytabine	Gemzar
Hydroxyurea	Hydrea, Droxia
Methotrexate	Amethopterin, Methotrexate
Mercaptopurine (6-MP)	Purinethol
Pentastatin (2-DCF)	Nipent

Generic name	Brand name
Raltitrexed	Tomudex
Thioguanine	Lanvis

Antineoplastics/Antibiotics

Amsacrine	AMSA
Altretamine	Hexalen
Arsenic trioxide	Trisenox
Bleomycin	Blenoxane
Dactinomycin	Cosmegen
Denileukin	Ontak
Diclofenac	Solaraze
Estramustine	Emcyt
Formifer	Photofrin
Imatinib	Gleevec
Irinotecan (CPT-11)	Camptosar
Mitomycin	Mutamycin
Mitoxantrone	Novantrone
Mithramycin	Mithracin
Pegaspargase	Oncaspar
Streptozocin	Zanosar
Temozolomide	Temodar
Teniposide (VM-26)	Vumon

Anti-Microtubule Taxanes

Doxataxel	Taxotere
Paclitaxel	Taxol

Retinoids/Psoralens

Altitretinoin	Panretin Gel
Bexarotene	Targretin
Methoxsalen	MOP, Oxsoralen
Tretinoin	Vesanoid

Anti-DNA Replication Drugs

Asparaginase	Elspar, Kidrolase
Topotecan	Hycamtin

Monoclonal Antibodies

Alemtuzumab	Campath
Gemtuzumab	Mylotarg
Rituximab	Rituxan
Trastuzumab	Herceptin

XX. Anticancer Adjunct Drugs

Levamisole	Ergamisol

(continued)

(continued)

Generic name	Brand name
Antiandrogens	
Bicalutamide	Casodex
Buserelin	Suprefact
Cyproterone	Androcur
Flutamide	Eulexin, Euflex
Nilutamide	Nilandron, Anandron
Triptorelin	Trelstar
Antiestrogens	
Anastrozole	Arimidex
Exemestane	Aromasin
Letrozole	Femara
Tamoxifen	Nolvadex, Tamofen, Tamone
Toremifene	Fareston
Antigonadotropic Drugs	
Goserelin	Zoladex
Leuprolide	Lupron, Viadur
Anti-Adrenal Drugs	
Aminoglutethamide	Cytadren
Mitotane	Lysodren

XXI. Antiviral Drugs

Generic name	Brand name
Anti-HIV	
Abacavir	Ziagen
Amprenavir	Agenerase, APV
Delavirdine	Rescriptor
Didanosine	ddI, Videx
Efavirenz	Sustiva
Indinavir	Crixivan, IDV
Lamivudine	Epivir, 3TC, Heptovir
Nelfinavir	Viracept, NFV
Nevirapine	Viramune
Ritonavir	Norvir, RTV
Saquinavir	Fortovase, Invirase
Stavudine	d4T, Zerit
Zalcitabine	ddC, Hivid
Zidovudine	AZT, Retrovir, Azidothymidine, ZDV
Anti-HIV Combinations	
Abacavir + lamivudine + zidovudine	Trizivir
Lamivudine + zidovudine	Combivir
Lopinavir + ritonavir	Kaletra

Generic name	Brand name
Anti-Cytomegalovirus (in HIV+)	
Cidofovir	Vistide
Fomivirsen	Vitravene
Foscarnet	Foscavir
Ganciclovir	Cytovene, Vitrasert
Valganciclovir	Valcyte
Anti-Influenza	
Amantadine	Symmetrel
Oseltamivir	Tamiflu
Rimantadine	Flumadine
Zanamivir	Relenza
Anti-Herpetic	
Acyclovir	Zovirax, Avirax
Idoxuridine	Herplex Liquifilm, Stoxil
Famociclovir	Famvir
Trifluridine	Viroptic
Valacyclovir	Valtrex
Vidarabine	Vira-A

XXII. Cytokines/Cell – Cell Signaling Drugs

Interferon-alpha	Alferon, Intron, Roferon, Wellferon
Interferon-beta	Avonex, Rebif
Interleukin-2	Proleukin, Aldesleukin
Denileukin	Ontak

XXIII. Neurological Drugs

Generic name	Brand name
Anticonvulsants	
Carbamazepine	Tegretol, Carbatrol, Epitol
Clonazepam	Klonopin, Clonapam, Rivotril
Ethosuximide	Zarontin
Gabapentine	Neurontin
Methsuximide	Celontin
Phenobarbital	Luminal
Phenytoin	Dilantin, Diphen
Primidone	Mysoline
Topiramate	Topamax
Valproic acid	Depakene, Depakote, Depacon, Epiject, Epival, Deproic
H3 Receptor Antagonist (Anti-Migraine) Drugs	
Almotriptan	Axert
Naratriptan	Amerge
Rizatriptan	Maxalt

(continued)

(continued)

Generic name	Brand name
Sumitriptan	Imitrex
Zolmitriptan	Zomig

Anti-Myasthenic Drugs

Ambenonium	Mytelase
Neostigmine	Prostigmin
Pyridostigmine	Mestinon, Regonal

Skeletal Muscle Relaxants/Anti-Spastics

Baclofen	Lioresal
Carisoprodol	Soma, Vanadom
Chlorphenesin	Maolate
Chlorzoxasone	Parafon, Paraflex, Remular, Strifon
Cyclobenzaprine	Flexeril
Dantrolene	Dantrium
Diazepam	Valium, Diastat
Metaxalone	Skelaxin
Methocarbamol	Robaxin, Carbacot, Skelex
Orphenadrine	Norflex
Tizanidine	Zanaflex

Antiparkinsonian Drugs
  Antidyskinetics

Amantadine	Symmetrel, Endantadine
Benztropine	Cogentin, Bensylate
Biperiden	Akineton
Ethopropazine	Parsidol, Parsitan
Procyclidine	Kemadrin
Selegiline	Eldepryl, Carbex, Deprenyl, Atapryl, Selpak
Trihexyphenidyl	Artane, Trihexane

  Dopaminergics

Bromocriptine	Parlodel
Levodopa	Laradopa
Levodopa/Carbidopa	Sinemet, Atamet, Levocarb
Pergolide	Permax
Pramipexole	Mirapex
Ropinirole	Requip

Anti-ALS (Amyotrophic Lateral Sclerosis) Drugs

Riluzole	Rilutek

XXIV. Multiple Sclerosis Antagonists

Glatiramer	Copaxone

Generic name	Brand name
XXV. Psychotropic Drugs	
Benzodiazepine Anxiolytics	
Alprazolam	Xanax
Clorazepate	Tranxene
Chlordiazepoxide	Librium
Diazepam	Valium, Vivol, E Pam
Estazolam	ProSom
Flurazepam	Dalmane, Somnol, SomPam
Lorazepam	Ativan
Oxazepam	Serax
Temazepam	Restoril
Triazolam	Halcion
Other Anxiolytics	
Buspirone	Buspar, Bustab, Buspirex
L-tryptophan	Tryptan
Promethazine	Promethazine
Sedatives/Hypnotics	
Chloral hydrate	Aquachloral Supprettes, Somnote, Noctec
Diphenhydramine	Benadryl, Banaril, Dephen, Sominex, Allerdryl, Allernix
Methotrimeprazine	Nozinan
Zaleplon	Sonata, Starnoc
Zolpidem	Ambien
Monoamine Oxidase Inhibitors (MAOIs)	
Isocarboxazid	Marplan
Phenelzine	Nardil
Tranylcypromine	Parnate
Stimulants	
Dexedrine	Dexedrin, Dextrostat
Methylphenidate	Ritalin, Methylin, Metadate, Concerta
Pemoline	Cylert
Anti-Mania Drugs	
Lithium	Lithane, Eskalith, Cibalith, Carbolith, Duralith
Tricyclic Antidepressants	
Amitriptyline	Elavil, Endep, Vanatrip
Amoxapine	Asendin
Clomipramine	Anafranil
Desipramine	Norpramin
Doxepin	Sinequan, Zonalon
Imipramine	Tofranil

(continued)

(continued)

Generic name	Brand name
Maprotilin	Ludiomil
Nortriptylin	Aventyl, Pamelor
Phenylzine	Nardil
Trimipramine	Surmontil, Rhotrimine

Serotonin Reuptake Inhibitor Antidepressants

Citalopram	Celexa
Fluoxetine	Prozac
Fluvoxamine	Luvox
Paroxetine	Paxil
Sertraline	Zoloft

Antidepressants—Other

Bupropion	Wellbutrin
Trazodone	Trazodone
Venlafaxine	Effexor

Tranquilizers/Anti-Psychotics

Chlorpromazine	Thorazine, Largactil
Clozapine	Clozaril
Flupenthixol	Fluanxol
Fluphenazine	Permetil, Prolixin, Modicate, Moditen
Haloperidol	Haldol
Loxapine	Loxitane, Loxapac
Mesoridazine	Serentil
Molindone	Moban
Olanzapine	Zyprexa
Pericyazine	Neuleptil
Perphenazine	Trilafon
Pimozide	Orap
Pipotiazine	Piportil
Promazine	Promazine
Quetiapine	Seroquel
Risperidone	Risperdal
Thioridazine	Mellaril
Thiothixene	Navane
Trifluoperazine	Stelazine

APPENDIX B

Effects of Medications on Heart Rate, Blood Pressure, the Electrocardiogram (ECG), and Exercise Capacity

Medications	Heart rate	Blood pressure	ECG	Exercise capacity
I. β-blockers (including carvediolol, labetalol)	↓*(R and E)	↓ (R and E)	↓ HR*(R); ↓ ischemia† (E)	↑ in patients with angina; ↓ or ↔ in patients without angina
II. Nitrates	↑(R); ↑ or ↔ (E)	↓(R); ↓ or ↔ (E)	↑ HR (R); ↑ or ↔ HR (E); ↓ ischemia† (E)	↑ in patients with angina; ↔ in patients without angina; ↑ or ↔ in patients with congestive heart failure (CHF)
III. Calcium-channel blockers				
Amlodipine Felodipine Isradipine Nicardipine Nifedipine Nimodipine Nisoldipine	↑ or ↔ (R and E)	↓ (R and E)	↑ or ↔ HR (R and E); ↓ ischemia† (E)	↑ in patients with angina; ↔ in patients without angina
Bepridil Diltiazem Verapamil	↓ (R and E)	↓ (R and E)	↓ HR (R and E); ↓ ischemia† (E)	
IV. Digitalis	↓ in patients with atrial fibrillation and possibly CHF Not significantly altered in patients with sinus rhythm	↔ (R and E)	May produce nonspecific ST-T wave changes (R) May produce ST segment depression (E)	↑ only in patients with atrial fibrillation or in patients with CHF
V. Diuretics	↔ (R and E)	↔ or ↓ (R and E)	↔ or PVCs (R) May cause PVCs and "false positive" test results if hypokalemia occurs May cause PVCs if hypomagnesemia occurs (E)	↔, except possibly in patients with CHF
VI. Vasodilators, nonadrenergic	↑ or ↔ (R and E)	↓ (R and E)	↑ or ↔ HR (R and E)	↔, except ↑ or ↔ in patients with CHF
Ace inhibitors	↔ (R and E)	↓ (R and E)	↔ (R and E)	↔, except ↑ or ↔ in patients with CHF
Alpha-adrenergic blockers	↔ (R and E)	↓ (R and E)	↔ (R and E)	↔
Antiadrenergic agents without selective blockade	↓ or ↔ (R and E)	↓ (R and E)	↓ or ↔ HR (R and E)	↔

Key: ↑ = increase; ↔ = no effect; ↓ = decrease; R = rest; E = exercise; HR = heart rate; PVCs = premature ventricular contractions.

*β-blockers with ISA lower resting HR only slightly.

†May prevent or delay myocardial ischemia (see chapter 6).

Medications	Heart rate	Blood pressure	ECG	Exercise capacity
VII. Antiarrhythmic agents	All antiarrhythmic agents may cause new or worsened arrhythmias (proarrhythmic effect)			
Class I				
Quinidine	↑ or ↔ (R and E)	↓ or ↔ (R) ↔ (E)	↑ or ↔ HR (R)	↔
Disopyramide			May prolong QRS and QT intervals (R) Quinidine may result in "false negative" test results (E)	
Procainamide	↔ (R and E)	↔ (R and E)	May prolong QRS and QT intervals (R) May result in "false positive" test results (E)	↔
Phenytoin Tocainide Mexiletine	↔ (R and E)	↔ (R and E)	↔ (R and E)	↔
Flecainide Moricicine	↔ (R and E)	↔ (R and E)	May prolong QRS and QT intervals (R) ↔ (E)	↔
Propafenone	↓ (R) ↓ or ↔ (E)	↔ (R and E)	↓ HR (R) ↓ or ↔ HR (E)	↔
Class II				
β-Blockers (see I)				
Class III				
Amiodarone	↓ (R and E)	↔ (R and E)	↓ HR (R) ↔ (E)	↔
Class IV				
Calcium-channel blockers (see III)				

Key: ↑ = increase, ↔ = no effect; ↓ = decrease; R = rest; E = exercise; HR = heart rate; PVCs = premature ventricular contractions.

*β-blockers with ISA lower resting HR only slightly.

†May prevent or delay myocardial ischemia (see chapter 6).

(continued)

Medications	Heart rate	Blood pressure	ECG	Exercise capacity
VIII. Bronchodilators	↔ (R and E)	↔ (R and E)	↔ (R and E)	↑ in patients limited by bronchospasm
Anticholinergic agents Methylxanthines	↑ or ↔ (R and E)	↔	↑ or ↔ HR May produce PVCs (R and E)	↔
Sympathomimetic agents	↑ or ↔ (R and E)	↑, ↔, or ↓ (R and E)	↑ or ↔ HR (R and E)	↔
Cromolyn sodium	↔ (R and E)	↔ (R and E)	↔ (R and E)	↔
Corticosteroids	↔ (R and E)	↔ (R and E)	↔ (R and E)	

Key: ↑ = increase, ↔ = no effect; ↓ = decrease; R = rest; E = exercise; HR = heart rate; PVCs = premature ventricular contractions.

*β-blockers with ISA lower resting HR only slightly.

†May prevent or delay myocardial ischemia (see chapter 6).

Reprinted, by permission, from American College of Sports Medicine, 2000, *ACSM's guidelines for exercise testing and prescription*, 6th ed., edited by B.A. Franklin, M.H. Whaley, and E.T. Howley.

APPENDIX C

Effects of Non-Cardiovascular and Non-Respiratory Drugs on Exercise Capacity

Generic Name	Effects on Exercise
I. Cardiovascular Anti-Atherosclerosis Drugs	
Anti-Hyperlipidemia Drugs	
Bile Acid Binding Resins	
Fibric Acid Derivatives	• Fibric acid derivatives have a synergistic potential to cause rhabdomyolysis when used together with an HMG CoA reductase drug.
HMG CoA Reductase Inhibitors	• HMG CoA reductase inhibitors can cause skeletal muscle rhabdomyolysis, which can be exacerbated by exercise.
Nicotinamides (niacin)	• Niacin can cause flushing, but this is not known to have an effect on exercise.
II. Anti-Thrombosis Drugs	
Platelet Aggregation Antagonists	
Cilostazol	• Cilostazol improves walking performance in intermittent claudication.
Antithrombotics/Anticoagulants	
Viscosity-Reducing Drugs	
Pentoxifylline	• Pentoxifylline reduces red cell rigidity, which is thought to improve walking performance in intermittent claudication.
III. Respiratory Drugs—Bronchodilators	
Sympathomimetic Bronchodilators	• Sympathomimetic bronchodilators and anticholinergic bronchodilators have similar effects on the pulmonary and right-heart responses to exercise.
Albuterol	• Albuterol and salmeterol improve exercise performance in some persons with chronic obstructive pulmonary disease (COPD).
Salmeterol	

(continued)

Generic Name	Effects on Exercise
Anticholinergic Bronchodilators Ipratropium	• Ipratropium increases exercise capacity in individuals with COPD who are limited by respiration, but not in those limited by non-respiratory mechanisms. • Ipatropium improves respiratory function in COPD after long-term treatment over 1 year.
Xanthine Bronchodilators Theophylline	• Theophylline increases angina threshold in men with syndrome X and in atherosclerotic coronary artery disease (CAD), probably by an adenosine-mediated mechanism. • Theophylline increases exercise capacity in some individuals with COPD.

IV. Respiratory Drugs—Anti-Asthmatics

Corticosteroid Anti-Inflammatory Anti-Asthmatics	• Corticosteroids suppress inflammation in the bronchial tree, which improves ventilation. They also may have an interactive effect with bronchodilators over the long term to further improve ventilation.
Asthma Prophylactic Drugs Cromolyn	• Cromolyn improves exercise by preventing exercise-induced asthma.
Anti-Leukotriene Anti-Asthmatics Montelukasat	• Montelukast prevents exercise-induced bronchospasm.
Zafirlukast	• Zafirlukast prevents exercise-induced bronchospasm but is associated with a post-treatment refractory period of up to 6 hours.
Mucolytics/Expectorants Combination Anti-Asthmatics	

V. Respiratory Drugs—Anti-Allergy

Antihistamines Cyproheptadine	• Cyproheptadine's antiserotonergic effects can improve walking performance in persons with spasticity.
Diphenhydramine	• Diphenhydramine, chlorpheniramine, and terfenadine (discontinued) have no effect on the acute response to exercise.
Terfenadine	• Terfenandine (discontinued) improves exercise-induced bronchoconstriction. • Antihistamines (terfenandine) do not alter exercise tolerance in chronic fatigue syndrome (CFS) despite immunologic symptoms in CFS.

Generic Name	Effects on Exercise
VI. Diabetes Drugs	
Sulfonylureas Biguanides Alpha-Glucosidase Inhibitors Thiazoladinediones Meglitinides Insulin (all rapidity of onset types) Glucagon	• Drugs to treat diabetes have the potential to alter the glycemic response to exercise, especially insulin, glucagon, and sulfonylureas.
VII. Weight-Loss Drugs	
Orlistat	• Orlistat inhibits fat absorption, but probably has little effect on the acute response to exercise.
Sibutramine	• Sibutramine has sympathomimetic effects that can increase resting HR and BP, and presumably exertional BP.
VIII. Gastrointestinal Drugs	
H-2 Receptor Blockers Gastric Secretion Inhibitors/Mucosa Protectors Gastrointestinal Motility Agents Metoclopramide	• Metoclopramide may decrease the BP response and increase the HR response to exercise.
Digestive Enzymes Amylase-lipase-pancrease	• Amylase-lipase-pancrease has no known direct effect on exercise, but improved digestion may improve muscle and substrate anabolism.
IX. Analgesic Drugs	
Non-Narcotic Analgesics Acetominophen	• Exercise does not affect the pharmacokinetic properties of acetaminophen.
Barbiturate Analgesics Narcotic Analgesics Morphine	• Morphine improves exercise tolerance in persons with COPD and is better tolerated when used in combination with promethazine.
Narcotics + Acetaminophen	
X. Analgesic/Anti-Inflammatory Drugs	
Nonsteroidal Anti-Inflammatory Drugs (NSAIDs) Prostaglandin Inhibitor NSAIDs	

(continued)

Generic Name	Effects on Exercise
Aspirin Diclofenac Ibuprofen Indomethacin Piroxicam Cyclooxygenase II Inhibitor (Cox II) NSAIDs	• Aspirin reduces EMG evidence of delayed-onset muscle soreness. • Aspirin reduction of pro-inflammatory cytokines may be partly responsible for the cardio-protective effect of aspirin. • Low-dose aspirin does not alter the prostaglandin response to exercise. • Ibuprofen reduces creatine kinase in blood after eccentric exercise, but not other markers of delayed-onset muscle soreness, probably by blockade of prostaglandin response. • Indomethacin can decrease leg blood flow in persons with CHF who have prostaglandin-dependent hyperemia during exercise. • Naproxen reduces delayed-onset muscle soreness. • Diclofenac reduces delayed-onset muscle soreness. • Piroxicam facilitates a more rapid return to exercise after ankle sprains, but may delay return to normal joint function.

XI. Anti-Inflammatory/Immunosuppressant Drugs

Glucocorticoid Immunosuppressants Prednisolone	• Anti-inflammatory drugs may improve exercise performance by a number of mechanisms, depending on the disease condition. The main mechanism would be reduction of pain and subsequent improvement in musculoskeletal function because of decreased inhibition of muscle contractions. • Prednisolone improves FVC, $\dot{V}_E$max (maximal minute ventilation), $\dot{V}O_2$max, and maximal HR in persons with COPD.

XII. Immunosuppressant Drugs

Immune Modulator Drugs (see also Anticancer Drugs, Anticancer Adjunct Drugs) Tacrolimus	• Tacrolimus appears to exacerbate abnormal pressor response in kidney transplant recipients.

XIII. Anti-Arthritis Drugs

Gouty Arthritis Osteoarthritis Hylauronic acid and derivatives Rheumatic Immunomodulating Drugs	• Exercise is relatively contraindicated in active crystal-induced arthritis. • Arthritis medications improve exercise performance by relieving the condition, but it is not known if they have other effects on exercise.

Generic Name	Effects on Exercise
	• Other arthritis moderating and mitigating drugs improve exercise function by relieving symptoms. In most cases, other effects on exercise are not known.

XIV. Osteoporosis Drugs

	• Osteoporosis drugs presumably improve the ability to achieve higher bone loading at reduced risk of fracture.
Bone Resorption Inhibitors (Bisphosphonates)	• Bisphosphonates have no known effect on exercise capacity.
	• Exercise in combination with bisphosphonates may help increase bone density above that of either exercise or biphosphonates alone. Bisphosphonates may have synergy with exercise training.
Parathyroid Hormones	
Estrogen Antagonists	

XV. Miscellaneous Metabolic Disease Drugs

Renal Failure Adjunctive Drugs	
Mydriatic Drugs	
Scopolamine	• Scopolamine may enhance exercise capacity and improve HR variability in CHF.
	• Scopolamine improves balance of sympathetic and parasympathetic drive, baroflex sensitivity, and exercise test performance in persons with CAD.
Anti-Glaucoma Drugs	

XVI. Sex Hormones

Androgens	• Androgens may decrease postexertional rhabdomyolysis and stress response to resistance exercise.
	• Testosterone probably increases muscle leanness, muscle mass, and bone density in men with AIDS wasting syndrome, or with COPD, and may increase muscle mass in elderly men with low testosterone levels.
	• Testosterone had no benefit on muscle mass, and was inferior to exercise training, in men with AIDS and normal blood testosterone levels.
	• Testosterone improves anginal threshold, probably through coronary artery relaxation.
	• Testosterone has not consistently been shown to increase strength or exercise capacity.
	• Androstenedione/androstenediol has no effect on strength during heavy resistance training in middle-aged men but does worsen cardiovascular risk factors.

(continued)

Generic Name	Effects on Exercise
Estrogens and Progesterones	
Conjugated estrogen	
Diethylstilbestrol	
Esterified estrogens	
Estradiol	
Estrone	
Estropipate	
Oral Contraceptives	• Oral contraceptives increase coagulation activation and blunt the fibrinolytic response to exercise, which may lead to a pro-thrombotic state during and/or after exercise.
Progestins for Non-Contraceptive Use	

XVII. Other Hormones

Human Growth Hormone	• No effect on HR or BP at rest or peak exercise.
	• Increases muscle fiber size but not strength.
	• Increases ventilatory threshold and decreases fatigue.
	• Increases $\dot{V}O_2$peak and time to exhaustion.
	• Improves cardiac indices and hemodynamics in CHF.
	• Decreases % body fat.
Hematopoietic Colony-Stimulating Factors	
Erythropoietin (r-HuEPO)	• r-HuEPO increases $\dot{V}O_2$peak, but not in proportion to hematocrit; also increases SVR and BP.
Melatonin	• Melatonin may improve exercise performance after jetlag.
Somatostatin Analogs	
Octreotide	• Octreotide improves cardiac indices and peak exercise capacity in persons with acromegaly; suppresses growth hormone response to exercise.
Thyroid	
Levothyroxine	• Levothyroxine improves resistance to fatigue in hypothyroidism.

XVIII. Anticancer Drugs

Anticancer drugs come in several classes, with some drugs belonging to more than one class. The list is not comprehensive.

Alkalating Agents	• Cancer chemotherapy, in general, has deleterious effects on exercise during treatment, mainly because of excessive fatigue.
	• Many chemotherapeutic agents can cause anemia, leading to exercise intolerance and fatigue.
	• Chemotherapy can also induce acute gout, preventing exercise (see Anti-Arthritis Drugs).

Generic Name	Effects on Exercise
Plant Alkaloids and Antibiotics	
Doxorubicin	• Anthracyclines, especially doxorubicin and daunorubicin, can cause a delayed-onset cardiomyopathy that is typically not reversible.
Daunorubicin	
Vincristine	• Vinca alkaloids, especially vincristine and vinblastine, cause peripheral neuropathy (risk of weakness and poor proprioception).
Vinblastine	
Anti-Microtubule Agents	
Antimetabolites	
Antineoplastics/Antibiotics	
Bleomycin	• Bleomycin can cause pulmonary fibrosis.
Synthetic Antineoplastics	
Mitoxantrone	• Mitoxantrone can cause cardiomyopathy.
Anti-DNA Replication Drugs	
Monoclonal Antibodies	

XIX. Anticancer Adjuvant Drugs

Retinoids/Psoralens	• See section on sex hormones.
Hormones and Steroids	• Adjuvant therapy with high-dose corticosteroids can cause myopathy.
Cytokines/Cell-Cell Signaling Drugs	• Prednisolone improves FVC, $\dot{V}_E$max (maximal minute ventilation), $\dot{V}O_2$max, and maximal HR in persons with COPD.
	• See Other Hormones for additional agents.

XX. Antiviral Drugs

Anti-HIV	• Direct effects of each agent on exercise are not well documented.
Anti-HIV Combinations	• Successful combination therapy with anti-HIV agents can improve exercise performance because of preventing the sarcopenia (muscle wasting) associated with AIDS.
Anti-Cytomegalovirus (in HIV+)	
Anti-Influenza	
Anti-Herpetic	

XXI. Neurological Drugs

Anticonvulsants	
Carbamazepine	• Carbamazepine and valproate may inhibit mineralization of bone in children, and have been associated with fractures.
Gabapentin	• Gabapentin has been reported to improve paroxysmal dystonia of unknown etiology (case report).
Valproic acid	• Valproate and carbamazepine can cause weight gain.

(continued)

Generic Name	Effects on Exercise
H3 Receptor Antagonist (Anti-Migraine) Drugs	
Sumatriptan	• Sumatriptan reduces exercise tolerance in normal men.
Anti-Myasthenic Drugs	
Ambenonium	
Neostigmine	
Pyridostigmine	
Skeletal Muscle Relaxants/Anti-Spastics	
Baclofen	• Baclofen may improve spasticity in denervation disorders.
Dantrolene	• Dantrolene may relieve cramping in persons with some congenital enzyme deficiencies.
Antiparkinsonian Drugs	
Antidyskinetics	
Selegiline	• Selegiline worsens BP response to orthostatic testing, and reduces the pressor response to isometric exercise.
Trihexyphenidyl	• Trihexyphenidyl is anecdotally reported to improve focal dystonias in musicians and athletes.
Bromocriptine	• Bromocriptine worsens BP response to orthostatic testing.
	• Bromocriptine has been reported to improve the pressor response in persons taking metoclopramide (Reglan).
	• Bromocriptine may alter the sweat response to exercise.
Levodopa	• Levodopa improves BP response to orthostatic testing, but has no effect on fatigability in normal men.
Levodopa/Carbidopa	
Anti-ALS (Amyotrophic Lateral Sclerosis) Drugs	
Riluzole	

XXII. Multiple Sclerosis Antagonists

Glatiramer

XXIII. Psychotropic Drugs

Benzodiazepine Anxiolytics	
Clonazepam	• Clonazepam improves chest pains symptoms in person with panic disorder (normal coronary arteries).
Lorazepam	• Lorazepam has been shown to decrease the cortisol response and increase the insulin response to exercise, although time to exhaustion was not affected (endurance exercise).

Generic Name	Effects on Exercise
	• Lorazepam decreases peak power output during Wingate bicycle testing.
Other Anxiolytics Promethazine	• Promethazine used in combination with morphine may improve exercise tolerance in persons with COPD.
Sedatives/Hypnotics Monoamine Oxidase Inhibitors (MAOIs)	• MAOIs, in combinations with catechol-O-methyltransferases, have no effect on the HR, BP, and catecholamine responses to exercise.
Tranylcypromine	• Tranylcypromine may have trophic effects on neural cells when combined with exercise. • Tranylcypromine can precipitate hypertensive crisis.
Sympathomimetic Drugs	• Sympathomimetic drugs markedly increase many acute responses to exercise, including HR and BP. • *Extreme caution* is needed when combined with exercise (potentially lethal effects).
Anti-Mania Drugs Lithium	• Lithium can cause weight gain.
Tricyclic Antidepressants	• Almost all tricyclic antidepressants can cause weight gain.
Imipramine	• Imipramine may have trophic effects on neural cells when combined with exercise.
Serotonin Reuptake Inhibitor Antidepressants	• Serotonin reuptake antagonist ritanserin (2A/2C receptor specificity) does not alter resistance to fatigue in normal men. • Selective serotonin reuptake antagonists have been associated with weight loss.
Tranquilizers/Anti-Psychotics	• Almost all anti-psychotic drugs can cause weight gain.
Loxapine	• Loxapine has been associated with weight loss.

APPENDIX D

Web Sites for Additional Resources on Chronic Diseases and Disabilities

There are many very high quality Web sites for chronic diseases and disabilities. Some have good information on exercise. The list presented here, compiled from recommendations by the authors of this text, is neither comprehensive nor a ranking.

For all-purpose Internet resources, the U.S. National Institutes of Health and the Centers for Disease Control have Web sites that are difficult to surpass for impeccably high quality of information, very fast transfer speeds, and many resources in both English and Spanish. There is a variable amount of information on exercise, but there is often some information on exercise in specific conditions. For general references on conditions discussed in this book, try the following sites:

National Institutes of Health
www.nih.gov

Centers for Disease Control and Prevention
www.cdc.gov

Although the authors of this book predominantly recommend the Web sites of the NIH and CDC, there are many non-profit organizations and for-profit companies that have excellent Web sites. Examples include the following:

American College of Sports Medicine
www.acsm.org

National Center on Physical Activity and Disability
www.ncpad.org

New York Public Library and New York Academy of Medicine
www.noah-health.org

CARDIOVASCULAR DISEASES

All Chapters

National Heart, Lung, and Blood Institute
www.nhlbi.nih.gov

American Heart Association
www.americanheart.org

Cardiac Transplant

International Society for Heart and Lung Transplantation
www.ishlt.org

Harrison Online
www.harrisononline.com

PULMONARY DISEASES

Chronic Obstructive Pulmonary Disease, Chronic Restrictive Pulmonary Disease, Asthma

National Heart, Lung, and Blood Institute
www.nhlbi.nih.gov

American Lung Association
www.lungusa.org

Cystic Fibrosis

Cystic Fibrosis Foundation
www.cff.org

Lung and Heart-Lung Transplant

Second Wind
www.2ndwind.org

International Society for Heart and Lung Transplantation
www.ishlt.org

METABOLIC DISEASES

Diabetes, Obesity

National Institute of Diabetes, Digestive, and Kidney Diseases
www.niddk.nih.gov

Hyperlipidemia

National Heart, Lung, and Blood Institute
www.nhlbi.nih.gov/chd/

Renal Failure

Life Options, Inc.
www.lifeoptions.org

Frailty

National Institute of Aging
www.nia.nih.gov

IMMUNOLOGICAL/HEMATOLOGICAL DISORDERS

Cancer

National Cancer Institute
www.nci.nih.gov

Acquired Immune Deficiency Syndrome (AIDS)

National Institute of Allergy and Infectious Diseases
www.niaid.nih.gov

Abdominal Organ Transplant

Life Options, Inc.
www.lifeoptions.org

Chronic Fatigue Syndrome

Centers for Disease Control
www.cdc.gov/ncidod/diseases/cfs/

Fibromyalgia

National Institute of Arthritis and Musculoskeletal and Skin Diseases
www.niams.nih.gov

American College of Rheumatology
www.rheumatology.org

ORTHOPEDIC DISEASES AND DISABILITIES

Arthritis, Lower Back Pain Syndrome

National Institute of Arthritis and Musculoskeletal and Skin Diseases
www.niams.nih.gov

Osteoporosis

National Institutes of Health, Osteoporosis and Related Bone Diseases Resource Center
www.osteo.org

National Osteoporosis Foundation
www.nof.org

Dairy Council of California
www.dairycouncilofca.org

Lower-Limb Amputation

National Disabilities Sports Alliance
www.ndsaonline.org

Centers for Disease Control
www.cdc.gov/safeusa/home/safehome.htm

NEUROMUSCULAR DISORDERS

Stroke and Brain Injury

National Disabilities Sports Alliance
www.ndsaonline.org

National Institute for Neurological Disorders and Stroke
www.ninds.nih.gov

Spinal Cord Disabilities: Paraplegia and Tetraplegia

National Disabilities Sports Alliance
www.ndsaonline.org

Michigan State (disability sports Web page)
ed-web3.educ.msu.edu/kin866/

National Center for Physical Activity in Disabilities
www.ncpad.org

AbleData (National Institute on Disability and Rehabilitation Research)
www.abledata.com

Muscular Dystrophy

Muscular Dystrophy Association
www.mdausa.org

Neuromuscular Disease Center (Washington University School of Medicine)
www.neuro.wustl.edu/neuromuscular/index.html

National Disabilities Sports Alliance
www.ndsaonline.org

Epilepsy

Epilepsy Foundation of Northeast Ohio
www.efneo.org

Maryland Epilepsy Center (University of Maryland Medical Center)
www.marylandepilepsy.com

Epilepsy Foundation of America
www.efa.org

Multiple Sclerosis

National Disabilities Sports Alliance
www.ndsaonline.org

Polio and Post-Polio Syndrome

National Institute for Neurologic Disorders and Stroke
www.ninds.nih.gov

National Institutes of Health (fact sheet with comments on exercise in post-polio syndrome)
www.ninds.nih.gov/health_and_medical/pubs/post-polio.htm

Amyotrophic Lateral Sclerosis

Amyotrophic Lateral Sclerosis Association
www.alsa.org

ALS Clinic at Baylor College of Medicine (Houston, Texas)
www.bcm.tmc.edu/neurol/struct/als/als60.html

Cerebral Palsy

National Disabilities Sports Alliance
www.ndsaonline.org

American Academy of Cerebral Palsy & Developmental Medicine
www.aacpdm.org/home.html

Parkinson's Disease

Organization for Movement Disorder Information and Education
www.wemove.org

The Parkinson's Institute
www.parkinsonsinstitute.org

COGNITIVE, PSYCHOLOGICAL, AND SENSORY DISORDERS

Mental Retardation

American Association of Mental Retardation
www.aamr.org

Special Olympics, Inc.
www.specialolympics.org

Mental Illness

Boston University Center for Psychiatric Rehabilitation
www.bu.edu/cpr

Alzheimer's Disease

Alzheimer's Disease Education and Referral Center (National Institute on Aging)
www.alzheimers.org

Deaf and Hard-of-Hearing

Michigan State (disability sports web page)
ed-web3.educ.msu.edu/kin866/

El Paso Center for the Deaf and Hard of Hearing
www.whc.net/epcdhh/deafsport.html

Montgomery County Association for the Deaf (Maryland)
www.mcad.org/dlsport.html

U.S.A. Deaf Sports Federation
www.usadsf.org

Visual Impairment

American Foundation for the Blind
www.afb.org

Helen Keller National Center for Deaf/Blind
www.helenkeller.org/

The Lighthouse
www.lighthouse.org/index.html

The italicized *t* following page numbers refers to tables.